T0332298

Benefit-Risk Assessment Methods in Medical Product Development

Bridging Qualitative and Quantitative Assessments

Chapman & Hall/CRC Biostatistics Series

Published Titles

Adaptive Design Methods in Clinical Trials, Second Edition
Shein-Chung Chow and Mark Chang

Adaptive Designs for Sequential Treatment Allocation
Alessandro Baldi Antognini and Alessandra Giovagnoli

Adaptive Design Theory and Implementation Using SAS and R, Second Edition
Mark Chang

Advanced Bayesian Methods for Medical Test Accuracy
Lyle D. Broemeling

Advances in Clinical Trial Biostatistics
Nancy L. Geller

Applied Meta-Analysis with R
Ding-Geng (Din) Chen and Karl E. Peace

Basic Statistics and Pharmaceutical Statistical Applications, Second Edition
James E. De Muth

Bayesian Adaptive Methods for Clinical Trials
Scott M. Berry, Bradley P. Carlin, J. Jack Lee, and Peter Muller

Bayesian Analysis Made Simple: An Excel GUI for WinBUGS
Phil Woodward

Bayesian Methods for Measures of Agreement
Lyle D. Broemeling

Bayesian Methods for Repeated Measures
Lyle D. Broemeling

Bayesian Methods in Epidemiology
Lyle D. Broemeling

Bayesian Methods in Health Economics
Gianluca Baio

Bayesian Missing Data Problems: EM, Data Augmentation and Noniterative Computation
Ming T. Tan, Guo-Liang Tian, and Kai Wang Ng

Bayesian Modeling in Bioinformatics
Dipak K. Dey, Samiran Ghosh, and Bani K. Mallick

Benefit-Risk Assessment in Pharmaceutical Research and Development
Andreas Sashegyi, James Felli, and Rebecca Noel

Benefit-Risk Assessment Methods in Medical Product Development: Bridging Qualitative and Quantitative Assessments
Qi Jiang and Weili He

Biosimilars: Design and Analysis of Follow-on Biologics
Shein-Chung Chow

Chapman & Hall/CRC Biostatistics Series

Benefit-Risk Assessment Methods in Medical Product Development

Bridging Qualitative and Quantitative Assessments

Edited by

Qi Jiang

Amgen Inc

Thousand Oaks, California, USA

Weili He

Merck & Co., Inc.

Rahway, New Jersey, USA

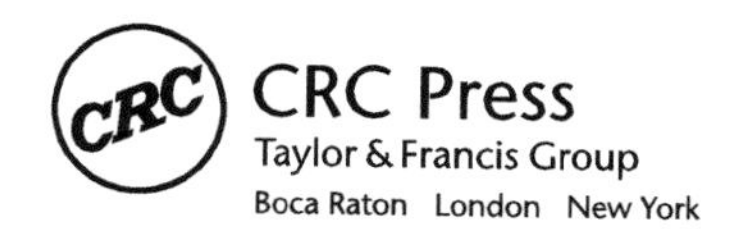

CRC Press is an imprint of the
Taylor & Francis Group, an **informa** business

A CHAPMAN & HALL BOOK

CRC Press
Taylor & Francis Group
6000 Broken Sound Parkway NW, Suite 300
Boca Raton, FL 33487-2742

Printed on acid-free paper
Version Date: 20160404

International Standard Book Number-13: 978-1-4822-5936-0 (Hardback)

Library of Congress Cataloging-in-Publication Data

Names: Jiang, Qui. | He, Weili (Statistician), editor.
Title: Benefit-risk assessment methods in medical product development : bridging qualitative and quantitative assessments / Qui Jiang and Weili He.
Description: Boca Raton : Taylor & Francis, 2016. | Series: Chapman & Hall/CRC biostatistics series | Includes bibliographical references and index.
Identifiers: LCCN 2015045977 | ISBN 9781482259360 (alk. paper)
Subjects: LCSH: Health risk assessment--Methodology. | Clinical trials--Evaluation.
Classification: LCC RA427.3 .J53 2016 | DDC 362.1072--dc23
LC record available at http://lccn.loc.gov/2015045977

Visit the Taylor & Francis Web site at
http://www.taylorandfrancis.com

and the CRC Press Web site at
http://www.crcpress.com

Contents

Section IV Benefit–Risk Assessment Methods and Visual Tools

Section V Benefit–Risk Assessment Case Studies and Lessons Learned

Preface

Evaluation of a new treatment has always required a benefit–risk (B–R) assessment. However, in the past, the assessment tended to be informal and was often subjective, involving judgments from separate assessments of efficacy and safety. Notably, a few regulatory submissions in the last few years failed to gain regulatory approval because of benefits that did not outweigh risks. Such failures speak to the importance of structured B–R assessments to improve consistency, transparency, communication, and objectivity. However, B–R assessment is multifaceted and complex, and the B–R landscape is still evolving. There is increased interest and effort from companies, regulatory agencies, and other governance bodies to further enhance structured B–R assessments. Amid numerous existing frameworks, metrics, estimation techniques, and utility survey techniques in B–R assessment, however, there is still no commonly accepted B–R approach. Guidance on how to select specific B–R frameworks and quantitative methods, along with case studies and best practice sharing, is still lacking.

This book aims to fill this void and serves as a resource for practitioners who wish to conduct B–R assessment in their clinical development and regulatory submission. The target audience is anyone involved, or with an interest, in the development and implementation of B–R evaluations. This could include statisticians, clinicians, pharmacoepidemiologists, outcome researchers, commercial personnel, and regulatory liaisons, working in academic or contract research organizations, government, and industry.

This book is composed of five sections: Section I focuses on the need for B–R assessment and future directions. Section II presents an overview of B–R assessment and the regulatory environment. Section III delineates considerations of B–R assessment in a product's life cycle management, while Section IV offers details of B–R assessment methods and visualization tools. Section V presents a rich collection of practical case studies. Our goal for this book is to provide, to the extent possible, a comprehensive and in-depth coverage of B–R evaluation overviews, methods, tools, and case studies.

Section I includes one chapter, which discusses the role of B–R assessments in medicine development and regulation, the need for a common B–R framework and patient input into B–R decisions, and future directions. Section II consists of two chapters. Chapter 2 provides a summary and discussion of legislative and regulatory policy initiatives related to medical product B–R assessment worldwide, the dynamics of B–R assessment in the postmarket setting, and regulatory science knowledge gaps and related challenges. Chapter 3 focuses specifically on the device area, covering Food and Drug Administration (FDA) decision making at the Center for Devices and Radiological Health (CDRH), the role of qualitative and quantitative methods in B–R assessments, factors for B–R determination, and the CDRH B–R Guidance document, and concluding with a groundbreaking case study on patient preference solicitation.

Section III contains four chapters. Chapter 4 deals with an important issue in B–R assessment: uncertainty evaluation and quantification by identifying sources of uncertainties and providing approaches for quantification. Chapter 5 provides a conceptual framework for quantifying patient B–R trade-off preferences, outlines procedures for eliciting valid preference weights for therapeutic benefits and harms, and reviews applications of these methods in two recent regulatory case studies. Chapter 6 gets to the issue of B–R analysis in subgroups and discusses ways to identify subgroups with the best B–R profiles, while

Chapter 7 describes various data sources and how the available data could be used to assist B–R assessment. Section IV comprises three chapters. To equip practitioners with tools to conduct B–R evaluations, Chapter 8 discusses B–R assessment methodologies and recommends a set of systematic methods for general use, while Chapter 9 proposes a quantitative joint modeling and joint evaluation framework for B–R evaluation via a Bayesian approach. Chapter 10 presents a thorough review of visual tools for B–R assessment along with real examples.

Putting it all together, Section V, featuring Chapters 11 through 13, presents a few illustrative case studies. Lessons learned and best practices drawn from these case studies should prepare practitioners with a much needed toolkit to embark on their journey to develop and conduct their B–R evaluations.

We would like to express our sincerest gratitude to all of the contributors who made this book possible. They are the leading experts in structured B–R assessment from industry, regulatory agencies, and academia. Their in-depth knowledge, thought-provoking considerations, and practical advice based on a wealth of experience make this book unique and valuable for a wide range of audiences. We hope that you will find this book helpful as well. We would also like to thank John Kimmel and Laurie Oknowsky of CRC Press, Taylor & Francis Group, for providing us with the opportunity for publication, as well as for their patience and help in guiding us through the production phase of the book. Finally, our immense thanks go out to our families for their unfailing support.

Qi Jiang, PhD
Weili He, PhD

Editors

Dr. Weili He is a director of Clinical Biostatistics at Merck & Co. She has a PhD degree in Biostatistics. She has extensive experience in drug development. Dr. He has been active in initiatives related to benefit–risk assessments and is the co-lead of the Quantitative Sciences in the Pharmaceutical Industry (QSPI) Benefit–Risk Working Group. She was a lead editor of a book on adaptive design and implementation that was published by Springer in 2014 and is an editor of this book. Dr. He has been serving as an associated editor of *Statistics in Biopharmaceutical Research* since January 2014. Her research and collaboration with colleagues in various disciplines has led to more than 50 publications in statistical and medical journals.

Dr. Qi Jiang is an executive director of Global Biostatistical Science at Amgen. In this role, she is biostatistical therapeutic area head for oncology and hematology and is the lead of the Center of Excellence for Safety and Benefit–Risk. In addition, she provides oversight to Amgen's biostatistical efforts in Asia. Before joining Amgen, Dr. Jiang worked at the Harvard School of Public Health, Merck, and Novartis. She has many years of clinical trial experience across a broad spectrum of therapeutic areas and has authored more than 60 peer-reviewed publications on method development, study design, and data analysis and reporting. Dr. Jiang is an editor of a book Quantitative Evaluation of Safety in Drug Development and an editor of this book. Dr. Jiang is a co-lead of the American Statistical Association Biopharmaceutical Section Safety Working Group and a co-lead of the Quantitative Sciences in the Pharmaceutical Industry (QSPI) Benefit–Risk Working Group. Dr. Jiang is an associate editor for *Statistics in Biopharmaceutical Research* and is a Fellow of the American Statistical Association.

Contributors

Ramin B. Arani, PhD, is the statistical science director of the Advanced Analytics Centre at AstraZeneca. He has more than 19 years of research experience in clinical trials and statistical methodologies. He has published numerous book chapters and articles in peer-reviewed scientific journals. His research interests are safety signal detection, survival analysis methods, multiplicity, artificial intelligence, survival change-point models, and quantitative benefit–risk methods.

Dr. Jesse A. Berlin received his doctorate in biostatistics from the Harvard School of Public Health (HSPH) in 1988. After spending 15 years as a faculty member at the University of Pennsylvania, Jesse left Penn to join Johnson & Johnson, where he is currently vice president and global head of epidemiology across pharmaceuticals, devices, and consumer products. He has more than 250 peer-reviewed publications in a wide variety of clinical and methodological areas. He was elected as a fellow of the American Statistical Association in 2004. In 2013, Dr. Berlin received the Lagakos Distinguished Alumni Award from the Department of Biostatistics at HSPH.

Dr. Daniel Bloomfield is vice president of Global Cardiovascular Clinical Research at Merck Research Laboratories. In this role, he led the team responsible for the FDA Advisory Committee and ultimate approval for ZONTIVITY (vorapaxar). Dr. Bloomfield is also responsible for the central coordination and strategic oversight of Merck's R&D organization in China across all therapeutic areas. Dr. Bloomfield joined Merck in 2003. Before joining Merck, he was an associate professor of medicine at the Columbia University College of Physicians and Surgeons.

Christy Chuang-Stein retired from Pfizer as vice president, head of the Statistical Research and Consulting Center in July 2015. She is a Fellow of the American Statistical Association (ASA) with more than 145 publications. Christy is a repeat recipient of Drug Information Association's Donald Francke Award for Excellence in Journal Publishing and Thomas Teal Award for Excellence in Statistics Publishing. She is a founding editor of *Pharmaceutical Statistics*. Christy received ASA's Founders' Award and the Distinguished Achievement Award of the International Chinese Statistical Association.

Dr. Scott Evans (Harvard University) teaches clinical trials and is the director of the SDMC for the Antibacterial Resistance Leadership Group. He is a member of an FDA Advisory Committee, the Board of Directors for the Society for Clinical Trials, and numerous DMCs/ECs. He is the Editor-in-Chief for *CHANCE* and for *Statistical Communications in Infectious Diseases*. He has received the prestigious Mosteller Statistician of the Year Award, the Robert Zackin Distinguished Collaborative Statistician Award, and is a Fellow of the ASA.

Bo Fu is a manager of Statistics in Data and Statistical Science at AbbVie Inc. Dr. Fu received his PhD in Biostatistics from the University of Pittsburgh. He serves as project statistician in new drug application (NDA) and supplemental NDA. He also serves as key statistician in clinical trials to provide functional area input to drug development and regulatory submission. Dr. Fu's interests in methodological development are statistical techniques for benefit and risk evaluation of clinical trial, advanced clinical trial design, and real-world health care data analysis. He has been a reviewer for peer-reviewed journals in the fields of clinical trials, medical research methodology, and biostatistics.

Dr. Tarek A. Hammad joined Merck in 2013 as an executive director (Pharmacoepidemiology). Before that, Dr. Hammad has had a distinguished career with the FDA, most recently as deputy director of the Division of Epidemiology, Center for Drug Evaluation and Research. He is nationally and internationally recognized as a drug safety and benefit–risk expert. He has authored many peer-reviewed publications and made many presentations in various scientific settings. He holds several academic appointments, spanning various medical disciplines. For more information, see his professional website at www.DrTarekHammad.com.

Martin Ho, MS, is a team leader reviewing neurological and dental devices at the Center for Devices and Radiological Health (CDRH). He was an investigator of the CDRH study of patient preference for weight loss devices and received the 2013 FDA Outstanding Achievement Award. He is the 2015 president-elect of the FDA Statistical Association and a voting member of the FDA Research Involved Human Subject Committee, FDA's IRB. He has also served on the CDRH Patient Preferences Initiative and the Patient-Centered Benefit–Risk Assessment Project Steering Committee of the Medical Device Innovation Consortium, a public–private partnership devoted to advance medical device regulatory science.

Telba Irony is currently the Deputy Director of the Office of Biostatistics and Epidemiology at the Center for Biologics Evaluation and Research at the FDA. She received her PhD from UC Berkeley, is a Fellow of the American Statistical Association, and is an elected member of the International Statistical Institute. She was instrumental in preparing the guidance documents for the Use of Bayesian Statistics in medical device clinical trials, on Factors to Consider when Making Benefit–Risk Determinations for medical devices, and on the submission of Patient Preference Information for evaluation of medical devices. Telba received the FDA Excellence in Analytical Science Achievement Award for spearheading innovative regulatory science studies culminating in the release of novel guidance documents, supporting complex policy decision making and changing the submission review paradigm.

Dr. F. Reed Johnson has more than 35 years of academic and research experience in health and environmental economics. He has served on the faculties of universities in the United States, Canada, and Sweden and as a Distinguished Fellow at the Research Triangle Institute. He is currently a Senior Research Scholar in the Duke Clinical Research Institute. He led the first FDA-sponsored study to quantify patients' benefit–risk trade-off preferences for new health technologies. The results are being used to inform regulatory reviews of device submissions.

Chunlei Ke received his PhD degree in Statistics from the University of California, Santa Barbara, in 2000 and is currently a biostatistician at Amgen working on late-phase drug development in Oncology.

Xuefeng Li is a mathematical statistician in the Division of Biostatistics at the Center for Devices and Radiological Health at the FDA. He received his PhD degree in Statistics at the University of Pennsylvania and then joined FDA as a statistical reviewer in 2004. He mainly works on therapeutic medical devices and has good experience with quantitative benefit–risk analysis.

Lawrence Liberti is the executive director of CIRS (the Centre for Innovation in Regulatory Science, Ltd). For the past 38 years, Mr. Liberti has worked in and with the pharmaceutical industry, in the fields of regulatory affairs and clinical R&D. Mr. Liberti has been actively involved in promulgating best practices in the regulatory aspects of medicines development, especially in the emerging markets. He lectures on regulatory issues concerning expediting patient access to medicines, new paradigms of drug development, and ways to improve communications between regulators, HTAs, and sponsors.

Haijun Ma is a senior biostatistician at Amgen Inc. with more than 9 years' industry working experience. She received her PhD training in Biostatistics at the University of Minnesota, Twin Cities, and Master in Science degree from the Department of Statistics at Iowa State University. She served in various working groups aimed at promoting good practices and developing statistical methodologies; collaborated with members across industry, academia, and regulatory agencies; invited to present and teach in professional meetings; and published in areas including clinical trial safety, pharmacoepidemiology, benefits and risks assessment, meta-analysis, and Bayesian statistics.

Yabing Mai is a principal scientist of Clinical Biostatistics at Merck & Co. Dr. Mai received his PhD degree in Mathematical Statistics from the University of Maryland in 2008. Since then, he has been actively engaged in drug development and leading statistical support to late-stage clinical development programs in therapeutic areas of cardiovascular and oncology. His primary research interests are Survival Analysis, Adaptive Design, and Benefit–Risk Assessment.

Neil McAuslane, BSc, MSc, PhD, is currently the scientific director of the Centre for Innovation in Regulatory Science (CIRS). Since joining CIRS in 1991, Dr. McAuslane has worked on and initiated a number of the CIRS key projects in the areas of regulatory strategy, quality of regulatory review, benefit–risk assessment, quality of decision making, and R&D performance, working with pharmaceutical companies and regulatory agencies both mature and evolving. He has edited and coauthored several publications and reports in these areas and has been involved in the supervision of the CIRS PhD students.

Jose Pablo Morales, MD, Division of Cardiovascular Devices, Center for Devices and Radiological Health, is a medical officer in the Division of Cardiovascular Devices at the Center for Devices and Radiological Health–FDA. Dr. Morales received his MD from Universidad Pontificia Bolivariana (Colombia). He did his specialty training in vascular and endovascular surgery at Guy's and St Thomas' Hospital in London, UK. After that, he joined the Department of Vascular Surgery at The Cleveland Clinic, Ohio, where he worked as a research fellow for 2 years. He has published more than 30 manuscripts in the field of vascular surgery and interventional radiology and has coauthored several book chapters. He joined the FDA as a medical officer in 2009 and his expertise is in aortic endovascular grafts, inferior vena cava filters, embolization devices, and dialysis grafts.

Dr. George A. Neyarapally formerly worked in the US Senate (Congressional Health Fellow), Office of the Secretary of the US Department of Health and Human Services (Health Policy Fellow), the US Agency for Healthcare Research and Quality, the US FDA, and the New Hampshire Department of Health and Human Services on public health, regulatory, and legislative issues pertaining to pharmaceutical, health, and legislative policy. Dr. Neyarapally is currently completing his law degree at the University of Maryland School of Law.

Jonathan Norton has been working as senior principal statistician at MedImmune since 2013. He graduated with a PhD degree in Statistics from Florida State University and then became part of the Center for Drug Evaluation and Research at the FDA, where he reviewed several new drug and biologics license applications in the following areas: oncology, pain, metabolism, and rheumatology therapeutics. Jon is the creator of the Individual Response Profile graphic for benefit–risk assessment.

Dr. George Quartey is an expert statistical methodologist at Roche-Genentech with more than 23 years of diverse experience in statistical research, quantitative safety sciences, risk–benefit modeling, comparative effectiveness research, observational trial design, evidence synthesis, and data mining. His research interests are primarily concerned with the development and application of innovative statistical methods to improve real-world data strategy, trial design, and health technology assessment. Dr. Quartey is currently the co-director of the IMI EU2P program on benefit–risk assessment of medicines.

John Scott is deputy director of the Division of Biostatistics at the FDA's Center for Biologics Evaluation and Research. Before joining the FDA in 2008, he worked in psychiatric clinical trials at the University of Pittsburgh Medical Center. He holds a PhD in Biostatistics from the University of Pittsburgh, an MA in Mathematics from Washington University in St. Louis, and a BA in Liberal Arts from Sarah Lawrence College.

Steven Snapinn is vice president of Global Biostatistical Science at Amgen. This department provides biostatistical and statistical programming support to all phases of Amgen's drug development programs. Dr. Snapinn has a PhD from the University of North Carolina at Chapel Hill and has more than 30 years' experience in the pharmaceutical industry. He is a former editor of *Statistics in Biopharmaceutical Research* and is a fellow of the American Statistical Association. He has approximately 100 publications in the statistical and medical literature.

Guochen Song is a senior scientific advisor in Quintiles' Quantitative Decision Strategies and Analytics department. He has supported Quintiles' partners and clients in designing streamlined development programs. He uses his statistics expertise to empower drug developers to make decisions that will bring treatments to market in a quick and reliable manner. He earned his Doctor of Public Heath degree in Biostatistics from UNC Chapel Hill. He was involved in designing and implementing a variety of phase I through phase IV clinical trials.

Kao-Tai Tsai received his PhD in Mathematical Statistics from University of California, San Diego. He joined AT&T Bell Laboratories to practice applied statistics and data analysis. He then worked at the US FDA and pharmaceutical companies to focus on biostatistics for drug discovery. Kao-Tai has extensive experience in pharmaceutical industry with research ranging from methodological and applied statistics. He is a member of ICSA and ASA, and is also an adjunct professor of Rutgers University and Georgia Southern University.

Professor Stuart Walker, BSc, PhD, MFPM, FRSC, FIBiol, FRCPath, is the founder of the Centre for Innovation in Regulatory Science and is a professor of Pharmaceutical Medicine, Cardiff University. During his research career in academia and industry, he has supervised many PhD programs in clinical development, regulatory policies, benefit/risk assessment of medicines, and health technology assessment, and has coauthored 300 research papers and edited 26 books. He is frequently involved in the organization of international meetings on key issues that concern the regulatory review of medicines and has lectured extensively throughout Europe, the United States, the Asia-Pacific Region, Latin America, and the Middle East.

Dr. Shihua Wen received his PhD in Statistics from University of Maryland, College Park. Currently, he is working in the Data & Statistical Science division at AbbVie Inc., leading/co-leading a number of cross-functional research initiatives, such as benefit–risk assessment, safety signal detection, and so on. Dr. Wen is also an active member of the Society for Clinical Trials (SCT)–sponsored QSPI Benefit–Risk Working Group. Moreover, Dr. Wen is an enthusiastic advocate of adaptive trial design and has served as DMC statistician in multiple clinical programs.

Mo Zhou is a PhD student in the Health Economics and Policy program at the Johns Hopkins Bloomberg School of Public Health. With extensive training in econometrics, her research focuses on using discrete choice analysis to estimate demand for health care and the application of conjoint analysis in medicine. She has been involved in stated-preference studies in areas such as diabetes and vaccination and is particularly interested in studying preference heterogeneity and market segmentation using various econometric techniques.

Section I

The Need for Benefit–Risk Assessment and Future Directions

1

The Need for and Future Directions of Benefit–Risk Evaluations

Neil McAuslane, Lawrence Liberti, and Stuart Walker

CONTENTS

ABSTRACT An effective benefit–risk (BR) assessment is core to both efficient product development and regulatory decision making, with the goal of being transparent, building trust, and enhancing communication across all stakeholders. Despite the diversity in tools and approaches used by stakeholders to assess and communicate a benefit–risk assessment, the use of a common BR approach can lead to better communication and optimal discussions. A common framework has been shown to improve the transparency, communication, and consistency of BR assessment, thereby making the underpinnings of implicit judgments and decisions more explicit. This is particularly important as value judgments and interpretations become more important in making not only regulatory decisions but also health technology assessment (HTA)/payer decisions. For a sponsor, a BR framework is a tool for planning the drug development process and a means for organizing, interpreting, and communicating the value proposition to various stakeholders, and a structured approach is also amenable to soliciting input from those stakeholders. The BR framework could also be used as a systematic means of building a database of regulatory decisions that can be accessed (beyond public assessment reports) by emerging agencies, HTA agencies, and patient groups. Because all parties seek clear guidance on the future use of BR assessment approaches, convergence is desired and achievable through activities such as the draft guidance developed by the International Conference on Harmonisation of Technical Requirements for Registration of Pharmaceuticals for Human Use (ICH) and shared experiences among stakeholders. A consistent BR framework provides one building block of quality decision making in pharmaceutical development and regulation upon which future practices and processes will be built that will facilitate and ensure that quality decisions are being made by all stakeholders.

1.1 The Role of Benefit–Risk Assessments in Medicine Development and Regulation

Benefit–risk (BR) assessment is an important dimension of medicine development, regulation, and clinical practice, and in the past decade, emphasis has been put on the refinement of structured approaches to these evaluations. An effective BR assessment is core to both efficient product development and regulatory decision making, contributing to the goals of being transparent, building trust, and enhancing communication across all stakeholders. The globalisation of medicine development requires the use of efficient tools to characterise the safety and efficacy profiles of new medicines in a manner that is aligned with international standards yet provides the flexibility for local BR assessment that takes into context specific factors that can influence the BR profile within a country or region.

The need for a structured BR approach was identified at the beginning of the last decade (Mussen et al. 2010), but it took time for both agencies and companies to see that there was a need to

- Gain a better understanding of why different agencies come to different conclusions when faced with essentially the same application data
- Create an approach sufficiently dynamic and flexible that it can include the views of a wider range of stakeholders including pharmaceutical reviewers, the pharmaceutical industry, physicians, payers, and patients
- Provide consistency to the current approaches not only for regulators whose decisions may appear to be inconsistent but also for companies whose data and submissions on benefits and risks may not always be presented in a coherent and well-structured manner
- Enable the articulation of the means by which a BR decision was made, to satisfy the increasing pressure on agencies to improve transparency and accountability and to establish a paper trail to explain how decisions are reached

The need for a consistent framework was documented in a survey conducted by the Centre for Innovation in Regulatory Science (CIRS) among 20 multinational research-based companies and 11 regulatory agencies regarding their interest in implementing structured BR frameworks (Leong et al. 2013). All of the companies and 82% of the agencies believed that there is a need for a BR framework for application by both parties. Both agencies and companies believed that a structured BR framework would enhance the quality (transparency and consistency) and could provide the documentation for a structured discussion among peers within and between organisations and their stakeholders. Preliminary findings from a more recent 2015 CIRS survey presented at the June 2015 CIRS Workshop indicate that approximately half of international pharmaceutical companies and almost 90% of regulatory agencies surveyed now use formal frameworks for BR decision-making processes.

The evolution of structured BR approaches over the last 5 years ensures that important aspects of a therapy's characteristics are considered systematically in reaching a BR decision, using a standardised approach that facilitates the balanced consideration of benefits and risks. In addition, a structured framework provides a consistent and systematic approach for development and regulatory decisions, which encourages good review practices and supports quality decision making across companies and agencies in the pre- and post-authorisation evaluation of medicines.

While BR assessments are predicated on the details available from clinical and real-world experiences, applying the principles of a systematic review to these elements ensures that the "big picture" is kept in mind during a complex, detailed review. A scientifically relevant approach addresses diverse incoming signals such as clinical data, experiential information, safety signals, and background 'noise'. These approaches allow for the processing of the facts, integration of values and risk attitudes and consideration of uncertainty, and communicate outgoing (re-)actions that modify behaviour of patients, prescribers, industry and other stakeholders (Eichler, June 2015 CIRS Workshop). In this manner, the use of a structured approach to BR assessment has several key benefits, among these being the ability to provide scientifically rigorous tools that enhance clarity and transparency around the communication of factors that contributed to the decision outcome. When transparency and relevance of BR decisions are clearly communicated, the result drives stakeholder acceptance.

In the ensuing chapters, we will learn more about the tools being developed by industry and regulatory agencies to accomplish BR assessments. The CIRS-Benefit–Risk Action Team (BRAT) (http://www.cirs-brat.org/) approach offers a flexible approach that can be readily tailored by sponsors to assess BR throughout a product lifespan, identifies and tabulates key benefits and harms using a decision-tree process and also generates easily interpretable graphics from the underlying data. Through the use of the European Medicines Agency (EMA) Effects Table (Pignatti 2014) and the US Food and Drug Administration (FDA) Benefit–Risk assessment table (Frey 2014), agencies are striving to ensure that their assessments of BR are both systematic and structured, resulting in better communication of the reasoning behind their decisions; integrating these approaches into their public assessment reports will serve to keep stakeholders better informed and participatory (Leong et al. 2015).

The evolution and future direction of establishing a systematic, structured approach to BR will be underpinned by three key areas:

- A common BR framework
- Patient input into BR decision making
- BR assessment as a key component of a quality decision-making process

1.2 A Common BR Framework

Despite the growing diversity in tools and approaches used by stakeholders to assess and communicate a BR assessment (IMI Protect Consortium 2015), there is little doubt that the use of a common BR approach can lead to better decision making. A common framework will improve transparency, communication and consistency, thereby making the supporting factors for implicit judgments and decisions more explicit. This is particularly critical as value judgments and interpretations become more important in making not only development and regulatory decisions but also health technology assessment (HTA)/payer decisions.

Establishing a common overarching framework provides the umbrella under which any number of specialised tools can be developed to undertake specific types of BR analyses, from highly quantitative techniques to interpret difficult clinical situations during development to routine BR analyses in the post-authorisation period (Figure 1.1).

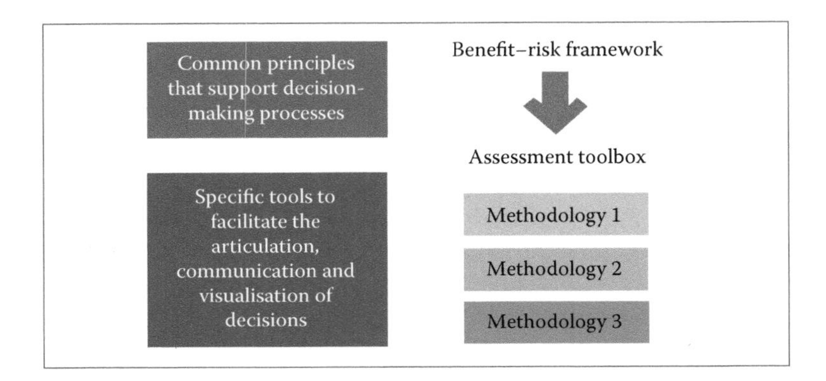

FIGURE 1.1
A BR framework contains the appropriate tools to make a range of decisions from simple assessments to complex analyses.

For a sponsor, common elements or steps that form the BR framework provide the platform that contains tools for planning the drug development process and that serves as a means for organising, interpreting and communicating the value proposition to various stakeholders. For agencies, irrespective of the specific process used, alignment with an overarching framework provides continuity, rigour and a commonality in the nature of the information that will be provided to characterise a product's BR profile. In addition to internal consistency, a common framework also enables cross-agency interpretations, as smaller agencies rely increasingly on mature agency decision making; adherence to the common elements will allow clarity of what has been considered, improving cross-agency understanding.

The approaches used by industry and regulators, while appearing diverse in their details, have been found to readily map to eight overarching process steps (Walker et al. 2015). These steps, which form the basis of the Universal Methodology for Benefit–Risk Assessment (UMBRA) framework (Figure 1.2), can provide a high-level guidance as to

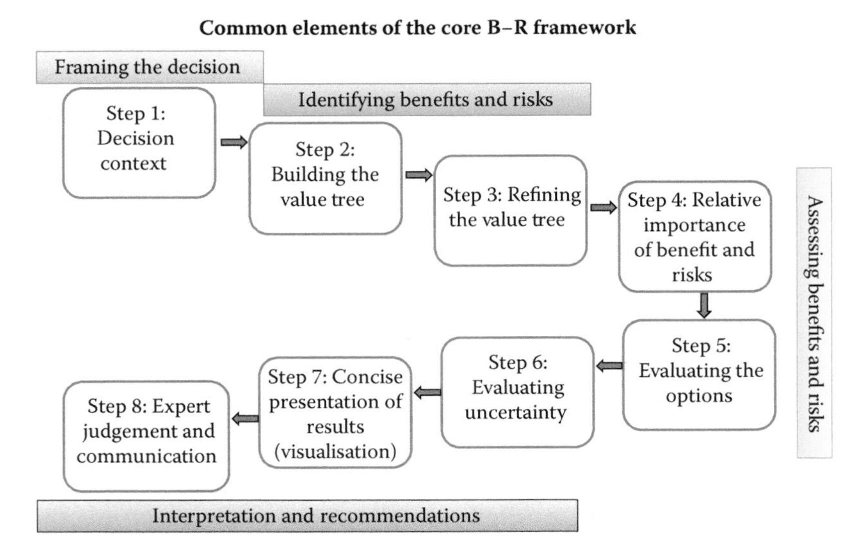

FIGURE 1.2
The eight steps of the CIRS UMBRA framework.

the core elements that characterise a robust BR assessment and communication process. Walker et al. have mapped the elements of the FDA, EMA, BRAT and other company- and agency-developed BR tools to these eight steps.

Using tools and methodologies that address the elements of the eight-step framework, irrespective of the order in which these are applied or the focus on specific features, provides the basis for a common overarching approach to BR assessment. When sponsors construct their marketing authorisation dossier BR sections in line with these eight steps, regulators will observe alignment with their respective approaches to BR assessment.

To this end, an International Conference on Harmonisation of Technical Requirements for Registration of Pharmaceuticals for Human Use (ICH) Expert Working Group is evaluating the current ICH Guideline M4E(R1) for the CTD Section 2.5.6 on BR assessment and to consider revising it to include greater detail on the format and structure of information presented therein. The goals of this activity will be the harmonisation of the presentation of the supportive information within regulatory submissions (ICH 2015).

Because each agency follows its own strategy in conducting a BR assessment and is guided by jurisdictional regulations and usual practices, the ICH Expert Working Group will appropriately not define a specific approach or process to be applied by regulators in conducting the BR assessment, such as specifying quantitative and qualitative methodologies, nor will it address how a regulator should reach a specific BR conclusion.

We support the concept that following a structured approach to the organisation, presentation and logical communication of BR information and addressing common precepts of a structured BR framework will facilitate the regulator's task of developing and communicating an assessment of a product's BR profile that is relevant to their agency's population and jurisdiction.

1.3 Patient Input into BR Decisions

All parties seek clear guidance on the future use of BR assessment approaches; convergence is desired and achievable through activities such as the ICH Working Group initiative and informed shared experiences among stakeholders. Importantly, a structured approach is amenable to soliciting input from multiple stakeholders, and patients are playing an ever-growing role in informing BR assessments. Involvement of patients from the earliest stages of medicine development assists in formulating the value proposition for a new medicine, defines the harms patients are willing to accept during different stages of their disease and, when appropriately integrated into an organisation's processes, can make decision-making processes more informed and robust.

Patients who live with a disease have a direct stake in the drug development and review process and are in a unique position to contribute to these. Consequently, sponsors and agencies are undertaking formal and informal initiatives to incorporate the patient voice into BR assessments.

Under the auspices of the Prescription Drug User Fee Act (PDUFA) V, the FDA has been provided with resources to expand activities dedicated to providing review divisions with patient input. Among these activities, FDA has been convening meetings with participation from review divisions, the relevant patient advocacy community and other interested parties (a total of 20 meetings over 5 years) to better understand patient perceptions of BR relevant to their specific disease. Through upcoming initiatives including the re-authorisation of PDUFA and the 21st Century Cures bill, the role of the patient in defining a product's BR profile will continue to grow.

In Europe, work is being undertaken at the centralised level to identify patient preferences and to determine how these stakeholders can inform and become more involved in the decision-making process (EMA 2014). This work is being echoed at the national level; for example, the Medicine and Healthcare Products Regulatory Agency (MHRA) plan for 2013–2018 has specified that BR decisions should be better informed by the perspectives and experiences of patients, patient representative groups, and the wider public (MHRA 2015). Additionally, greater patient participation in clinical decision making must be accompanied by increased understanding of the BR decisions that are being taken by regulators.

We are confident that over the next 5 years, all mature agencies and many growing agencies will begin to implement or continue to expand their patient-focused initiatives.

1.4 BR Assessment as a Component of Quality Decision Making

Making good decisions is critical to successful research and development and to ensure efficient access to innovative medicines. This is the case whether these are decisions to undertake additional work to develop a new medicine, to submit a dossier for review or to approve a new medicine. Further, good decision making is essential for HTA agencies to make a positive recommendation to list, list with restriction or not list new medicines as these are the critical decisions that affect sponsors and patients.

A systematic, structured BR framework provides one of the key building blocks for a quality decision-making process in pharmaceutical development, regulation, and access. As discussed above and further detailed in this book, the overarching elements of a framework for BR assessment have been well documented, revealing commonalities in the steps taken by both companies and agencies to assess a medicine's BR profile, irrespective of the tools or methodologies applied. Indeed, many companies are now internally using tools such as the CIRS-BRAT framework in order to better articulate the BR profile of a new medicine during development and to key stakeholders. As agencies and companies embed their BR framework into their decision-making processes to evaluate medicines during the key development, submission and review decision stages, the extent to which these frameworks have a positive real-world impact on BR decision making and communication remains an open question.

To this end, research is being conducted by CIRS to investigate the elements of different stakeholders' decision processes, with the objectives of identifying the strengths and weaknesses of these processes and determining the principles required for building quality into critical decision making in the development, review and reimbursement of new medicines.

1.5 Future Directions

The past 15 years have seen growing international interest among all healthcare stakeholders regarding how to best approach the BR assessment of medicines and to evolve structured systematic frameworks (Leong et al. 2015). This robust legacy of scientific groundwork in this field has paved the way to the future. What will be the challenges and opportunities for BR assessment over the next 5 years?

While the common elements of a structured, systematic framework for the assessment of BR have been identified, we expect that the next 5 years will see the refinement in the use of specific tools and techniques by regulators around the world. Some agencies may focus on descriptive approaches to categorising and communicating BR while others will explore novel approaches integrating more quantitative analyses and descriptive visualisations. For some, developing more comprehensive guidances on how to reflect the expression of values and trade-offs will be key. The role of descriptive and quantitative methods such as textual descriptions, value trees and numerical or categorical ratings in addressing the related issues of valuing and weighting the component factors of the BR profile will continue to be investigated.

New methodologies that more fully integrate the assessment of uncertainty pertaining to benefit and harms expected from a particular therapy for a defined treated population will be developed. There will be a continued growing emphasis on patient-focused drug development. To this end, the use of outcomes from patient preference studies to better characterise the risk tolerance and trade-offs associated with a new therapy will inform the value proposition of these therapies. As a growing number of disease-specific regulatory and HTA guidances are developed, there will be an increasing role for BR to inform these development approaches. Furthermore, clinical treatment guidelines will begin to address ways that both the clinician and patient can assess, communicate and agree on the BR profile of a treatment option.

Medicine development is a global endeavor. Sponsors therefore seek a consistent degree of process predictability across target jurisdiction regulatory agencies, and in the BR arena, this can come from the use of a globally acceptable, standardised, systematic approach to BR assessment, irrespective of the specific tools and methodologies that each employs to describe the BR profile of a product in support of its regulatory approvability.

As has been observed with the piloting of a simple template approach to BR assessment by the Health Sciences Authority (Singapore), Therapeutic Goods Administration (Australia), Swissmedic and Health Canada, a structured process can facilitate work sharing and the potential for joint reviews and improve information sharing with industry partners and other stakeholders such as patient groups and HTA agencies. This process can also provide a clearer understanding of rationales for different marketing and labelling decisions in different jurisdictions, such as clinical context and the practice of medicine, and enhanced collaboration in the post-market setting through, for example, the alignment of risk management plans and Periodic Safety Update Reports (B. Sabourin, presentation made at CIRS Workshop, Taipei, Taiwan, February 2015).

Other regional initiatives such as the International Summary Approach to Benefit–Risk Evaluation (iSABRE) project (McAuslane 2014) and the ICH Working Group activities will further align technical requirements and communication tools for more transparent BR assessments and outcomes communication. The next 5 years will also see the growing use of standardised BR assessment by HTA agencies as a component of their decision-making processes to determine the pharmacoeconomic value of medicines, both at the time of initial approval and as real-world evidence (RWE) accumulates post-authorisation. In all of these cases, whether interacting with regulatory or HTA agencies, establishing a dialogue with the stakeholders early during medicine development can contribute to effective, ongoing communications with a more consistent understanding and implementation of the expectations from each stakeholder.

In this regard, the use of novel data sources for the assessment of BR throughout a product's lifespan will continue to expand. As RWE becomes the new information currency in healthcare, decision makers will be challenged by the use of these new types of data sets. Over the next 3 to 5 years for particular therapeutic areas, there may be a shift to the use of robust proof-of-concept studies based on both earlier-stage clinical trial data and RWE. As development progresses, RWE will enhance the understanding of the product's safety profile and will be used to confirm clinical efficacy and real-world effectiveness.

The use of RWE for BR assessment will not be without challenges. The methodologies to assess the robustness and uncertainty around factors that confound the interpretation of RWE are only now being more fully explored. Disappointing evidence could result in the potential for early commercial failure and the risk of increasing liability; these events after an early launch could result in a loss of reputation for the companies, regulators and payers, especially when product withdrawals occur. A scenario of a low reimbursement level at launch based on a less well-defined BR profile could develop, which is not followed by a continuously increased reimbursement level, despite the collection of real world-effectiveness experience (Rönicke et al. 2015). RWE evidence collection will need to encompass a global view or, at the least, focus on key markets and jurisdiction experiences. Global pharmacovigilance strategies will need to become more sophisticated in their ability to collect, verify, analyse and report internationally collected RWE.

Transparency of the decision process is currently not optimal in terms of the elements of the framework that are in the public-facing assessment reports (Leong et al. 2014, 2015). However, as agencies look to evolve their assessment reports to mirror their BR assessment, this will provide greater insight into their decision-making processes. These insights will become valuable for HTA agencies and other stakeholders to inform a value decision.

Lastly, accountable and documented BR assessment will be the cornerstone on which current and new facilitated regulatory pathways (FRPs), that is, regulatory pathways designed to accelerate submissions, reviews and patient access to medicines for serious diseases where there is an unmet medical need by providing alternatives to standard regulatory review routes, will be accepted. FRPs may increase the communication and level of commitment between the developer and the agency, can give a larger role to effects on surrogate end points and may move some of the burden of evidence generation from the pre- to the post-authorisation phase (Liberti et al. 2015). FRPs will, therefore, require a move towards BR assessment techniques that address smaller experience numbers, shorter exposure durations and greater uncertainty around the parameters assessed. Experience is developing in this arena through the use of FRPs such as Breakthrough Therapy, Accelerated Approvals (in the United States), Conditional Marketing Authorisation (in the European Union) and the newly available scheme for the accelerated review and conditional authorisation of regenerative medical products and the Sakigake designation system for the rapid authorisation of unapproved medicines (Japan). The communication of how agencies have made their decision on the basis of these facilitated routes will become paramount, not only in terms of the initial decision but also regarding what has changed when a disinvestment decision is required post-authorisation.

The following chapters will expand on the concepts we have introduced. Understanding the role of BR assessments in the regulatory environment sets the stage for considerations of how BR assessments can be implemented across different clinical development settings to meet regulatory and HTA goals. While underpinned by a common framework, BR assessment methods need to be flexible, adapting to the stage of development, therapeutic area and stakeholder among other variables. Implementing BR assessments contributes to more effective and transparent communications with stakeholders throughout the product lifespan.

References

European Medicines Agency (2014). EMA Press release patients to discuss benefit–risk evaluation of medicines with the Committee for Medicinal Products for Human Use. Available at http://www.ema.europa.eu/ema/index.jsp?curl=pages/news_and_events/news/2014/09/news_detail_002172.jsp&mid=WC0b01ac058004d5c1. Accessed July 27, 2015.

Frey P: Benefit–risk framework implementation: FDA Update (2014) CIRS Workshop June 2014. Available at http://cirsci.org/sites/default/files/CIRS_June_2014_Workshop_report.pdf. Accessed July 27, 2015.

ICH: Final Concept Paper. M4E(R2): Enhancing the Format and Structure of Benefit–Risk Information in ICH. M4E(R1) Guideline. Revised on March 23, 2015. Available at http://www.ich.org/fileadmin/Public_Web_Site/ICH_Products/CTD/M4E_R2_Efficacy/M4E_R2__Final_Concept_Paper_27_March_2015.pdf. Accessed July 27, 2015.

IMI Protect Consortium: IMI-PROTECT Benefit–Risk Group—Recommendations Report. Recommendations for the methodology and visualisation techniques to be used in the assessment of benefit and risk of medicines. Available at: http://www.imi-protect.eu/documents/HughesetalRecommendationsforthemethodologyandvisualisationtechniquestobeusedinthe assessmento.pdf. Accessed July 27, 2015.

Leong J, Salek S, Walker S: *Benefit–Risk Assessment of Medicines—The Development and Application of a Universal Framework for Decision-Making and Effective Communication.* 2015; Switzerland: ADIS-Springer International Publishing.

Leong J, Salek S, Walker S: Strategy for communicating benefit–risk decisions: A comparison of regulatory agencies' publicly available documents. *Front Pharmacol Pharmacol.* 2014; 5:269. http://dx.doi.org/10.3389/fphar.2014.00269.

Leong J, McAuslane N, Walker S, Salek S: Is there a need for a universal benefit–risk assessment framework for medicines? Regulatory and industry perspectives. *Pharmacoepidemiol Drug Saf.* 2013; 22:1004–1012.

Liberti L, Stolk P, McAuslane N, Somauroo A, Breckenridge AM, Leufkens H: Adaptive licensing and facilitated regulatory pathways: A survey of stakeholder perceptions. *Clin Pharmacol Ther.* 2015 Accepted article, doi: 10.1002/cpt.140.

McAuslane N: An evaluation of the application of UMBRA to ensure a systematic documentation of benefit–risk in non-ICH countries. CIRS Workshop, June 2014. Available at http://cirsci.org/sites/default/files/CIRS_June_2014_Workshop_report.pdf. Accessed July 27, 2015.

Medicines and Healthcare Products Regulatory Agency. Corporate plans 2013–2018. Available at: https://www.gov.uk/government/uploads/system/uploads/attachment_data/file/350879/con261796__1_.pdf. Accessed July 27, 2015.

Mussen F, Salek S, Walker S: *Benefit–Risk Appraisal of Medicines: A Systematic Approach to Decision-Making.* Wiley & Blackwell, 2010.

Pignatti F: EMA framework development and pilot study, CIRS Workshop, June 2014. Available at http://cirsci.org/sites/default/files/CIRS_June_2014_Workshop_report.pdf. Accessed July 27, 2015.

Rönicke V, Ruhl M, Solbach T: Revitalizing pharmaceutical R&D: The value of real world evidence. Strategy&/PWC (Formerly Booze & Company). 2015. Available at: http://www.strategyand.pwc.com/media/file/Revitalizing-pharmaceutical-RD.pdf. Accessed July 2015.

Walker S, McAuslane N, Lawrence L, Leong J, Salek S: A universal framework for the benefit–risk assessment of medicines: Is this the way forward? *Ther Innov Reg Sci.* 2015; 49:17–25.

Section II

Overview of Benefit–Risk Assessment and Regulatory Environment

2

Regulatory and Legislative Policy and Science Considerations in the Era of Patient-Centeredness, Big Data, and Value

Tarek A. Hammad and George A. Neyarapally

CONTENTS

ABSTRACT Benefit–risk (B–R) assessment underpins premarket drug development, regulators' decisions to approve drugs for marketing as well as attendant postmarket regulatory actions, and payers' coverage decisions. In 2012, the Institute of Medicine highlighted the need for a transparent, continuous, and integrated assessment and reassessment of a drug's B–R profile throughout its life cycle. In the past 10 years, important legislative and policy initiatives pertaining to B–R assessment have been enacted or initiated throughout the world. These initiatives have supported the approval of innovative medical products while increasing the need to study both safety and effectiveness in the postmarket setting owing to the increasing paucity of evidence on these medical products before market approval. In this vein, regulators have withdrawn indications due to a negative shift in the B–R balance in light of emergent evidence, introduced risk mitigation strategies in the postmarket setting to ensure the safe use of drugs that have been associated with serious harm, and scaled back risk management programs when safety issues did not pan out after further study. Further, even if a drug is approved for marketing and stays on the market after safety-related regulatory actions, payers may not support the initial or ongoing coverage of the drug based on their own B–R and value assessment. These developments underscore the uncertainty regarding a drug's B–R profile over time and the importance of regulatory science initiatives designed to enhance the ongoing assessment and management of a drug's benefits and risks. The ability to reduce the uncertainty regarding the benefits and risks of drugs in the postmarket setting stems initially from the premarket evidence base and the ability to evaluate both benefits and risks in the postmarket setting via valid and accepted approaches. This chapter discusses recent regulatory policy and science initiatives, opportunities, and challenges related to B–R assessment, as well as current regulatory B–R assessment considerations for structured B–R evaluation in medical product development across clinical development phases and beyond. The focus is on policies and initiatives in the United States and Europe, as they substantially influence those in other parts of the world and generally drive the field, although initiatives from other regions are important and are mentioned in brief.

2.1 Introduction

The volume and complexity of health data and the challenges associated with integrating these data have increased exponentially from the development of information theory in the middle of the 20th century to the modern era of meaningful use of health information technology, including increased adoption of electronic health records (EHRs) and e-prescribing as well as health reform in the United States.[1–5] Further, de-identified patient data from clinical trials may also be much more widely available in light of recent industry initiatives and impending legislative and policy changes as well as the establishment of distributed research networks that support the learning health system.[6–9] This deluge of big data has stimulated the development of health analytics and methodologies in the United States and globally to leverage these data for the advancement of population health and personalized medicine.[2,10] These new methodologies strive to account for patients' genotypes and phenotypes and enhance the development and evaluation of drugs (and attendant risk management programs) to treat both rare and prevalent conditions. The mapping of the human genome and the development of targeted therapies have produced a tension between personalized drug therapy and the traditional paradigm that is based on mean population-level drug effects. Additionally, increased investments have been made in comparative effectiveness research (CER), also sometimes referred to as patient-centered outcomes research (PCOR) in the context of patient-focused CER, with a focus on outcomes important to patients.[11,12]

Opportunities and challenges that arise from these changes both enrich and complicate the assessment of the benefit–risk (B–R) profiles of drugs,* which underpins premarket drug development, regulators' decisions to approve drugs for marketing as well as

* For purposes of this chapter, the terms *medical product* and *drug* are used interchangeably and refer to medical products, including drugs, biologics, and/or devices.

attendant postmarket regulatory actions, and payers' coverage decisions. Further, the development and approval of biosimilars will contribute to challenges in drug development, evaluation, and uncertainty in the context of interchangeability of germane data on benefits and risks.[13] Thus, in recent years, stakeholders have emphasized the importance of developing structured B–R assessment approaches, including those that employ explicit qualitative or quantitative frameworks, which may transparently address the way of handling the uncertainties stemming from the aforementioned evolving landscape.

In this vein, in 2012, the Institute of Medicine (IOM) highlighted the need for a transparent, continuous, and integrated assessment and reassessment of a drug's B–R profile throughout its life cycle.[14] The stakes for the industry cannot be overstated in light of the increasing focus on the value of health care interventions owing to increasing health care costs, as well as challenges stemming from the evolving regulatory and payers' policies aimed at evaluating medical products' value on an ongoing basis both before and after approval.[15–17] There will likely be more variation in the approval status of medical products as a result of this increasing focus on value, which may be defined as the benefits, i.e., positive health and other patient-centered outcomes associated with a medical product relative to its costs.[18] These costs may include direct monetary as well as indirect clinical costs (i.e., adverse reactions caused by the medical product). For example, regulators have withdrawn indications owing to a negative shift in the B–R balance in light of emergent evidence, introduced risk mitigation strategies in the postmarket setting to ensure the safe use of drugs that have been associated with serious harms, and scaled back risk management programs when safety issues did not pan out after further study.[19] However, critical challenges in removing medical products from the market, a form of de-innovation, need to be addressed.[20]

The increasing biopharmaceutical industry investment in, and approval of, high-cost specialty drugs for more prevalent conditions such as hepatitis C and cancer, along with rare, orphan diseases, has provided more impetus to focus on interventions' value, including the need to reconcile short-term, annual government budgets with long-term, potentially substantial, associated cost savings.[21–24] This has fueled the ongoing development of health technology assessment, adaptive licensing (AL), comparative effectiveness, and value-based purchasing policies to fulfill the triple aim of better population health, better health care quality, and lower costs.[25,26] In the United States, health care delivery system reforms such as accountable care organizations and bundled payments, and the recent commitment of the US Department of Health and Human Services (HSS) to shift away from fee-for-service payments for health care services to global payments for a package of services based on value,[17] will affect the types of data needed for B–R evaluation and potentially enhance the perceived value of interventions in at-risk systems because these interventions can prevent costly hospital readmissions and physician visits and lower costs if patients are adherent.[27–30]

In the future, health insurance companies will differ from their current form[31] and thus the data needed to assess benefits and risks will be different. In addition, even if a medical product is approved for marketing and stays on the market after safety-related regulatory actions, payers may not support the initial or ongoing coverage on the basis of their own B–R and value assessment. Importantly, payer interventions are playing an increasingly influential role in the use of drugs and biosimilars in the United States.[32,33] These dynamics underscore the uncertainty regarding the perception of a medical product's B–R profile over time and the importance of regulatory policy and science initiatives designed to enhance the ongoing assessment and management of benefits and risks over a product's life cycle. Further, the increasing focus on patient engagement in research and in medical product development,[34–36] decreased economic returns on new drugs,[37] and postapproval decision making in the context of shared decision making with patients and their prescribers[38] constitutes a more challenging and dynamic environment for the industry in the context of B–R assessment.

This chapter discusses recent regulatory policy and science initiatives, opportunities, and challenges related to B–R assessment, as well as current regulatory B–R assessment considerations for structured B–R evaluation in medical product development across clinical development phases and beyond. The focus is on policies and initiatives in the United States and Europe, as they substantially influence those in other parts of the world and generally drive the field, although initiatives from other regions are important and are mentioned in brief.

2.2 Legislative and Regulatory Policy Initiatives Related to Medical Product B–R Assessment

In the past 10 years, important legislative and policy initiatives pertaining to B–R assessment have been enacted or initiated throughout the world. These initiatives have supported the approval of innovative medical products while increasing the need to study both safety and effectiveness in the postmarket setting owing to the increasing paucity of evidence on these medical products before market approval. This section will discuss these initiatives as they pertain to B–R assessment during drug development, approval, and use (Table 2.1).

2.2.1 United States

With respect to drug development, the Food and Drug Administration (FDA) Amendments Act (FDAAA) of 2007 included important statutory mandates pertaining to drug B–R assessment.[39] The law required the registration and posting of results of all Phase II–IV clinical trials conducted for FDA approval. This is important from a B–R assessment perspective as it increases awareness of all relevant trials evaluating the benefits and risks of drugs moving forward, thus negating publication bias stemming from trials unpublished because of null or negative findings. However, this mandate only pertained to new trials and does not address previously conducted trials, which constitute most of the evidence for certain indications. The mandate also required summary information to be posted, which means it does not inform patient-level analyses and may preclude meaningful adverse event analyses across trials.[44] Late in 2014, a draft rule was published by the HHS discussing the final data submission requirements for the provision of trial summary data.[45] HHS proposed in the draft rule to add unapproved medical product–related trials to approved ones, which would expand the summary data available on drug trials, increasing the available evidence on the benefits and risks of drugs in the premarket setting.[45] The reasons underpinning this decision include the need to address publication bias and facilitate the robust evaluation of drug classes via increased awareness of all evidence on benefits and risks.[46] Further, individual companies and the US and European regulatory and research agencies have increased access to de-identified patient level data in recent years, which will facilitate more robust meta-analyses for the assessment of drug benefits and risks.[47] Although increased access to clinical trial data is generally positive as it supports B–R

TABLE 2.1

Timeline for Regulatory and Legislative Policy and Science Initiatives for B–R Assessment and Pertinent Aspects

Year	Initiative
2007	FDA Amendments Act (FDAAA)/PDUFA IV
2008	Innovative Medicines Initiative (IMI)
	EU-ADR Project
	EMA Benefit Risk Methodology Project[40]
	Australia Risk Management Program Requirement Initiation
2009	HITECH Act, American Recovery and Reinvestment Act (ARRA)
	FDA-EMA Parallel Scientific Advice Program
	Chinese FDA Priority Review Regulatory Pathways
2010	EU Pharmacovigilance Legislation
	Patient Protection and Affordable Care Act
	EU Net HTA-EPAR Initiative
	India's National Pharmacovigilance Program
2011	FDA-CMS Parallel Review Program: Devices
2012	FDA Safety and Innovation Act (FDASIA)/PDUFA V
	Institute of Medicine (IOM) Report: Ethical and Scientific Issues in Studying the Safety of Approved Drugs
	White House Big Data Initiative: New R&D Investments
	NIH Genomic Data Initiative
2013	FDA Periodic Benefit–Risk Evaluation Report (PBRER) Guidance
	FDA Structured Approach to Benefit–Risk Assessment in Drug Regulatory Decision Making
	NIH Big Data Initiative
	EMA-EUNet Data Collection Initiative
	Japanese Pharmaceutical Affairs Act
2014	US Department of Health and Human Services: Clinical Trials Summary Data Rule
	ICH Working Group Formation: M4E R2
	CIOMS Guidance on Risk Management
	EMA Adaptive Licensing Project
	Health Canada: Guidance Document for Developing a Post Market Benefit–Risk Assessment[41]
	FDA CBER/CDRH: Benefit–Risk Factors to Consider When Determining Substantial Equivalence in Premarket Notifications [510(k)] with Different Technological Characteristics. Draft Guidance for Industry and Food and Drug Administration Staff[42]
	IOM report: Characterizing and Communicating Uncertainty in the Assessment of Benefits and Risks of Pharmaceutical Medical Products
2015	US Department of Health and Human Services: Payment Reform Administrative Rule
	FDA Medical Device Innovation Consortium (MDIC) Patient Centered Benefit–Risk Project[43]
	21st Century Cures Act Discussion Draft
2017	PDUFA VI (Forthcoming)

assessment, it may also be used to spuriously identify unfounded harm-related associations with drugs, which may cause patients to stop taking beneficial drugs.[48] Nonetheless, recently discussed legislative proposals in the United States in 2015, along with a recent IOM report recommendation,[49] would make de-identified clinical trial data available for meta-analyses.[50] Thus, the future of US policy in this area is in flux.

Further, the FDAAA conferred the FDA with the ability to require Risk Evaluation and Mitigation Strategies (REMS) to manage serious drug risks of harm as a prerequisite of drug approval, in addition to the postmarket setting as safety issues arise. The FDA is increasingly requiring REMS for new drugs and biologics,[51] and the more restrictive REMS, which have Elements to Assure Safe Use (ETASU), may decrease access to drugs in some situations (e.g., by allowing only certified health care professionals to prescribe a drug) to ensure safe use. REMS may be increasingly required in the future to manage serious risks associated with high-cost specialty orphan drugs, which are approved with less evidence and increasing in use.[51] A recent study using pharmacy and medical claims data demonstrated that an ETASU REMS can successfully be used to limit off-label prescribing,[52] which is prevalent in the real-world setting. In a similar vein, although not conferred by name, experts have construed the combination of FDA's REMS, postmarket safety monitoring, and accelerated approval/fast track review processes as tantamount to an AL authority as the FDA might approve some drugs with less evidence associated with a restrictive REMS and then require postmarket studies to evaluate the situation further. The REMS can then be relaxed in the subsequent years of a medical product's life cycle as warranted.[53]

Another development that will have a major impact on the ongoing assessment of medical products' B–R profiles is the utilization of distributed research network data models by the Health Maintenance Organization Research Network, the Agency for Healthcare Research and Quality (AHRQ), the FDA, the Centers for Disease Control and Prevention, and the Observational Medical Outcomes Partnership, which has clear utility in enabling the use of large amounts of data for postmarket evaluation of drug risks and benefits.[54–56] Considering legal issues pertaining to patient privacy and data ownership[57] and recent changes to the Health Insurance Portability and Accountability Act,[58] the practical approach was to operationalize these endeavors by building common data models (CDMs) using anonymized distributed data.

FDAAA also supported the Mini-Sentinel pilot project, which spanned dozens of partners consisting of mostly claims but also some EHR data and supported several drug safety evaluations.[39] This active surveillance system employs a distributed research network of health plan claims and EHR data in a standardized format for drug safety evaluation purposes. As of September 2013, more than 150 million lives and 4 billion drug claims are included and millions are added each month.[59] Several drug safety evaluations have been completed and some have been published and discussed in FDA drug safety communications and informed drug label changes.[60] Also, a sequential testing tool called PROMPT has been created to facilitate the periodic monitoring of medical product safety, which eventually will affect the B–R profiles of these medical products.[61] The thresholds selected to indicate that a particular safety signal should be further assessed will be important to inform the ability to tease out signals of concern from noise. Also, integrating findings from this system with other evidence sources to inform regulatory decision making is an ongoing challenge, as was the case with findings from dabigatran and bleeding evaluations.[60,62] Recent efforts to develop a consistent framework for quality regulatory decision making may assist in this process.[63]

Although Mini-Sentinel focused exclusively on drug safety per the statutory mandate, in the future, the full Sentinel system may be leveraged by various stakeholders for effectiveness and other evaluations as more EHR data source nodes are added to the distributed network. Increased availability of richer data sources and linkage of these sources, including EHR and patient-related data sources, such as personal health records (PHRs), along with Veterans Affairs (VA), Centers for Medicare and Medicaid Services (CMS), and Department of Defense data, may address concerns of regulators who believe that only randomized controlled trials can be used to discern drug benefits and help address the imbalance between evidence on drug risks and benefits in the postmarket setting.[64] Further, many of the same observational research methods included in AHRQ and the Patient Centered Outcomes Research Institute (PCORI) guidance documents and the final FDA guidance on conducting these studies, which was completed as part of a Prescription Drug User Fee Act (PDUFA) IV commitment/FDAAA, will apply to the studies conducted using the Mini-Sentinel and future Sentinel network.[65]

It is worth noting that despite the increased focus on observational studies to evaluate postmarket drug safety, it is noteworthy that in recent years spontaneous reports have contributed to the majority of safety-related regulatory actions, including labeling changes.[66,67] Further, the spontaneous adverse event surveillance system will likely continue to play a role in drug risk assessment in the postmarket setting and complement other evidence sources.

The American Recovery and Reinvestment Act (ARRA) of 2009 appropriated several billion dollars to support the uptake, adoption, and meaningful use of EHRs for the enhancement of the quality and safety of health care.[68] This has largely been successful in increasing the ability of most office-based physician practices to access and use EHRs with basic functionalities, although efforts are ongoing to build in more advanced functions such as clinical decision support.[3] ARRA also provided $1.1 billion funding to HHS, AHRQ, and the National Institutes of Health (NIH) for the conduct of CER on medical interventions, including drugs. In the process, the ARRA funds have increased the availability of e-health resources for the evaluation of drugs in the premarket setting (EHR-based clinical trials), as well as the evaluation of drugs in the postmarket setting with enriched information beyond claims, including critical variables such as weight, body mass index, blood pressure, blood test results, and others, which have historically constituted important unmeasured confounders in postmarket US administrative claims-based observational studies.

In 2010, the passage of the Affordable Care Act in the United States concluded the long quest for comprehensive national health reform.[4] PCORI, an independent funding organization, was created under this law and is mandated to fund research on outcomes important to patients. The leadership of PCORI defines patient-centered outcomes research as "the evaluation of questions and outcomes meaningful and important to patients and caregivers."[69] PCORI is required to engage patients and incorporate their input in the research it funds. In fact, half of the review teams that evaluate study proposals are patients, ensuring that their input is included in the decisions about which studies to fund.[69] The research will affect drug development in the context of which patient-centered outcomes to target as well as comparative drug evaluation. Although this type of comparative evaluation may be seen by some as a substantial risk to medical product viability (i.e., there will be winners and losers), the increased focus on patient outcomes may increase the perceived value of products if the patient impact is properly accounted for versus more traditional evaluations that are based on surrogate measures. In contrast to the United Kingdom and other European countries, historically there has not been a US national agency or organization that evaluates the cost-effectiveness of drugs, and PCORI is specifically prohibited from evaluating drugs using quality-adjusted life years, as the National Institute for Health and Clinical Excellence (NICE) does in the United Kingdom. PCORI also recently launched an initiative to support the development of a patient-centered research network to provide infrastructure for the conduct of pragmatic trials.[70] This may facilitate the evaluation of drug benefits and risks in the premarket setting and expedite the determination of the impact of approved drugs on outcomes important to patients. Additionally, some US private health insurers, such as Aetna, plan to evaluate the postmarket effectiveness and safety of weight loss drugs used as part of a comprehensive weight loss program to inform future coverage decisions.[71]

The Affordable Care Act also created an approval process for biosimilars in the United States.[4] Unique B–R assessment and comparative effectiveness and safety challenges may be associated with biosimilars in the postmarket setting depending on naming conventions employed—debates are ongoing about whether or not biosimilars will retain the same generic name as biologics and how they will be distinguished. The FDA has published guidance documents on the development and approval of biosimilars and B–R assessment considerations.[72] In Europe, biosimilars have the same nonproprietary name as approved biologic counterparts, although in addition to stating that a medical product is a biosimilar, in some European countries such as the United Kingdom, additional notation in the form of a black triangle is required to indicate that close monitoring of risks is recommended.[73] Substitution rules differ in different European countries. Further, many US states have developed bills to restrict the substitution of biosimilars for biologics, potentially superseding FDA's imprimatur in the development of regulatory policy for drugs.[74] However, the experiences from other regions including Europe may be instructive as biosimilars have been available in these countries for several years.

In 2011, the FDA initiated a pilot parallel review process with a large US government insurance program that is predominantly for the elderly, Medicare, for the joint review of devices.[75] The purpose of this pilot was to support collaboration between a federal payer and regulator to expedite device approval by incorporating the payer's perspective in the context of premarket evidentiary requirements for devices, including B–R assessments and the integration of these requirements into the FDA's regulatory approval requirements to the extent practicable. However, this process will not likely apply to drugs as most Medicare coverage decisions pertaining to drugs are made at the local level (local coverage decisions) versus national coverage decisions to which the parallel review process would apply.[76] Further, national coverage decisions have become more parsimonious in recent years, with less positive decisions about medical products based on the same extent of evidence on benefits and risks of harm.[77]

In 2012, the US White House announced a holistic big data initiative across several aspects of government, including the NIH, the largest US government funder of medical and scientific research. The NIH initiative, the 1000 Genomes Project, will provide large amounts of free genomic data to researchers who will only be charged for use of computing services.[78] Further, in 2013, the NIH pioneered the Big Data to Knowledge Initiative to "enable the biomedical research community to use the various types of big data for research."[79] This may stimulate the development of methods to use big data for premarket and postmarket medical product B–R assessment.

The Food and Drug Administration Safety and Innovation Act (FDASIA) of 2012, including the PDUFA V reauthorization, included several provisions relevant to drug development and evaluation in the context of B–R assessment.[80] The law created a new breakthrough therapy pathway that enables drugs with preliminary evidence of a substantial benefit to be approved[81]—this is analogous to previous authorities designed to achieve the same purpose, including accelerated approval, but enhances FDA's ability to communicate with and support the industry in obtaining approval for drugs with early evidence of substantial benefit. This also introduces challenges in the evaluation of the benefits and risks of these drugs in light of the limited evidence available at the time of approval.[82] Since its inception, many applications for such drugs have been received and some drugs have been approved as breakthrough therapies. In fact, FDA already received 92 requests for breakthrough therapy status by September 2013 and granted the designation for approximately

29% of these requests.[83] This dovetails with the increasing number of orphan drugs and medical products approved in recent years as both of these types of drugs tend to have limited evidence on benefits and risks at the time of approval in light of the small target patient populations in many cases.

FDASIA also mandated the inclusion of patients in the drug development process, eventually weighing in on the desired B–R balance, and efforts are ongoing to implement this mandate, including the solicitation of comments from the public on how to better incorporate the patient input in regulatory decision making related to the benefits and risks of drugs and drug approval status.[35] FDA held several patient-focused drug development meetings in 2014 and 2015 and will hold more in 2016.[84] Further, PDUFA V required FDA to develop guidance on the policies underpinning the decisions to require REMS as well as on the evaluation of REMS programs' effectiveness.[85] Stakeholders have called for FDA to leverage the increasing availability of e-health data (big data) for the evaluation of REMS, in addition to patient-centered resources such as online web portals.[86] The creation of a framework for patient consent will help ensure that patient autonomy is respected while supporting the participation of patients in current and future comparative effectiveness and real-world–based research.[87]

The PDUFA V included a plan for the implementation of FDA's structured B–R assessment framework.[87] The framework consists of the following decision factors in the assessment of a drug's benefits and risks: analysis of the condition of interest, current treatment options, benefits, risks, and risk management. The framework also highlights that evidence and uncertainties within these factors should be reflected in the summary of the evidence and also includes the final step of conclusions and reasons for the findings and implications for the regulatory decision.[88] The B–R assessment framework implementation timeline indicates that the framework will be applied in a stepwise fashion, to eventually apply to all original New Drug Applications (NDAs) by FY 2017. This qualitative framework is designed to provide more consistency and transparency to FDA's B–R assessment and attendant regulatory decisions on the basis of this assessment. The impact of the FDA framework on B–R assessment and decisions remains to be seen in the upcoming few years. The framework focuses more on communication than quantification and thus qualitatively supports consistent decision making. However, the framework does not fully tease out the evidentiary challenges and complexity that underpin B–R assessments, especially when they are made in light of substantial uncertainty about risks and benefits. Specifically, although uncertainties are included as part of the qualitative framework, quantitative approaches to assess B–R and uncertainty and associated assumptions are not explicitly part of the framework. It is worth noting that the proposed 21st Century Cures Act would also mandate that the patient's input be included in the B–R framework to further incorporate the patient input into medical product regulatory decision making in a consistent manner.[9] However, the FDA framework does not explicitly offer a regulatory pathway for the capture and incorporation of patient preferences and trade-offs in the decision-making process.

Further, the FDA published a guidance document in 2013 regarding the provision of postmarket periodic safety reports in the International Conference on Harmonization (ICH) E2C (R2) Format (Periodic Benefit–Risk Evaluation Report [PBRER]).[89] The required frequency of periodic reporting on B–R evaluation is every 6 months for the first 3 years and then annually thereafter. The focus of the PBRER is on new safety information placed in the context of "pertinent" effectiveness information that may have arisen in the postmarket setting. This provides a structured, qualitative framework for postmarket B–R assessment although there is a lack of guidance on a common standard for periodic B–R evaluation reporting on marketed medical products across ICH regions.[89]

In 2014, FDA awarded a 3-year contract to Credible Meds to support the use of clinical decision support (CDS) for safe prescribing of antibiotics.[90] This and future initiatives will integrate identified risks and benefits from periodic B–R assessments into prescribing via electronic approaches such as CDS, consistent with the meaningful use incentives provided by the Affordable Care Act to use EHRs to enhance patient safety and care. Further, in 2014, FDA promulgated a solicitation for the creation of an electronic medical record (EMR) database that would allow FDA to mine connected EMRs, which include data on typically missing confounders.[91]

Despite the significant increase in federal funding in recent years for CER/PCOR, it is likely, owing to the high cost and time burden of randomized clinical trials, that these funds may be used mostly for observational studies or pragmatic trials. In the future, these studies may contribute toward the postmarket evaluation of medical products' B–R profiles.[92] EHR data may also be leveraged in a linked fashion for public health surveillance and evaluation such as the use of the MDPHnet for the detection of influenza-like illness and rapid epidemiological investigations.[93] Relatively recently, the director of the US FDA Center for Drug Evaluation and Research emphasized the need for new methods to evaluate the comparative effectiveness of drugs, biologics, and devices that are sufficiently reliable but may not need to be as robust for regulatory purposes.[92] In light of the increased focus on value, some have suggested that FDA should require a higher standard of comparative evidence, mandating comparative effectiveness via active comparators at the point of approval for drugs[15]—as more CER studies are published, this may become a possibility although it would require legislation.

As in the United States, there is no national entity that evaluates medical product safety, clinical effectiveness, and cost-effectiveness in order to make decisions or recommendations about coverage and payment of medical products (e.g., for Medicare); the terms *comparative effectiveness* and *cost-effectiveness* are often used in the context of federal health policy in the United States and the term *health technology assessment* (HTA) is often reserved for private insurance companies in the United States and others that perform these types of holistic evaluations.[94] However, there are US state-based or regional entities that evaluate both clinical and cost-effectiveness, such as the California Technology Assessment Forum, now part of the larger Institute for Clinical and Economic Review (ICER), which recently evaluated the relatively new hepatitis C drugs.[95] This is in contrast to Europe in which there are many national HTA agencies that make recommendations or decisions for national health payers.

2.2.2 Europe

Similar to the United States, there have been several legislative and policy initiatives in Europe in the past 10 years or so related to drug B–R assessment in the premarket and postmarket setting. In 2008, the European Commission funded the EU-Adverse Drug Reaction (ADR) project to develop a system that leverages EHR data from the Netherlands, Denmark, the United Kingdom, and Italy.[96] This system has been used to identify and assess drug safety signals, enhancing postmarket drug risk assessment. This project ended in 2013[96] and its results demonstrate that EHR-based systems may be able to detect more safety signals and to better ascertain more adverse events of interest that are relatively more prevalent in the general population, such as myocardial infarction. Spontaneous reporting systems often are not able to identify these types of signals.[96] In 2009, FDA and

EMA initiated a parallel scientific advice program for drug sponsors, which facilitate discussions around B–R assessment (among other issues associated with drug development) and alignment of evidentiary requirements for this assessment to obtain drug approval.

New pharmacovigilance legislation in the European Union (EU), on a scale comparable to the substantial drug safety authorities conferred to FDA in the United States in 2007, was passed in 2010, along with attendant implementing regulations in 2012.[97] The major aspects of the legislation included "proactive and proportionate risk management, higher quality of safety data, stronger link between safety assessments and regulatory action, strengthened transparency, communication and patient involvement… improved EU decision-making procedures, and the establishment of the Pharmacovigilance Risk Assessment Committee (comparable to the US Drug Safety and Risk Management Advisory Committee)."[98] This legislation became applicable to medicines in Europe in July of 2012. Additional changes to the pharmacovigilance legislation were made in 2012 to facilitate the "prompt notification and assessment of safety issues" after the withdrawal of Mediator (benfluorex).[98] This pharmacovigilance legislation also allows for the requirement of postmarket medical product safety and effectiveness studies, akin to AL paradigm[53] in that the regulatory approval status and required risk management program and risk minimization strategies can be altered in the future based on real-world evidence. Further, in 2013, a black symbol was added to medical products that require additional monitoring to alert prescribers, health care professionals, and patients—this is similar to the black triangle required in the United Kingdom for new medical products—indicating that there is uncertainty about the safety and effectiveness of the new drug when used in the broader real-world population after approval.[99]

With respect to clinical trials, in 2010, the EMA promulgated a transparency policy allowing third parties to request and obtain access to information, including clinical trial data (and clinical trial reports pertaining to studies conducting outside of the EU), submitted to EMA in support of marketing authorization.[100] Since the inception of this regulatory policy, several requests for access to clinical trial data have been granted. Most of these decisions have been supported, and two out of the three cases involving company disputes about data releases were resolved after the companies accepted the EMA's approach to selectively releasing data.[100] In EMA's 2010 to 2015 roadmap report published in 2010, EMA emphasized the plan to focus clinical trials on "good" responders, which not only can make expensive clinical trials more efficient but also will result in less generalizable evidence when medical products are used more broadly in the postmarket environment. Also in 2010, EMA and HTAs initiated a parallel review process similar to the CMS-FDA/CDRH (devices) agreement. This is a voluntary program and this process may grow further in the future in light of the increasing focus on the need for evidence of additional drug benefit relative to drugs currently approved to treat the disease of interest.

Further, in 2012, legislation was passed in the United Kingdom to reform the British National Health Service and emphasized the need to achieve better value and patient-focused outcomes, and in January 2014, a new value-based pricing model was implemented to try to better reflect value in drug pricing.[53] In 2014, the EU passed clinical trial regulations that create a single drug application and authorization procedure, facilitate the conduct of clinical trials, increase the transparency regarding such trials (but not clinical trial reports for studies conducted outside of the EU), and require the creation of a clinical trial portal and database by EMA.[101] The evolving policies and regulations may facilitate the confirmation of study findings as well as the enhancement of future study designs and use of biomarkers, which may in turn bolster evidence-based drug B–R assessment.

The Innovative Medicines Initiative is a Public–Private Partnership whose first phase spanned from 2008 to 2013 with an approximately 2 billion pound budget. This endeavor is considered one of the largest public–private initiatives in drug development and evaluation. In April 2013, the comprehensive IMI report on drug B–R assessment methodologies was published. The report included several methods for the evaluation and communication of drug benefits and risks to prescribers, other health care professionals, patients, and other stakeholders.[102] These methods fall under one of four domains including frameworks (qualitative, e.g., BRAT; quantitative, e.g., MCDA), metric-based indices (threshold, health, and trade-off indices), estimation techniques (PSM, MTC), and utility survey techniques (DCE). Although many approaches were identified, importantly, the report authors stated that they "…did not find widespread applications to real-life B–R decision-making."[103] Nonetheless, this report will be the basis for forthcoming discussions around the choice and implementation of various B–R assessment methodologies.

In 2014, the Council for International Organizations of Medical Sciences (CIOMS) published a guidance document on risk management.[104] This guidance emphasizes that the goal of risk management is to improve patient health outcomes and reduce the frequency of harm as much as practicable, although entirely eliminating it is normally not possible.[104] The authors emphasize balancing benefits and risks, risk mitigation, and preservation of access to medicines, including considerations of the burden to patients and the health care system. The importance of tailoring risk management tools to be commensurate with the relevant risks over the medical product's life cycle and obtaining patient perspectives in the development and design of risk management programs is emphasized, consistent with the aforementioned increased patient-focused US initiatives. In contrast to traditional B–R assessment, CIOMS guidance recommends use of the RE-AIM framework for risk management program assessment, including the following dimensions: reach, effectiveness, adoption, implementation, and maintenance.[105] The guidance also recommends prior development of an analysis plan, which may enhance risk management program evaluation in the future as there are many limitations in the evaluation of these programs.[106] Future modalities for the implementation and evaluation of risk management programs include electronic audit and feedback to rapidly implement and assess health care professional knowledge, web-based physician checklists integrated into workflow via decision support tools, simulations, and web-based strategies.[104]

Regarding the patient input, the EMA recently revised the framework for interacting with patients and consumers to better incorporate their values and preferences into evaluations and regulatory decision making.[100] Specific provisions include establishing disease-specific patient experts to facilitate obtaining the patient input in medical product–related activities and training patients to facilitate their integration into EMA's work.[100] The IMI2's new proposal includes initiatives to elicit patient's perspectives on drug benefits and risks for the supplementation of "benefit–risk assessments by regulations and HTAs from development through the entire life cycle."[107]

In late 2014, the EMA discussed critical issues for the Agency in 2015 and 2016, including facilitating early stages of drug development, continuing implementation of pharmacovigilance and clinical trials legislation, and increasing transparency and access to data.[108] EMA also expects an increased provision of parallel advice with HTA bodies to facilitate timely access to drugs. In contrast to the United States, many European countries have their own national entities that evaluate drug cost-effectiveness and make recommendations on insurance coverage of drugs based on drug B–R and cost assessments. For example, NICE in the United Kingdom is one of the most famous of these entities. As mentioned above, future collaborations with payers by EMA and other regulatory agencies will enhance the coverage of drugs immediately after approval as the evidence provided will be more relevant for payers than in the past. Further, similar to regulatory agencies, HTA agencies are testing risk sharing and coverage with evidence development initiatives that may provide for conditional approval contingent on further B–R assessment studies.[93] As a matter of fact, in 2010 and 2013, two important initiatives started; the EMA and European Network for Health Technology Assessment (Eunet HTA) EPAR (European Public Assessment Report) initiative started in 2010 to better address payer evidentiary requirements and, in 2013, the EMA and Eunet data collection initiative started to shorten HTA review time by coordinating regulatory and payer data collection; however, it is still too early to evaluate these initiatives.[70] These initiatives are designed to streamline B–R assessment requirements between regulators and payers and to expedite access to drugs. Unique approaches to link payment for drugs and B–R assessment–related evidence (e.g., the linkage of a future rebate on pazopanib, indicated for the treatment of patients with advanced renal cell carcinoma, on the results of a future head-to-head clinical trial) are emerging and will increase the impetus to comparatively assess the benefits and risks of medical products in the same class by linking coverage to such postmarket evidence generation.[70]

Further, many AL proposals have arisen in recent years based on the fact that, as aforementioned in this chapter, the evidence base on drug benefits and risks evolves over time.[31] Through "iterative phases of evidence gathering to reduce uncertainties," AL focuses on maximizing "the positive impact of new drugs on public health by balancing timely access for patients with the need to assess and to provide adequate evolving information on benefits and harms so that better-informed patient-care decisions can be made." Drivers of AL include increasing patient demand for rapid access to drugs to address unmet medical needs, especially during the window of opportunity during which they may benefit. Enablers of AL include better knowledge management, improved clinical trial approaches, incorporation of patient acceptability of uncertainty, and targeted prescribing, among other enablers.[109] Under these approaches, evidence would be more limited at the initial time of approval but the drug's use would be restricted initially via some risk minimization measure. Over time, as evidence is made available in a preplanned fashion via mandated randomized controlled trials and other evidence sources including observational studies and others, the indication would be expanded, pursuant to the plan, on the basis of the emergent evidence.[30]

The AL paradigm is consistent with the PBRER approach of periodically collecting data on benefits and risks over time, although the PBRER does not link this periodic evaluation directly with the approval and coverage of drugs. Collection of robust postmarket evidence for the AL paradigm would necessarily require the support from members of the health care team other than prescribers as well as other stakeholders such as payers, regulators, and health care organizations.[70] Recently, the term *medicines adaptive pathways to patients* (MAPPs) has been coined to reflect that all aspects to increase access, including regulatory, must be addressed (e.g., use in the real-world clinical setting). Ideally, postmarket evidentiary requirements would be defined a priori and aligned with payers under a managed entry agreement (MEA)/CED approach. Importantly, patients' willingness to accept uncertainty under this model needs to be determined and incorporated into regulatory decisions to approve with or without specific restrictions.[109] From the payer perspective, the increasing use of performance-based risk sharing agreements fits hand in glove with AL as they are based on the premise that reimbursement can change over time in the postmarket setting, as more evidence on the B–R profile evolves and in light of uncertainty at the time of approval.[53] Adaptive licensing will not apply to all drugs and may be most useful for rare disease drugs for which risks of harm are presumed not to exceed benefits or when there is substantial regulatory and payer uncertainty.[110] Simulation models can inform drug company decisions to develop particular products under an AL paradigm and patients should be engaged as drugs approved under this model may entail increased risk of harm in light of uncertainty.[110]

In 2014, EMA launched an AL project and is collaborating with HTA agencies, patient organizations, and guideline developers to build on existing regulatory processes and explore "the strengths and weaknesses of all options for development, assessment, licensing, reimbursement, monitoring, and utilization pathways in a confidential manner and without commitment from either side." Findings from this project will inform the development of the AL pathway in Europe for different types of medical products and indications and the nature of iterative drug B–R assessments over time to support drug marketing authorization and also coverage by health care payers.[111]

2.2.3 Asia

2.2.3.1 India

In July of 2010, India's national pharmacovigilance program, implemented by the Drug Controller General of India, was reinitiated as the Pharmacovigilance Program of India (PVPI). PVPI will be expanded in the upcoming years and the goal is to establish 350 ADR centers. This will enhance medical product risk assessment in India at the national level. In contrast to the United States and the EU, which changed aspects of their risk management systems in the past 10 years as aforementioned, India does not have specific guidelines pertaining to risk management systems.[112] In short, the pharmacovigilance system in India is still developing, although adverse drug reactions are increasingly being reported in India under the auspices of the PVPI.

2.2.3.2 China

In 2009, the Chinese FDA created regulatory pathways for the priority review of drugs with the potential to provide substantial benefit. This pathway focuses on drugs to treat serious conditions such as AIDS or cancer, or rare diseases.[113] Further, a risk control plan is required under this pathway, which is comparable to the ICH E2E pharmacovigilance plan and must include a summary of risks and attendant uncertainties. Similar to India, the Chinese drug regulatory system and B–R assessment related requirements are rapidly evolving, although structured B–R assessment frameworks are not in place at this time.

2.2.3.3 Japan

The Pharmaceuticals and Medical Devices Agency (PMDA) established a Science Board in 2012 that supports the advancement of regulatory science in Japan and the evaluation of new medical products. Further, the revised Pharmaceutical Affairs Act was passed in Japan in 2013 and strengthens mechanisms to ensure the safety of drugs and devices.[114] In 2013, risk management plans (RMPs) and plans of postmarket studies were required in Japan for new drugs. The RMPs must be approved by the PMDA and a summary is published on the PMDA website for the public to view.[104] In addition, PMDA is currently developing a medical information database that will have data ready on more than 10 million patients to facilitate postmarket drug risk assessment by PMDA and inform safety-related regulatory actions. Of note, Japan is a voting member of various committees of the ICH, which is tasked to harmonize regulatory requirements for drug approval submissions across various regulatory agencies.

2.2.4 Australia

Australia started requiring risk management plans for selected applications in 2008.[104] In 2009, the Australian Therapeutic Goods Administration started to incorporate the EMA guidelines on risk management plans, which formalizes the requirement to provide robust evidence on risks associated with drugs and facilitate ongoing B–R assessment and management of risks. By 2013, 131 risk management plans were required. Further, recently Australia has attempted to address the underreporting of adverse events by supporting community pharmacy software that facilitates reporting on the safety of drugs and vaccines—this effort has already started to enhance drug risk assessment, and in 2014, many more reports from community pharmacists were received.[115]

2.2.5 ICH M4E (R2) B–R Assessment Guidance

Under the current ICH Guideline finalized in September 2002, the first revision of Module number 4 on Efficacy (M4E, R1), medical product applicants are expected to include their conclusions about drug benefits and risks in the Clinical Overview of Module 2 of the Common Technical Document (CTD) under section number 2.5.6 (Benefits and Risks Conclusions). The Clinical Overview is primarily intended for use by regulatory agencies in the review of the clinical section of a marketing application. As described in M4E (R1), the purpose of section number 2.5.6 is to integrate the multiple conclusions reached in previous sections to provide an overall appraisal of the benefits and risks in clinical use within the context of the indication as well as other available treatments.

However, although the guidance provided general recommendations regarding the expected content of the section, it did not suggest a particular format that could aid applicants in structuring B–R assessment write-ups. Consequently, there is a high level of variability in the approaches taken by various applicants in presenting this information, ranging from unstructured to structured, descriptive or quantitative frameworks. Further refinement of the ICH guidance was needed to promote the original concept of the CTD, that is, reduce regulatory and industry burden and enhance transparency in communication between stakeholders. Therefore, in November 2014, a new ICH Expert Working Group (M4E, R2) was formed to revise section number 2.5.6 of the CTD. The goal of the working group is to provide greater specificity on the format and structure of B–R information in the CTD in order to standardize the presentation of B–R assessment information in regulatory submissions. Such standardization would encompass the information inputs as well as the industry views on those inputs that make up the B–R assessment.[116] The tide is clearly turning as stakeholders (both regulators and payers) increasingly focus on explicit product B–R profiles with a focus on ongoing evaluation over time. The revised section 2.5.6 will constitute a convenient location in the CTD to succinctly discuss the value of medical products in one place without requiring reviewers and assessors to search for disparate components of the needed evidence throughout the submission. This will definitely have an impact on the planning for applicants' submissions and the ability to optimize holistic B–R assessments.

Some notable aspects in the guidance for the revised section include providing the option for applicants to incorporate information about patients' input, which might be descriptive information on patient attitudes toward their disease or information on methodologies intended to elicit patient preferences regarding trade-offs between specific benefits and risks. Although the guidance does not prescribe a specific methodology, it states that "an applicant may choose to use methodologies that quantitatively express the underlying judgments and uncertainties in the assessment," which opens the door for the utilization of more sophisticated methodologies. The use of the terms *key benefits* and *key risks* in the guidance is intended to be consistent with other B–R relevant ICH guidelines (e.g., PBRER). In effect, the document encourages the continuity in the assessment between the pre- and postmarket phases. Suggestions are provided in the guidance for the types and characteristics of benefits and risks to consider when characterizing the B–R profile. Further, strengths, limitations, and uncertainties pertaining to benefit and risk information are expected to be explicitly identified and discussed in this section. Applicants may also, at their discretion, use summary tables or graphical displays to communicate the clinical importance of the key benefits and key risks, as well as the resulting B–R assessment. This implies that tools like "effects tables" and other sophisticated graphical representations might be used to facilitate the visualization of B–R profiles. Finally, the guidance for the revised section stipulates that key benefits may also encompass important characteristics of the medicinal product, which might not have been traditionally characterized as "study end points," including its convenience (e.g., a more convenient dosing regimen or route of administration), that may lead to improved patient adherence, functional or quality-of-life improvement, or benefits that affect those other than the patient (e.g., population benefits of a vaccine owing to herd immunity).

2.3 The Dynamics of B–R Assessment in the Postmarket Setting

Medical product benefits and risks are initially assessed in the premarket setting, starting from the preclinical studies and human clinical trials (Phase I–III trials). This section specifically focuses on characterizing the context for the postmarket medical product risk assessment as it relates to the B–R profile of such products because (1) more medical products are being approved based on evidence in smaller populations with less information on medical product benefits and risks via accelerated approval pathways, (2) information on how well medical products work and how safe they are in real-world use is increasingly dependent on postmarket evidence, and (3) several new regulatory policy and science initiatives to assess B–R, as mentioned earlier, are calling for ongoing B–R assessment in the postmarket setting.

Postmarket product risk assessment is a multidimensional paradigm, reflecting the interaction between multiple sources of evidence and many stakeholders. There are three basic dimensions to postmarket medical product risk assessment: evidence generation, evidence interpretation and integration, and regulatory decision making; each dimension has its own unique set of considerations (Figure 2.1).[44] In a nutshell, the first dimension, evidence generation, involves the identification and assessment of a safety signal that may arise from one or more pre- or postmarket evidence sources. Often, analysis of the quality and strength of the evidence behind the initial signal is followed by other studies or evaluations designed to refine the signal. The scope of these additional studies is dictated

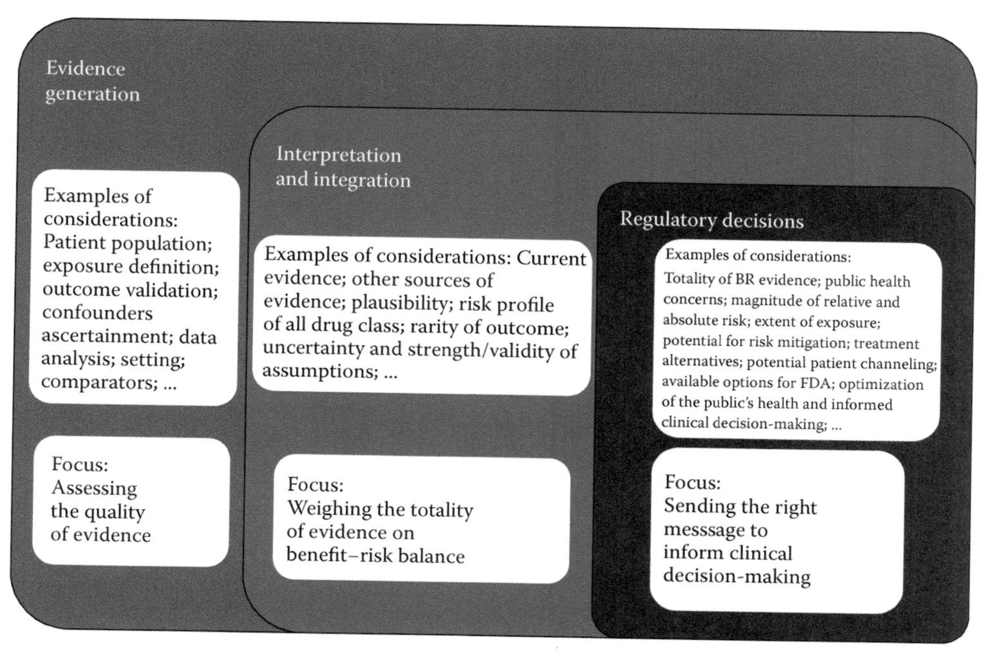

FIGURE 2.1
Dimensions of postmarket drug safety assessment. (From Hammad TA et al. *Clin Pharmacol Ther.* 2013;94:349–358.)

by the information needed for an accurate understanding of the potential risks of harm in a relevant patient population in order to support a meaningful B–R evaluation of the medical product.

After the evidence from each source is assessed, the second dimension entails the interpretation and integration of evidence from all sources regarding the safety issue of interest. This dimension involves weighing the totality of evidence regarding the risks of harm as well as assessing the level of residual uncertainty concerning this risk at the time of evaluation. The third dimension is the decision to take a specific action to address the safety concern based on whether the evidence unfavorably shifts the already established B–R balance. In this complex dimension, regulators consider, among other factors, the totality of the evidence of the product's benefits and risks, the unmet medical need, the availability of alternate therapies, and the available risk management tools that can mitigate the risk of harm. The critical goal under this dimension is to communicate an accurate and meaningful message to patients and health care professionals on the product safety issue in a timely fashion and thus inform evidence-based clinical decision making to manage products' harms in light of their benefits. More details about the specifics of this paradigm can be found elsewhere.[44]

It is worth noting that the evaluation of various sources of evidence supporting a particular safety concern, and attendant actions, does not progress in a linear fashion from the lower-level evidence to the higher-level evidence, but rather may be done in sequence or in parallel (Figure 2.2). The utility of any evidence source is evaluated within the context of the other sources and all the aforementioned considerations, not in a vacuum. Additionally, depending on the strength of the available evidence and the importance of the safety issue to the public's health, at any point in the evaluation process, a more in-depth formal study of a given safety signal can be initiated or a regulatory action can be undertaken. Therefore,

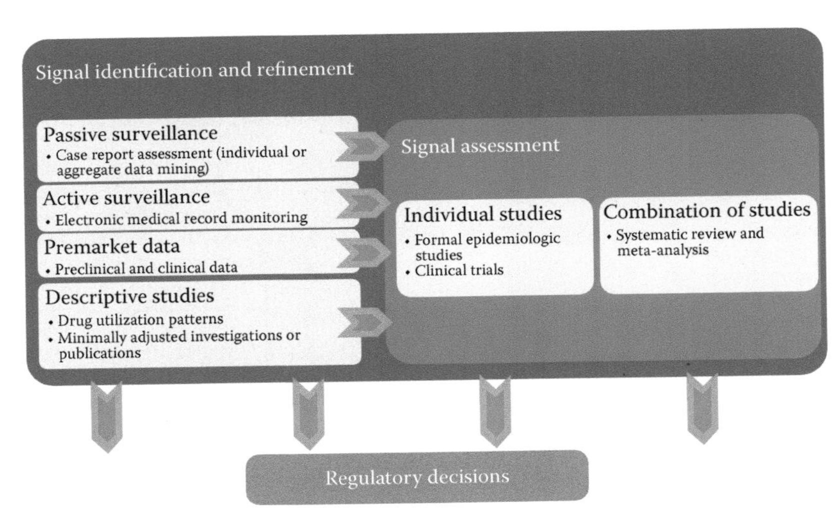

FIGURE 2.2
Postmarket medical product safety signal evaluation dynamics.

it is crucial to appreciate that a particular type/level of evidence might not play the same role or have the same contribution every time, even for situations with apparently similar safety concerns. As such, the strength of evidence for product safety is a continuum with shifting boundaries that are sometimes difficult to discern for those not involved in the day-to-day evaluations of safety concerns. Importantly, as new information emerges over time, the totality of evidence is reevaluated on an ongoing basis, making it a dynamic, iterative process. The implication of the dynamic nature of the evaluation process is that multiple regulatory actions on the same product safety issue may take place over time and this might have a significant impact on the perception of the B–R balance.[44]

One of the main challenges in establishing an ongoing pattern of B–R assessment lies in the source of the information (Figure 2.3). Efficacy data (i.e., can a product work?) are mostly obtained from premarket clinical trials, whereas a more complete picture of safety might emerge from postmarket sources that complement what is known from the premarket phase. Effectiveness data (i.e., does a product work in the real-world clinical setting?), on the other hand, are harder to gauge in the postmarket phase. Relying on premarket data for benefit while accruing data on safety on an ongoing basis in the postmarket setting dictates that the postmarket B–R evaluation is influenced only by the new safety data and thus that B–R balance can only become less favorable than the initial one over time. Although this is a perennial challenge, new initiatives funded by entities such as the US-based PCORI may support the development and use of methods to improve confidence in findings regarding benefits from real-world evidence. More details about the specific challenges encountered with the information used in the pre- and postmarket B–R evaluations can be found elsewhere.[44,117] Further, because some adverse reactions of special interest occur infrequently, even a few cases can drastically change the risk estimates and related B–R balance, underscoring inherent uncertainties associated with dealing with sparse data.

These realities underscore the need to recast the paradigm of how postmarket B–R evaluations should optimally be undertaken, for example, what are the optimal data sources and whether the evaluation should be carried out on a quantitative or a qualitative basis taking into consideration some of the challenges depicted in the following section about

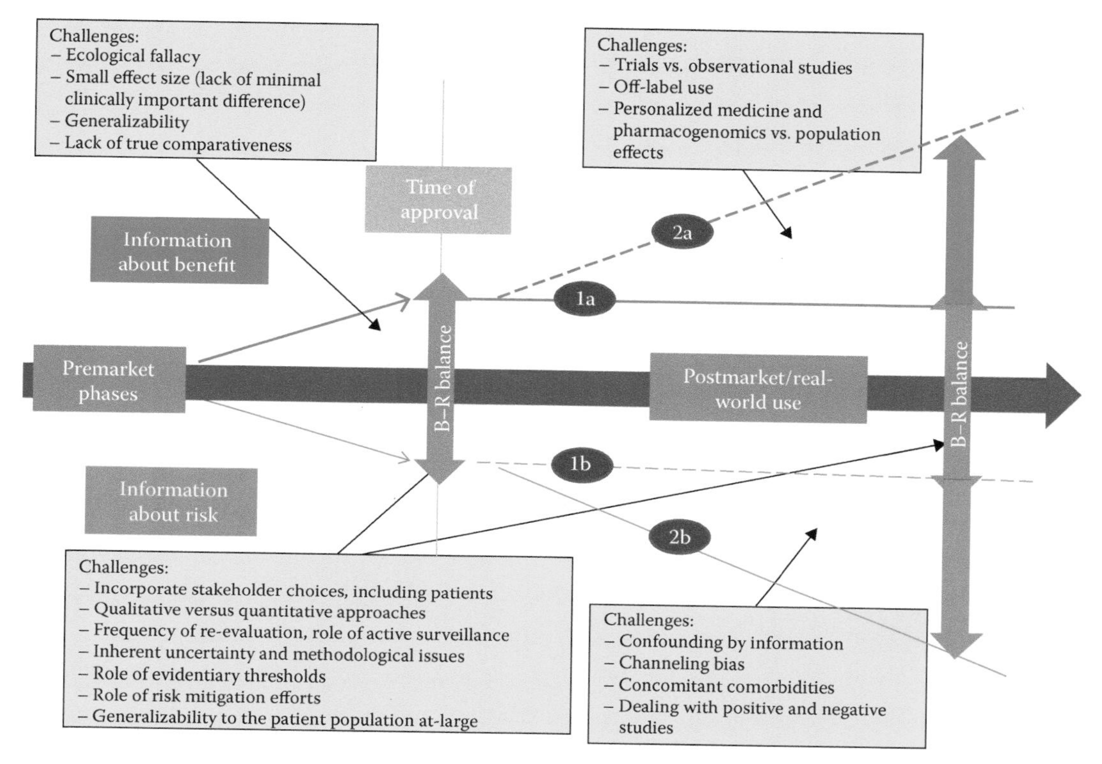

FIGURE 2.3
Select challenges in population-based benefit–risk assessment. The horizontal red and green lines (1a and 1b) in the postmarket setting reflect the level of information "carried over" from the premarket setting regarding benefit and risk. The sloped lines (2a and 2b) in the postmarket setting reflect the accrued (for safety) and the desired (for benefit) information. The knowledge gap pertains to approaches for addressing the difference between the solid and dashed lines within the context of the listed challenges. The nature of the knowledge gaps related to benefits and risks in the postmarket setting are not similar since it is inevitable to collect (and accept) more safety information postmarket, although the data on benefits are harder to gauge.[44] (From Hammad TA et al. *Clin Pharmacol Ther.* 2013;94;349–358.)

current regulatory science knowledge gaps. Regulators are working with stakeholders to develop approaches to enhance the evaluation of benefits and risks in the pre- and postmarket settings, which should optimize the regulatory decision-making process.

2.4 Regulatory Science Knowledge Gaps and Related Challenges[44]

Several regulatory science knowledge gaps related to our ability to assess medical products' benefits and risks, in the pre- and postmarket stages, will be identified in this section, many of which are consistent with the gaps formerly identified by Hammad et al.[44] Regulators and payers should continue the ongoing dialogue with multiple stakeholders to address relevant critical knowledge gaps regarding managing evidentiary uncertainty in all the regulatory science domains involved with B–R assessment.

In a nutshell, these gaps include the following:

- Better methods to link and leverage the increasingly available electronic health and patient-centered data for B–R evaluations are needed, especially pertaining to following individual patients across the continuum of care. This linkage will support the conduct of timelier postmarket drug B–R evaluations to inform clinical decision making and future shared savings models that may provide savings to patients and health care professionals based on the selection of drugs or other interventions that provide comparable value at a lower cost.[118]
- A dialogue about the need for the development and validation of acceptable thresholds for safety concerns and related actions should be initiated as this aspect has a major impact on the perceived B–R balance of various products.
- Novel approaches need to be further developed for the integration of evidence from disparate sources, while addressing conflicting findings, along with ensuring that all evidence is given appropriate weight in the evaluation of overall B–R balance.
- There is a need to develop methodologies to assess the impact of various risk mitigation programs, for example, REMS; perhaps in the future, regulators may leverage EHRs for the implementation and evaluation of REMS and similar strategies intended for enhancing the B–R balance.[119]
- More attention should be paid to develop approaches to manage uncertainty in the evidence behind benefits and risks. The impact of potential over-adherence to the precautionary principle should be assessed as this may not be consistent with patients' perspectives about their disease.
- The role of patient engagement in B–R assessment should be further refined. Novel quantitative and qualitative approaches are being identified and piloted to capture the patient input in the assessment of benefits and risks in the premarket and postmarket settings. This will facilitate the incorporation of patient views into regulatory decision-making processes.
- With respect to the potential role of personalized medicine in the B–R assessment process, more than 150 FDA-approved drugs include some pharmacogenomics information in their label but there is very limited information on the clinical utility of related tests,[120] and thus in many cases, the tests are not covered by insurance companies. Innovative future efforts to develop the evidence base on the clinical utility of these tests will increase their value and use.
- Policies and approaches to implement AL, in collaboration with relevant stakeholders, are being piloted and, in the future, might fill some of the important knowledge gap pertaining to the adaptability of the drug regulatory approval and postapproval coverage process to ever-changing evidence on drugs benefits and risks.

More details on some of these knowledge gaps are included in Sections 2.4.1 through 2.4.6.

2.4.1 Data Sources

Data collected in the postmarket period of medical products' life cycles play an integral role in the ongoing evaluation of B–R profiles. Over the past several decades, there has been increasing use of electronic health care data, including administrative claims data and EHRs, to evaluate medicines (see Section 4.2, Data Sources Chapter in this book). Some of these data are collected primarily for billing and patient management and using it to evaluate B–R balance represents a secondary use, or repurposing, of the data. The increasing experience with use of large health care databases to study drug-related outcomes has led to the identification of certain systematic gaps in these data sources. For example, there is a general lack of methods to routinely link multiple types of US electronic health data, although this might be changing in light of PCORI and other initiatives in this area.[121,122] The needs for linking health data in these databases fall under one or more of the following scenarios (Figure 2.4):[44] (1) data on individual patients to evaluate postmarket drug-related outcomes longitudinally across the continuum of care (e.g., subjective and objective clinical information and results of lab work, inpatient and outpatient treatments in the same health system, data from multiple payers, e.g., private insurance as well as Medicare, Medicaid, or VA, and data from the multiple health plans that the patient might enroll in over time), (2) data to evaluate the effect of drug exposure of one patient on a related patient (e.g., mothers and babies), and (3) data on different patients from a distributed network of multiple sites of care (e.g., across various regions and countries). The challenge in dealing with these scenarios is that they are often intertwined as several scenarios might be encountered at the same time when investigators try to enhance their study power by gathering information on as many patients as possible.

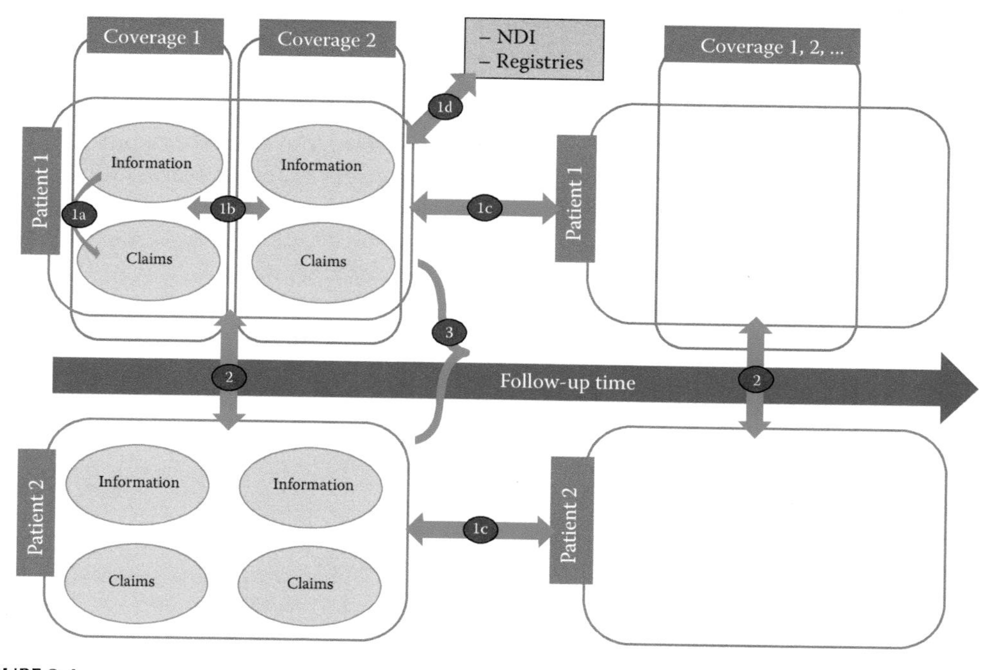

FIGURE 2.4
Data linking and pooling. 1a, Link contemporaneous patient information within the same health insurance coverage. 1b, Link contemporaneous patient information under different simultaneous health insurance coverage. 1c, Link patient information over time, within and across various health insurance coverage. 1d, Link patient information to stand-alone sources like registries and National Death Index (NDI). 2, Link information for two related patients, for example, mother and baby. 3, Pool information on different patients from distributed network of databases.[44] (From Hammad TA et al. *Clin Pharmacol Ther.* 2013;94;349–358.)

In the United States and some other countries, the first gap arises from the fact that, in practice, patients enroll into and disenroll from health plans at discrete time points, a practice that often precludes the capture of all relevant episodes of care over time. Additionally, at a given point in time, some episodes of care may be captured by an electronic health care data source, while other episodes may not be captured or captured only in paper format. Further, there is often a lack of complete data on some key determinants of health, such as relevant medical history, smoking, body mass index, and use of over-the-counter medical products. Lack of longitudinal data that capture all care interferes with interpretation of the a given product's association with a long-latency outcome such as cancer, which is increasingly reported as a potential concern with the use of some products.[123] This aspect is particularly missing from many clinical trials that are often not long enough to provide accurate depiction of such outcomes. The aforementioned features of electronic health care data create an ongoing challenge for generating evidence that would be incorporated in an ongoing B–R assessment. For example, when evaluating combined hormonal contraceptives (CHCs) and the risk of thromboembolism,[124] some studies took these factors into account while others could not, resulting in somewhat conflicting findings regarding the evaluated risk of harm, as reflected in the updated CHC drug labels.[125] This implies slightly different B–R profiles based on the respective studies. Studies of the association between tumor necrosis factor alpha blockers and the risk of cancer have also led to conflicting results possibly for similar reasons.

Nonetheless, the increasing adoption and use of electronic health (e-health) records, PHRs, mobile devices, and patient-centered websites, and the development and use of data-rich health information exchanges (HIEs) for patient care and medical intervention evaluations, may alleviate some of these problems in the future. For example, projects to link claims data from multiple payers (e.g., CMS with private payers, outpatient claims with inpatient billing data) may mitigate limitations on the ability to study patients' complete continuum of care over time.[126] HIEs[127] are also being developed in some US states to provide access to holistic data on patients across insurers and providers. HIEs are platforms that can connect all types of users together and can be used to link EMR, prescriptions, administrative claims, patient portable device, and other data sources,[128] resulting in more informed B–R assessment and timelier actions by stakeholders.[128] These resources would enable health care practitioners to use population-based data in a more refined way in individual patient care, furthering the goals of personalized medicine. Along these lines, increased use of electronic prior authorization (ePA) by insurers[129] will inform the study of off-label drug uses if the reason for prescribing is a mandated field in the ePA submission process, which it is for some drugs for select ePA platforms. A related initiative may improve the production of evidence on the off-label use of cancer drugs, which account for the highest proportion of the increasing cost of specialty drugs. This initiative would do this by encouraging the use of coverage with evidence development and creating a Targeted Agent and Profiling Utilization Registry for patients who fail conventional regimens and have genetic mutations, identifiable with validated tests. These patients can then be targeted by a drug approved by the FDA for another indication.[130]

Data linking would also leverage efforts initiated through registries to study drug safety in the context of the ongoing evaluation of B–R profiles. Drug manufacturers have established registries to examine certain outcomes in patients taking their drug in the postmarket setting. These registries typically enroll patients taking the manufacturer's drug and only follow these patients while they are taking that drug. Even if long-term outcomes can be ascertained, such drug-based registries are often inefficient in capturing the therapies that a patient may switch to or from, along with changes in medical conditions over time, all of which can be determinants of the ultimate clinical outcome of interest. An alternative approach has been the development of disease-based registries to assess adverse drug outcomes that may be more efficient than multiple, independent drug-based registries pertaining to the same indication and are important for the evaluation of rare conditions.[131,132] These registries could play an important role in postmarket B–R assessment, especially for drugs indicated for orphan conditions,[133] which may be approved based on a relatively small number of patients in the preapproval safety database. Further, linkage of registries to large e-health databases and others such as cancer registries will facilitate evaluating drug effects in the real world.

Ethical and patient-related considerations prohibit studying drug exposure effects on pregnant women, which in turn creates another knowledge gap in many medical products' B–R profiles. Linking medical data for related patients, such as mother–child pairs, facilitates the examination of certain drug safety situations that cannot be examined otherwise. The Medication Exposure in Pregnancy Risk Evaluation Program (MEPREP) is an example of a novel program, funded by the FDA, designed to link data from mothers and their babies across multiple population-based data sources. In addition to the aforementioned issues around linking individual patient data, two other challenges were encountered: (1) valid linkage of the pregnant woman's data with that of her baby and (2) building a CDM to combine data from a network of multiple sources to enable statistical analyses of pooled data, while preserving patient privacy. A 2012 paper describes the steps taken to build this unique system, which expanded the capacity to examine drug use in pregnancy and will facilitate the study of health outcomes in babies after maternal exposure to drugs.[134] More effort is needed to expand these types of linkages even further to enable studies to have enough statistical power to quantify or rule out important pregnancy-related drug exposure safety signals aiding the accurate depiction of B–R profiles for various medical products.

It is important to note that CDMs, which are required for any distributed research network data models (e.g., MEPREP, Sentinel, OMOP, etc.), come with their own set of structural and analytic challenges. Often, CDMs are tailored structurally for the least amount of common information available across sites within a network to amass information on as many patients as possible. However, this approach might deprive investigators of the ability to utilize the more detailed information available in one or more sites, while adding another layer of variability stemming from the heterogeneity across sites; this heterogeneity can arise because of differences between sites in patient populations, formulary restrictions, enrollment criteria, level of clinical outcomes ascertainment and validation, coding practices, availability of key health determinants such as smoking and medical history in the medical record, and other factors. In certain instances, this could have a significant impact on the ability to use data in the CDM to investigate or interpret drug safety findings. For example, in the studies of attention deficit hyperactivity disorder medications and the risk of serious cardiovascular events, risk estimates differed between Medicaid and non-Medicaid populations.[135] On the other hand, attempting to maximize the use of available data in all sites might mean that risk estimates could be adjusted for different sets of covariates within each site, which might complicate the interpretation of pooled findings of the safety investigation across sites. A more general challenge related to pooling data across multiple sites is the need to develop methodologies to analyze and interpret conflicting findings among sites within a network or an overall finding that is driven by one or a few sites that happened to be large enough to influence the results. Finally, CDMs are rarely compatible across research networks, thus limiting their utility to only one network. However, it is true that several efforts are ongoing to connect distributed research networks and this could be a game changer. While a universal CDM might not be practicable, an effort to examine the feasibility of establishing the minimal common elements of a universal CDM for various data networks might be warranted.

2.4.2 Threshold for Safety Concerns and Impact on B–R Balance

The issue of whether to use a risk estimate threshold in the assessment of B–R profiles requires further exploration to determine if it is possible to develop and evaluate actionable and evidence-based risk estimate thresholds that enable the minimization of inherent uncertainty encountered in various drug safety evaluation scenarios, especially in the postmarket setting. The significance of this issue is heightened because of the increased focus on the ongoing value-based B–R assessment and reassessment of a drug's B–R profile throughout its life cycle.[14]

The assessment of a medical product's B–R profile entails a judgment on the level of acceptable risk of harm versus the extent of anticipated benefits. The source of information makes a difference in considering the thresholds used for making this judgment. Traditional evidentiary hierarchies, which designate RCTs as the highest quality evidence, may not always be applicable or appropriate for studying postmarket drug safety.[136] Because of limitations in capturing safety information in some clinical trials[117] and the relatively low frequency of certain serious adverse drug reactions, observational studies may be a more informative source of drug safety evidence in some situations (see Data Sources Chapter in this book, Section 4). Furthermore, the lack of generalizability to the real-world setting of some safety data from premarket RCTs may have important implications for postmarket (B–R) evaluation and decision making.[137] However, because of the absence of treatment randomization between the exposure and comparator groups, observational studies are vulnerable to potential confounding and bias, as measured and unmeasured health determinative factors associated with prescribing the drug may lead to spurious associations or a change in the strength of the observed association between some drug exposures and adverse clinical outcomes.[138] In addition, the ability to access data on large numbers of patients in electronic health care databases increases the likelihood of statistically significant associations that may not always be clinically relevant. Therefore, there is often an interest in utilizing a threshold of risk estimate to account for the potential impact of these challenges in the evaluation of observed associations between drug exposure and health outcomes in the postmarket setting.

The threshold of a relative risk estimate of 2.0 (which means the risk is doubled because of drug exposure) has been posited in the past by some as a minimum bar for the use of observational evidence for regulatory decision making,[139] although others point out that the threshold should be developed on a case-by-case basis depending on the drug and the safety issue of interest and might be much higher in some scenarios.[140] The concern over risk estimates between 1.0 and 2.0 is that statistical adjustment techniques cannot control completely for confounding and that relative risk estimates below 2.0 may still represent the effects of residual confounding or bias, although very large studies with strong controls for confounding in place may constitute valid evidence.[140] However, the absolute risk corresponding to the relative risk in this range could have a considerable public health importance; if the absolute risk is high in the general population, even a small relative risk increase owing to drug exposure can be consequential on a population level. On the other hand, taking an action based on a small absolute risk might deprive some patients of the beneficial effects of drugs. The lack of consensus on the appropriate risk estimate threshold, if any, from the societal and public health burden point of view, warrants further dialogue among stakeholders.

The careful development of thresholds is also gaining importance with the increased focus on active surveillance, which may include continuous and sequential monitoring for specific types of drug safety concerns. This is because active surveillance is anticipated to be an ongoing source of information that will affect the perception of B–R balance of many medical products. Methods to address the impact of using sequential multiple testing on threshold determination will be important in understanding active drug safety surveillance evaluations. Some have proposed the development of an alerting algorithm tailored to particular features of a drug–outcome pair, including the expected event frequencies.[140] Others suggested avoidance of traditional scenario-based measures of accuracy, such as sensitivity and specificity, and instead have proposed an event-based classification approach that explicitly accounts for the accuracy in alerting, the timeliness in alerting, and the trade-offs between the costs of false-negative and false-positive alerting.[142]

2.4.3 Integration of Information from Multiple Sources

Information related to benefits and risks may be gathered from a multitude of sources and it is essential to leverage the best science for integration (see Section 6 in Data Sources Chapter in this book). However, there is a lack of evidence-based approaches to optimally integrate information from multiple sources.[144] Under the auspices of the Innovative Medicines Initiative, focused on strengthening the biopharmaceutical enterprise in Europe, drug safety monitoring projects were recently undertaken to address multiple regulatory science knowledge gaps, including the integration of information, which should enlighten efforts around the world regarding B–R evaluation. Methods to integrate information within a particular evidence source, for example, differing results from multiple studies of similar design attributes, are also a critical regulatory science knowledge gap.[145] Perhaps the development and application of Bayesian approaches may facilitate the use and integration of prior knowledge, such as clinical pharmacologic and other data, in drug risk assessments and subsequently in B–R evaluations.[146] A related aspect is the need to improve the adjudication of conflicting findings from different evidence sources.[14] The previously mentioned IOM report highlighted different FDA scientists' interpretations of the conflicting evidence on the association between rosiglitazone and cardiovascular risks and underscored the importance of transparency and consistent approaches to address conflicting findings, along with ensuring that all evidence is given appropriate weight in the evaluation of drug safety; methods to address these issues need to be further developed.

The use of novel computer-based modeling and systems approaches may leverage multiple data sources and types of data for the evaluation of the safety, effectiveness, and quality of medical interventions in the postmarket setting.[147,148] In addition, methods continue to be developed and evaluated (e.g., a case-centered logistic regression of angioedema and renin–angiotensin–aldosterone system drugs) for the synthesis and use of evidence from multiple distributed network sites used in postmarket drug safety surveillance evaluations,[60] as well as evidence from multiple observational safety studies. CIOMS Expert Working Group X, which brings together experts from industry, academia, and regulatory agencies, is developing a guidance document on the meta-analysis of studies for drug safety evaluation.

2.4.4 Managing Evidentiary Uncertainty

B–R assessment lies at the intersection of three domains of regulatory science: (1) the evaluation of benefits, including efficacy (i.e., can a drug work?) and effectiveness (i.e., does a drug work in the real-world clinical setting?); (2) risk assessment and mitigation, which entails the identification and characterization of risks associated with the prescribing and use of medications and the selection of mitigation strategies to optimize the B–R balance; and (3) approaches to evaluate the B–R balance in the pre- and postmarket stages on an ongoing basis.[44] Each one of these scientific fields is associated with its unique sources of uncertainty, which compounds the overall uncertainty challenge. In general, additional scientific knowledge gaps remain, pertaining to how to (1) best address the uncertainty stemming from the heterogeneity of drug benefits and risks in the pre- and postmarket settings and (2) operationalize population group-level evidence to optimize individual patient therapy.

It is a challenge to strike the right balance between the precautionary principle, which entails taking substantial steps to limit or avoid potential serious risks in light of uncertainty (i.e., the first do no harm mantra), and eschewing or minimizing the potential impact of such risks in order to maximize access to helpful drugs.[149] After all, the over-adherence to the precautionary principle may be conflating two different sources of uncertainty: the uncertainty about the extent of the risk with uncertainty about the willingness of the patient to accept the risk. A patient's willingness to accept risk is likely to change over time depending on the stage of life and the severity of disease, which adds to the complexity of drug regulatory decisions.[150] This is especially challenging in light of the nature of ever-emerging evidence on the benefits and risks of drugs.[44] Regulators and payers should continue the ongoing dialogue with multiple stakeholders to address the relevant critical knowledge gaps.

Areas of uncertainty that require additional attention were as highlighted in the FDA's B–R assessment implementation plan. To address these areas of uncertainty, the US IOM supported a workshop, in 2013, on drug B–R assessment focused on characterizing and communicating uncertainty in the assessment of the benefits and risks of drugs.[150] Regulatory policy decisions pertaining to drug approval status and attendant risk management programs, made on the basis of B–R assessments in the pre- or postmarket settings, are laden with uncertainty and an inability to assess counterfactual outcomes, which is a key challenge in many other policymaking arenas.[151] The workshop highlighted the specific areas of debate around B–R assessment, including metrics employed (qualitative vs. quantitative), timing/frequency of evaluation (static vs. sequential), perspectives/preferences (differential preference based on stakeholder), contents, format, and frequency of communications to stakeholders, and the best choice for comparators in the evaluation of B–R profiles of products. Sources of uncertainty were characterized as clinical, statistical, and methodological; more details can be found in the workshop summary.[150]

With respect to biosimilars, despite the FDA's guidance documents, in the ensuing months, criteria will need to be developed by regulators for the B–R assessment requirements, which would suffice to establish interchangeability of medical products, a task that will likely be very challenging.[73]

2.4.5 Risk Management and Minimization Assessment

The Food and Drug Administration Amendments Act of 2007 gave FDA the authority to require REMS plans from manufacturers to ensure that the benefits of a drug or biological medical product outweigh its risks of harm. Regulators evaluating the impact of REMS, or risk minimization strategies, and similar strategies employed by other regulatory agencies on B–R profiles face many challenges across the different REMS evaluation domains. These challenges include the following: (1) for many drugs, the requirement for a REMS is often imposed at the time of initial approval and thus it is not feasible to compare outcomes between a drug with a REMS and the hypothetical counterfactual scenario of that same drug without a REMS; (2) there are often no appropriate comparator drugs, in the same or similar class, without a REMS; (3) it is difficult to evaluate REMS' impact on the actual health outcomes (vs. surrogate measures of these outcomes) and patient burden as well as access; (4) for many drugs with a REMS with ETASU, the patient populations are relatively small, limiting statistical power to characterize meaningful changes; and (5) many REMS manage risks that are difficult to ascertain, such as teratogenicity.

Many previous evaluative studies for the impact of regulatory actions have not been robust. In addition to FDA's forthcoming PDUFA V–mandated guidance on REMS evaluation and the new CIOMS guidance, the development and validation of rigorous methodologies for the evaluation of REMS and other regulatory actions are essential to ensure REMS effectiveness. As aforementioned, perhaps in the future, regulators may be able to leverage EHRs for the implementation and evaluation of REMS and similar strategies intended for enhancing the B–R balance through risk mitigation.[119] This is especially important because these strategies may be increasingly required for specialty drugs and biologics to restrict their use in light of limited evidence on safety and effectiveness that is available in the premarket setting.

2.4.6 The Role of Patient Engagement in B–R Assessment

In addition to premarket drug development, there is an increasing need to better capture and incorporate the patient input into the regulatory decision making. Although, in recent years, one patient representative has typically been included on FDA advisory committees to opine and provide advice on drug approval and postmarket regulatory actions, the patient representatives' contributions have generally been limited. Further, patients who speak in open public hearings during advisory committee meetings provide an important point of view, although if the speakers have benefitted from the drug at issue in the clinical trial setting, their views may not be representative of all relevant patients with the condition of interest. Stakeholders increasingly believe that more scientific and evidence-based approaches to account for patients' input in regulatory decision making and the B–R assessment as well as risk minimization strategies would enhance these assessments and decisions during the development of pharmaceutical medical products as well as in the approval and postapproval settings. The robustness and transparency of pharmaceutical development as well as the regulatory approval process will be improved through facilitating patient involvement and input. In general, such input can, for illustrative purposes, fall in one of three operational aspects across the medical product development life cycle: patient perspectives, patient preferences, and patient-centered choices (Figure 2.5).

Evaluating the patient perspectives entails gathering insights into the day-to-day living with the disease and its major symptoms and struggles. This aspect aids in understanding the nature of the challenge that the patient faces, specific unmet needs, and what is known as the minimal clinically important difference, defined as the minimal change in the disease that patients perceive as beneficial. Characterizing this aspect would inform targeting the appropriate disease attributes, end point selection, and trial design and conduct. However, the value gleaned from the effort is limited by the features of the available

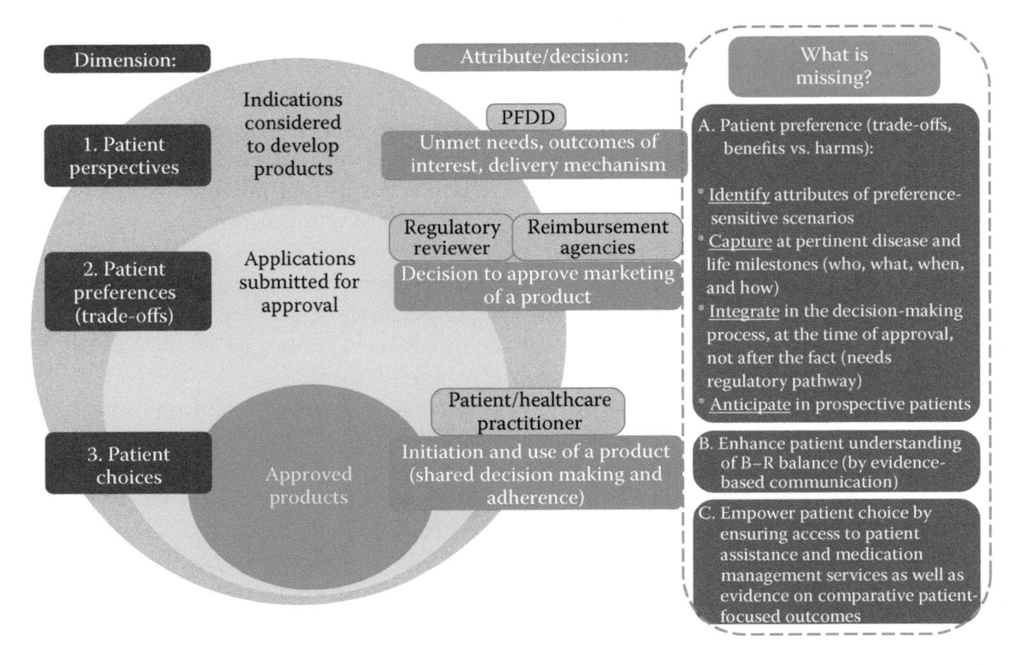

FIGURE 2.5
Patient-focused drug development, regulatory decision making or real-world drug use: perspectives, preferences, and choices.

medical products regarding the ability to tackle identified patient struggles. In other words, after collecting information about how a particular disease really affects patients from their perspectives, there is no guarantee that there will be available medical products to address patients' needs, although they may be developed in the future.

Patient preferences ascertainment entails an elicitation of how patients feel about recognized benefits and risks. This aspect aids in understanding and characterizing sources of heterogeneity in patient preferences, which reflects the extent to which preferences differ among patients regarding benefits, risks, costs, and patient willingness to accept uncertainty about benefits and risks. In this context, it could help identify the minimum required knowledge, regarding the key benefits and risks, before patients can decide on specific trade-offs, as well as the most appropriate and practical platform to collect these data (e.g., in-person surveys vs. Internet-based approaches). Characterizing this aspect should inform the decision making by regulatory authorities and HTA bodies through better appreciation of the individual patient views based on an understanding of factors underpinning differences among patients as well as those influencing patients' willingness to accept uncertainties around adverse effects in light of recognized benefits. Eventually, the effort should enhance the ability to identify and communicate a more accurate and balanced depiction of B–R balance of various medical products, which is in the best interest of all stakeholders. It is worth noting that patient preferences ascertainment, in some scenarios, might provide at least a partial solution to the potential for over-adherence to the precautionary principle, which, as aforementioned, conflates the uncertainty about the extent of the risk with the uncertainty about the willingness of patients to accept the risk. However, we should take into consideration that, when we try to operationalize the information we gather, there is a difference between finding the subgroup of patients with a favorable B–R profile and the subgroup of patients that a particular B–R profile is acceptable to them. The implication is that for the former, we try to find predictors of when a patient will benefit with minimal risk, but for the latter, we need to be able to predict the individual patients' preferences when they are faced with several choices among interventions with varied B–R balance, which is more difficult.

Patient-centered choices refer to the choices made after licensure among medical products and services. This entails collecting pertinent information to prepare the appropriate answers for patients' questions during the discussion that takes place with them when it is time to make a choice of which drug to take. Characterizing this aspect aids in understanding the drivers behind patient choices as well as eventual adherence to take helpful drugs regularly and should inform the effort for more effective patient education and resource utilization for marketed medical products. Further, it is necessary to empower patient choice by further ensuring access to patient assistance and medication management services as well as germane evidence on comparative patient-focused outcomes. However, the domain of available choices would be limited by the subset of medical products that made it to market, which underscores the significance of engaging patients earlier in the process to understand their preferences, as depicted previously, to make sure patients have more choices to satisfy their needs at the point of care. An important knowledge gap here stems from need to develop approaches to ensure that patients, at the point of care, appreciate how patient preferences, if any, were used in the approval process and how these preferences may or may not necessarily be acceptable to them.

More effort is warranted to develop methods and approaches to better characterize each one of the three patient input aspects (perspectives, preferences, and choices). These approaches should take into consideration how to capture the aforementioned variation in patient input driven by the stage of life at diagnosis (younger vs. older patients) as well as the stage of disease (mild vs. advanced). The data collected should be compatible with the nature of the group-level data used in medical product development; anecdotal and narrative data are much harder to consistently integrate in the development process. An integral effort is also needed to develop approaches to enhance patients' understanding of the vocabulary used to discern B–R balance by enhancing the science of evidence-based communication. Along these lines, studies have pointed out that current B–R communication vehicles are not optimal.[152]

2.5 Conclusion

This chapter provided a background on the drug B–R assessment landscape, discussed recent policy initiatives pertaining to B–R assessment, and highlighted key knowledge gaps that should be addressed in the upcoming months and years to enhance B–R assessment on an ongoing basis and attendant regulatory decision making.

In conclusion, rapid changes in regulatory policy and science across the world are taking place and will affect drug B–R assessments. Efforts are ongoing to develop robust innovations that will link disparate data sources to potentially inform a variety of evaluations on comparative drug value.[153] Further, proposed legislation, such as the 21st Century Cures Act in the United States as well as similar efforts in other countries, may increase the number of medical products for which there is greater uncertainty about benefits and risks in the premarket setting and a greater need for robust postmarket evaluations of benefits and risks. Nonetheless, advances in predictive analytics, regulatory science, personalized genomic information, and related digital tools may enable the prediction of adverse events associated with drugs and other medical interventions.[154] Additionally, the recent initiative by President Obama in precision medicine, launched early 2015, and comparable global efforts are likely to support the development of more targeted therapies that benefit smaller subsets of patient populations. These initiatives may inform the forthcoming sixth reauthorization of the PDUFA in the United States in 2017, along with other global policy and scientific initiatives. Enhanced data sources and capture on the basis of the aforementioned initiatives may in fact ensure that both personalized and population health can be realized simultaneously in the not so far future.[153] Collaboration among the biopharmaceutical industry, regulators, payers, patients, academics, health care professionals, and health care organizations will increasingly be required in the future to optimize drug B–R assessments and related linkages to health technology assessments and coverage status, and fill important knowledge gaps in this value-focused era.

References

1. James Gleick. 2011. The Information: A History, A Theory, A Flood. New York: Random House.
2. Jason Burke. 2013. Health Analytics: Gaining the Insights to Transform Health Care: Hoboken, New Jersey: John Wiley & Sons.
3. National Center for Health Statistics. No. 143. Use and Characteristics of Electronic Health Record Systems Among Office-based Physician Practices: United States, 2001–2013. 8 pp. (PHS) 2014–1209. January 2014.
4. Patient Protection and Affordable Care Act (PPACA) of 2010, Pub. L. 111–48.
5. Meghan Hufstader Gabriel & Matthew Swain, Office of the National Coordinator for Health Information Technology. E-Prescribing Trends in the United States. July 2014.
6. Hughes S, Wells K, McSorley P. Preparing individual patient data from clinical trials for sharing: The GlaxoSmithKline approach. *Pharm Stat.* 2014 May–Jun;13(3):179–83.
7. Krumholz HM, Peterson, ED. Open access to clinical trials data. *JAMA* 2014;312(10):1002–3.
8. Friedman C, Rubin J, Brown J et al. Toward a science of learning systems: A research agenda for the high-functioning Learning Health System. *J Am Med Inform Assoc.* 2014 Oct 23. pii: amiajnl-2014-002977. doi: 10.1136/amiajnl-2014-002977. [Epub ahead of print]
9. 21st Century Cures Act. United States House of Representatives Discussion Draft. 2015.
10. Marc L. Berger, Craig Lipset, Alex Gutteridge et al. Optimizing the leveraging of real-world data to improve the development and use of medicines. *Value Health* 2015;18:127–30.
11. PPACA at Section 6301.
12. O'Leary TJ, Slutsky JR, Bernard MA. Comparative effectiveness research priorities at federal agencies: The view from the Department of Veterans Affairs, National Institute on Aging, and Agency for Healthcare Research and Quality. *J Am Geriatr Soc.* 2010 Jun;58(6):1187–92.
13. Barlas S. FDA accepts its first biosimilar applications: However, the agency's requirements are still unclear. P&T. 2014 Oct;39(10):660.
14. Institute of Medicine. 2012. Ethical and Scientific Issues in Studying the Safety of Approved Drugs. Washington, DC: The National Academies Press.
15. Huseyin Naci and G. Caleb Alexander. Regulators should better leverage effectiveness standards to enhance drug value. *Pharmacotherapy* 2014; doi: 10.1002/phar.1467.
16. A Sisko, S. Keehan, G. Cuckler et al. National health expenditure projections, 2013–23: Faster growth expected with expanded coverage and improving economy. *Health Aff.* 2014;33: 1841–50.

17. United States Department of Health and Human Services. Better, Smarter, Healthier: In historic announcement, HHS sets clear goals and timeline for shifting Medicare reimbursements from volume to value. January 26, 2015. Available at: http://www.hhs.gov/news/press/2015pres/01/20150126a.html (accessed on February 14, 2015).
18. E.M. Kolassa. 2009. The Strategic Pricing of Pharmaceuticals. USA: The Pond House Press.
19. Rose S. FDA pulls approval for avastin in breast cancer. *Cancer Discov.* 2011;1:OF1–OF2.
20. Peter A. Libel and David A. Asch. Creating value in health by understanding and overcoming resistance to de-innovation. *Health Aff.* 2015;34(2):239–44.
21. Brennan T and Shrank W. New expensive treatments for hepatitis C infection. *JAMA* 2014;312(6):593–4.
22. James C. Robinson and Scott Howell. Specialty Pharmaceuticals: Policy initiatives to improve assessment, pricing, prescription, and use. *Health Aff.* 2014;33(10):1745–50.
23. EvaluatePharma. Budget Busters: The shift to high-priced innovator drugs in the USA, September 2014.
24. Bo Wang, Steven Joffe, and Aaron Kesselheim. Chemotherapy Parity Laws: A remedy for high drug costs? *JAMA Int Med.* 2014;174(11):1721–2.
25. Maureen Bisognano and Charles Kenney. 2012. Pursuing the Triple Aim Seven Innovators Show the Way to Better Care, Better Health, and Lower Costs. San Francisco: John Wiley & Sons.
26. Lee JL, Maciejewski M, Raju S et al. Value-based insurance design: Quality improvement but no cost savings. *Health Aff.* 2013;32(7):1251–7.
27. Congressional Budget Office. Offsetting Effects of Prescription Drug Use on Medicare's Spending for Medical Services. November 29, 2012.
28. Susan DeVoire and R. Wesley Champion. Driving population health through accountable care organizations. *Health Aff.* 2011;30:41–50.
29. Swaminathan S, Mor V, Mehrotra R, Trivedi A. Medicare's payment strategy for end-stage renal disease now embraces bundled payment and pay-for-performance to cut costs. *Health Aff. (Millwood)* 2012;31:2051–8.
30. H-G Eichler, K Oye, LG Baird et al. Adaptive licensing: Taking the next step in the evolution of drug approval. *Clin Pharmacol Therap.* 2012;91:426–37.
31. Ezekiel Emanuel. Reinventing American Health Care: How the Affordable Care Act will Improve our Terribly Complex, Blatantly Unjust, Outrageously Expensive, Grossly Inefficient, Error Prone System. 2014. USA: Public Affairs.
32. Rahul Nayak and Steven D. Pearson. The ethics of 'fail first': Guidelines and practical scenarios for step therapy coverage policies. *Health Aff.* 2014;33(10):1779–85.
33. Benjamin P. Falit, Surya C. Singh, and Troyen A. Brennan. Biosimilar competition in the United States: Statutory incentives, payers, and pharmacy benefit managers. *Health Aff.* 2015;34(2):294–301.
34. Section 1137, FDA Safety and Innovation Act (FDASIA) of 2012 (Pub. L. 112–144). Available at: http://www.gpo.gov/fdsys/pkg/FR-2014-11-04/html/2014-26145.htm (accessed on November 22, 2014).
35. Food and Drug Administration Activities for Patient Participation in Medical Product Discussions: Establishment of a Docket (Docket FDA-2014-N-1698). 79 Fed. Register 65410-11 (November 4, 2014).
36. Rachael Fleurence, Joe Selby, Kara Odom-Walker et al. How the patient-centered outcomes research institute is engaging patients and others in shaping its research agenda. *Health Aff.* 2013 Feb;32(2):393–400.
37. Ernst Berndt, Deanna Nass, Michael Klienrock et al. Decline in economic returns from new drugs raises questions about sustaining innovations. *Health Aff.* 2015;24:245–52.
38. Tammy C. Hoffman, Victor M. Montori, and Chris Del Mar. The connection between evidence-based medicine and shared decision making. *NEJM* 2014;312:129506.
39. FDA Amendments Act of 2007, Pub. L. 110–85.

40. EMA Benefit Risk Methodology Project, 2008: http://www.ema.europa.eu/ema/index.jsp?curl=pages/special_topics/document_listing/document_listing_000314.jsp&mid=WC0b01ac0580665b63. Accessed October 3, 2015.
41. Health Canada: Guidance Document for Developing a Post Market Benefit-Risk Assessment. Draft Version Date: 2014-02-14. http://www.fdanews.com/ext/resources/files/04/04-28-14-Canada.pdf. Accessed 10/3/2015.
42. FDA CBER/CDRH: Benefit-Risk Factors to Consider When Determining Substantial Equivalence in Premarket Notifications [510(k)] with Different Technological Characteristics. Draft Guidance for Industry and Food and Drug Administration Staff, July 15, 2014. http://www.fda.gov/RegulatoryInformation/Guidances/ucm282958.htm. Accessed October 3, 2015.
43. FDA Medical Device Innovation Consortium Patient Centered Benefit-Risk Project: https://www.youtube.com/watch?v=vZgsbUo9zEw&feature=youtu.be. Accessed October 2, 2015.
44. Hammad TA, Neyarapally GA, Iyasu S et al. The future of population-based postmarket drug risk assessment: A regulator's perspective. *Clin Pharmacol Ther.* 2013 Sep;94(3):349–58.
45. Kathy Hudson and Francis Collins. Sharing and Reporting the Results of Clinical Trials. JAMA. 2014 Nov 19. doi: 10.1001/jama.2014.10716. [Epub ahead of print]. Notice of proposed rulemaking: Clinical trials registration and results submission. *Fed Register* 2014;79:69599–69680.
46. Deborah A. Zarin, Tony Tse, and Jerry Sheehan. The Proposed Rule for U.S. Clinical Trial Registration and Results Submission. *NEJM* 2014; December 24, 2014. doi: 10.1056/NEJMsr1414226.
47. Strom BL, Buyse M, Hughes J et al. Data sharing, year 1–access to data from industry-sponsored clinical trials. *N Engl J Med.* 2014 Nov 27;371(22):2052–4.
48. Jeffrey K. Francera and Natalie A. Turnera. Responsible clinical trial data sharing: Medical advancement, patient privacy, and incentives to invest in research. *J Health Life Sci. L.* 2014;8:66–99.
49. Institute of Medicine. 2015. Sharing Clinical Trial Data: Maximizing Benefits, Minimizing Risks. Washington, DC: National Academies Press.
50. 21st Century Cures Act. Discussion Document. 114th Congress. Available at: http://energycommerce.house.gov/sites/republicans.energycommerce.house.gov/files/114/Analysis/Cures/20150127-Cures-Discussion-Document.pdf (accessed on February 16, 2015).
51. Kesselheim AS, Tan YT, Darrow JJ et al. Existing FDA pathways have potential to ensure early access to, and appropriate use of, specialty drugs. *Health Aff.* 2014;33(10):770–778.
52. A Sarpatwari, JM Franklin, J Avorn et al. Are risk evaluation and mitigation strategies associated with less off-label use of medications? The Case of Immune Thrombocytopenia. *Clin Pharmacol Ther.* 2015;97(2):185–93.
53. Shannon G. Gibson and Trudo Lemmens. Niche markets and evidence assessment in transition: A critical review of proposed drug reforms. *Med Law Rev.* 2014;22(2):200–220.
54. Robb MA, Racoosin JA, Sherman RE et al. The US Food and Drug Administration's Sentinel Initiative: Expanding the horizons of medical product safety. *Pharmacoepidemiol Drug Saf.* 2012;21 Suppl 1:9–11.
55. Toh S, Platt R, Steiner JF, Brown JS. Comparative-effectiveness research in distributed health data networks. *Clin Pharmacol Ther.* 2011;90:883–87.
56. Overhage JM, Ryan PB, Reich CG, Hartzema AG, Stang PE. Validation of a common data model for active safety surveillance research. *J Am Med Inform Assoc.* 2012;19:54–60.
57. McGraw D, Rosati K, Evans B. A policy framework for public health uses of electronic health data. *Pharmacoepidemiol Drug Saf.* 2012;21 Suppl 1:18-22. doi: 10.1002/pds.2319.:18–22.
58. HHS. Modifications to the HIPAA Privacy, Security, Enforcement, and Breach Notification rules under the Health Information Technology for Economic and Clinical Health Act and the Genetic Information Nondiscrimination Act. 1-25-2013. 78 Fed. Register 5565.
59. Bruce Psaty and Alasdair Breckenridge. Mini-sentinel and regulatory science—Big data rendered fit and functional. *NEJM* 2014;370:2165–2167.
60. Toh S, Reichman ME, Houstoun M et al. Comparative risk for angioedema associated with the use of drugs that target the renin-angiotensin-aldosterone system. *Arch Intern Med.* 2012;172(20):1582–9.

61. Mini-Sentinel Methods: Prospective Routine Observational Monitoring Program (PROMPT) User's Guide. Available at: http://www.mini-sentinel.org/work_products/Statistical_Methods/Mini-Sentinel_PROMPT_Users-Guide.pdf (Accessed on January 10, 2016).
62. Rita F. Redberg. The importance of postapproval data for dabigatran. *JAMA Int Med.* 2015;175(1):25.
63. Ronan Donelan, Stuart Walker, and Sam Selek. Factors influencing quality decision-making: Regulatory and pharmaceutical industry perspectives. *Pharmacoepidemiol Drug Saf* 2015; online early.
64. Robert Temple. A regulator's view of comparative effectiveness. *Clinical Trials* 2011;0:1–10.
65. AHRQ. Effective Healthcare Program. Developing a Protocol for Observational Comparative Effectiveness Research: A User's Guide. February 12, 2013; FDA. Guidance for Industry. Best Practices for Conducting and Reporting Pharmacoepidemiologic Safety Studies Using Electronic Healthcare Data. May 2013.
66. Lester J, Neyarapally GA, Lipowski E, Graham CF, Hall M, Dal PG. Evaluation of FDA safety-related drug label changes in 2010. *Pharmacoepidemiol Drug Saf* 2013;22:302–305.
67. Evans SJ and Leufkens G. Regulatory decision-making: Are we getting it right? *Pharmacoepidemiol. Drug Saf* 2014 Oct; 23(10):1012–6.
68. The Health Information Technology for Economic and Clinical Health (HITECH) Act, enacted as part of the American Recovery and Reinvestment Act of 2009. Pub. L. 111-5.
69. Lori Frank, Ethan Basch, Joe Selby et al. The PCORI perspective on patient-centered outcomes research. *JAMA* 2014;312:1513–14.
70. Sebastian Schneeweiss. Learning from big health care data. *NEJM* 2014;370:2161–2162.
71. LB Baird, R Banken, H-G Eichler et al. Accelerated access to innovative medicines for patients in need. *Clin Pharmacol Therap* 2014;online August 13, 2014.
72. FDA. Biosimilars Guidances. Available at: http://www.fda.gov/Drugs/GuidanceComplianceRegulatoryInformation/Guidances/ucm290967.htm (accessed on February 16, 2015).
73. Francis Megerlin, Ruth Lopert, Ken Taymor et al. Biosimilars and the European experience: Implications for the United States. *Health Aff.* 2013;32:1803–10.
74. Adriana Lee Benedict. State-level legislation on follow-on biologic substitution. *J Law Biosci* (2014). doi: 10.1093/jlb/lsu005. First published online: May 2, 2014.
75. Parallel Review of Medical Products, 75 Fed. Register, 57045 (2010).
76. George A. Neyarapally. A review of recent federal legislative and policy initiatives to enhance the development and evaluation of high value drugs in the United States. 14 DePaul *J Healthcare L.* 2013;503:524.
77. James D. Chambers, Matthew Chenowerth, Michael J. Cangelosi et al. Medicare is Scrutinizing Evidence More Tightly for National Coverage Decisions. *Health Aff.* 2015;253–60.
78. The Office of Science and Technology Policy. Obama Administration Unveils "Big Data" Initiative: Announces $200 Million in New R&D Investments. Available at: https://www.whitehouse.gov/sites/default/files/microsites/ostp/big_data_press_release_final_2.pdf (accessed on May 3, 2015).
79. NIH. Centers of Excellence for Big Data Computing in the Biomedical Sciences (U54). Available at: http://grants.nih.gov/grants/guide/rfa-files/RFA-HG-13-009.html (accessed on May 3, 2015).
80. FDA Safety and Innovation Act of 2012, Pub. L. 112–44.
81. FDA. Guidance for Industry: Expedited Programs for Serious Conditions: Drugs and Biologics. May 2014.
82. Kesselheim AS, Gagne JJ. Strategies for postmarketing surveillance of drugs for rare diseases. *Clin Pharmacol Ther.* 2014 Mar;95(3):265–8.
83. Darrow JJ, Avorn J, Kesselheim AS. New FDA breakthrough-drug category—Implications for patients. *N Engl J Med.* 2014 Mar 27;370(13):1252–8.
84. Regulatory Affairs Professionals Society. Patient-Focused Drug Development Tracker. December 19, 2014. Available at: http://www.raps.org/Regulatory-Focus/News/2014/12/19/19640/Patient-Focused-Drug-Development-Tracker/ (accessed on January 2, 2015).

85. Prescription Drug User Fee Act Reauthorization Performance Goals and Procedures Fiscal Years 2013 through 2017. Available at: http://www.fda.gov/downloads/ForIndustry/UserFees/PrescriptionDrugUserFee/UCM270412.pdf (accessed on February 16, 2015).
86. FDA. Standardizing and Evaluating Risk Evaluation and Mitigation Strategies (REMS). Available at: http://www.fda.gov/downloads/ForIndustry/UserFees/PrescriptionDrugUserFee/UCM415751.pdf (accessed on February 16, 2015).
87. Elizabeth Alexandra Gray and Jane Hyatt Thorpe. Comparative effectiveness research and big data: Balancing potential with legal and ethical considerations. *J. Comp. Eff. Res.* 2015;4:61–74.
88. FDA. Structured Approach to Benefit-Risk Assessment in Drug Regulatory Decision-Making. Draft PDUFA V Implementation Plan. February 2013. http://www.fda.gov/downloads/ForIndustry/UserFees/PrescriptionDrugUserFee/UCM329758.pdf. Accessed October 3, 2015.
89. FDA. Guidance for Industry: Providing Postmarket Periodic Safety Reports in the ICH E2C(R2) Format (Periodic Benefit-Risk Evaluation Report). Draft Guidance. April 2013.
90. CredibleMeds Awarded Three-Year FDA Contract To Support The Safe Use Of Antibiotics. Available at: https://www.crediblemeds.org/blog/crediblemeds-awardedthree-year-fda-contract-support-safe-use/ (accessed on January 2, 2015).
91. FDA. Solicitation; FDA-SOL-1128556. Available at: https://www.fbo.gov/index?s=opportunity&mode=form&id=78470dda7d4be10ce24f9e23459354d4&tab=core&tabmode=list (accessed on February 14, 2015).
92. Woodcock J. Comparative effectiveness research and the regulation of drugs, biologics and devices. *J Comp Eff Res.* 2013;2:95–97.
93. Joshua Vogel, Jeffrey Brown, Thomas Land et al. MDPHnet: Secure, distributed sharing of electronic health record data for public health surveillance, evaluation and planning. *AJPH* 2014;104:2265–70.
94. Gerry Fairbrother, Ellen O'Brien, Rosina Pradhananga et al. Improving Quality and Efficiency in Health Care Through Comparative Effectiveness Analyses: An International Perspective. Academy Health, 2014.
95. California Technology Assessment Forum (CTAF). Newest Treatments for Hepatitis C. Genotype 1. Available at: http://ctaf.org/reports/newest-treatments-hepatitis-c-genotype-1 (accessed on May 3, 2015).
96. Vaishali K. Patadia, Preciosa Coloma, Martijn J. Schuemie, et al. Using real-world healthcare data for pharmacovigilance signal detection—The experience of the EU-ADR project. *Expert Rev Clin Pharmacol.* 2015;8(1):95–102.
97. 2010/84/EU Amending Directive 2001/83/EC and Regulation (EU) No 2135/2010 Amending Regulation (EC) No 726/2004; Commission Implementing Regulation No 520/2012 of 19 June 2012.
98. EMA. Pharmacovigilance legislation. Available at: http://www.ema.europa.eu/ema/index.jsp?curl=pages/special_topics/general/general_content_000491.jsp&mid=WC0b01ac058058f32d (accessed on January 1, 2015).
99. EMA. Pharmacovigilance legislation. Available at: http://www.ema.europa.eu/ema/index.jsp?curl=pages/special_topics/general/general_content_000491.jsp&mid=WC0b01ac058058f32d (Accessed on January 1, 2015). See also, Institute of Medicine, The Future of Drug Safety. National Academy Press. 2006.
100. Sergio Bonini, Hans-Georg Eichler, Noël Wathion et al. Transparency and the European Medicines Agency—Sharing of Clinical Trial Data. *NEJM* 2014;371:2452–55.
101. Regulation EU No 536/2014.
102. IMI Protect. Available at: http://www.imi-protect.eu/ (accessed on February 16, 2015).
103. Mt-Isa et al. Balancing benefit and risk of medicines: A systematic review and classification of available methodologies. *Pharmacoepidemiol. Drug Saf.* 2014;23(7):667–78.
104. CIOMS. Practical Approaches for Risk Minimisation for Medicinal Medical products. Report of the CIOMS Working Group IX. 2014.
105. Glasgow RE, Vogt TM, Soles, SM. Evaluating the public health impact of health promotion interventions: The RE-AIM framework. *AJPH* 1999;89:1322–7.

106. Banerjee, AK, Zomerdijk, IM, Wooder, S, Ingate, S, Mayall, SJ. Post-approval evaluation of effectiveness of risk minimisation: Methods, challenges and interpretation. *Drug Saf.* 2014;37:33–42.
107. Innovative Medicines Initiative2 topic: Patient perspective elicitation on benefits and risks of medicinal products, from development through the entire life cycle, to inform the decision-making process by regulators and health technology assessment bodies. http://www.imi.europa.eu/content/stage-1-16. Accessed October 2, 2015.
108. EMA. EMA Management Board: Highlights of December 2014 meeting: The Board adopts EMA work programme 2015–2016. December 18, 2014.
109. H-G Eichler, LG Baird, R Barker et al. From adaptive licensing to adaptive pathways: Delivering a flexible life-span approach to bring new drugs to patients. *Clin. Pharm. Ther.* 2015; online publication.
110. Don Husereau, Chris Henshall, and Jamil Jivraq. Adaptive approaches to licensing, health technology assessment, and introduction of drugs and devices. *International Journal of Technology Assessment in Health Care* 2014;30(3):241–249.
111. EMA. European Medicines Agency launches adaptive licensing pilot project. Available at: http://www.ema.europa.eu/ema/index.jsp?curl=pages/regulation/general/general_content_000601.jsp&mid=WC0b01ac05807d58ce (accessed on December 28, 2014).
112. Atul Khurana, Rajul Rastogi, and Hans-Joachim Gamperl. A New Era of Drug Safety – New EU Pharmacovigilance (PV) Legislation and Comparison of PV in EU, US, and India. *International Journal of Pharmacy and Pharmaceutical Sciences* 2014.
113. Ling Su. Drug Development Models in China and the Impact on Multinational Pharmaceutical Companies. FDLI Update. September/October 2013. Available at: http://www.sidley.com/~/media/Files/Publications/2013/09/Drug%20Development%20Models%20in%20China%20and%20the%20Impact%20__/Files/View%20Article/FileAttachment/FDLI%20article%20%20Ling%20Su%20%202013 (accessed on January 10, 2016).
114. PMDA. Available at: http://www.pmda.go.jp/english/index.html (accessed on January 2, 2015).
115. Dr Tony Hobbs, Principal Medical Adviser, Therapeutic Goods Administration. Pharmacy Australia Congress, October 10, 2014.
116. ICH new Expert Working Group for benefit risk section (2.5.6), 2015. http://www.ich.org/fileadmin/Public_Web_Site/ICH_Products/CTD/M4E_R2_Efficacy/M4E_R2__Final_Concept_Paper_27_March_2015.pdf. Accessed 10/3/2015.
117. Hammad TA, Pinheiro SP, Neyarapally GA. Secondary use of randomized controlled trials to evaluate drug safety: A review of methodological considerations. *Clin Trials* 2011;8:559–570.
118. Schmidt H and Emanuel EJ. Lowering medical costs through the shared savings by physicians and patients: Inclusive shared savings. *JAMA Intern. Med* 2014;174:2009–13.
119. Fotsch EJ. Electronic health records: The new vehicle for drug labeling, safety, and efficacy. *Clin Pharmacol Ther.* 2012;91:917–19.
120. Bo Wang, William J. Canestaro, Niteesh K. Choudhry. Clinical evidence supporting pharmacogenomic biomarker testing provided in us food and drug administration drug labels. *JAMA Int Med* 2014;174:1938–44. doi: 10.1001/jamainternmed.2014.5266.
121. Hall GC, Sauer B, Bourke A, Brown JS, Reynolds MW, LoCasale R. Guidelines for good database selection and use in pharmacoepidemiology research. *Pharmacoepidemiol Drug Saf.* 2012;21:1–10.
122. Fleurence R, Whicher D, Dunham K, et al. The patient-centered outcomes research institute's role in advancing methods for patient-centered outcomes research. *Medical Care* 2015;53:2–7.
123. Rendell M, Akturk HK, Tella SH. Glargine safety, diabetes and cancer. *Expert Opin. Drug Saf.* 2013;12:247–263.
124. Sidney S, Cheetham TC, Connell FA et al. Recent combined hormonal contraceptives (CHCs) and the risk of thromboembolism and other cardiovascular events in new users. *Contraception* 2012.
125. FDA Drug Safety Communication: Updated information about the risk of blood clots in women taking birth control pills containing drospirenone. FDA [serial online] 2012.
126. CMS. Multi-Payor Claims Database. *CMS, Solicitation Number: RFQ-MPCD-2010-DRCG03* [serial online] 2011.

127. NORC. The State HIE Program Four Years Later: Key Findings From Grantees' Experiences from a Six-State Review. Case Study Report, December 2014.
128. Niam Yaraghi. A Sustainable Business Model for Health Information Exchange Platforms: The Solution to Interoperability in Healthcare IT. Center for Technology Innovation at Brookings. January 2015.
129. Douglas Hillblom, Anthony Schueth, Scott Robertson et al. The impact of health information technology on managed care pharmacy: today and tomorrow. *JMCP* 2014;20(11):1073–9.
130. Mark B. McClellan, Gregory W. Daniel, Dane Dickson et al. Improving evidence developed from population-level experience with targeted agents. *Clin Pharmacol Therap.* 2015. Accepted article, doi: 10.1002/cpt.90.
131. Bates KE, Vetter VL, Li JS et al. Pediatric cardiovascular safety: Challenges in drug and device development and clinical application. *Am Heart J* 2012;164:481–92.
132. Aaron S. Kesselheim and Joshua J. Gagne. Introduction to a Supplement on Innovative Approaches to Studying Health Outcomes in Rare Diseases. *J Gen Intern Med* 2014;29(Suppl 3):S709–11.
133. Woodcock J. The future of orphan drug development. *Clin Pharmacol Ther.* 2012;92:146–148.
134. Andrade SE, Davis RL, Cheetham TC et al. Medication Exposure in Pregnancy Risk Evaluation Program. *Matern Child Health J* 2012;16:1349–54.
135. Cooper WO, Habel LA, Sox CM et al. ADHD drugs and serious cardiovascular events in children and young adults. *N Engl J Med* 2011;365:1896–904.
136. Rawlins M. De testimonio: On the evidence for decisions about the use of therapeutic interventions. *Lancet* 2008;372:2152–61.
137. van Staa TP, Smeeth L, Persson I, Parkinson J, Leufkens HG. Evaluating drug toxicity signals: Is a hierarchical classification of evidence useful or a hindrance? *Pharmacoepidemiol Drug Saf.* 2008;17:475–84.
138. Grimes DA, Schulz KF. Bias and causal associations in observational research. *Lancet* 2002;359:248–252.
139. Temple R. Meta-analysis and epidemiologic studies in drug development and postmarketing surveillance. *JAMA* 1999;281:841–4.
140. Weed DL. Higher standards for epidemiologic studies—Replication prior to publication? *JAMA* 1999;282:937–8.
141. Austin B. Frakt. An observational study goes where randomized trials have not. *JAMA* 2015;313(11):1091–2.
142. Gagne JJ, Rassen JA, Walker AM, Glynn RJ, Schneeweiss S. Active safety monitoring of new medical products using electronic healthcare data: Selecting alerting rules. *Epidemiology* 2012;23:238–46.
143. Gagne JJ, Walker AM, Glynn RJ, Rassen JA, Schneeweiss S. An event-based approach for comparing the performance of methods for prospective medical product monitoring. *Pharmacoepidemiol Drug Saf.* 2012;21:631–39.
144. Dal Pan GJ, Arlett P. The Role of Pharmacoepidemiology in Regulatory Agencies. Pharmacoepidemiology. Fifth ed. Wiley-Blackwell; 2012.
145. Goldman M. The innovative medicines initiative: A European response to the innovation challenge. *Clin Pharmacol Ther* 2012;91:418–425.
146. Zhichkin PE, Athey BD, Avigan MI, Abernethy DR. Needs for an expanded ontology-based classification of adverse drug reactions and related mechanisms. *Clin Pharmacol Ther* 2012;91:963–5.
147. Lesko LJ, Zheng S, Schmidt S. Systems approaches in risk assessment. *Clin Pharmacol Ther.* 2013;93:413–24.
148. Eddy DM, Adler J, Morris M. The 'Global Outcomes Score': A quality measure, based on health outcomes, that compares current care to a target level of care. *Health Aff (Millwood)* 2012;31:2441–50.
149. Hans-Georg Eichler et al. The risks of drug aversion in drug regulation. *Nature Rev Drug Discovery* 2013;12:907–16.

150. Institute of Medicine (IOM). 2014. Characterizing and communicating uncertainty in the assessment of benefits and risks of pharmaceutical products: Workshop summary. Washington, DC: The National Academies Press.
151. Charles Manski. Public Policy in an Uncertain World: Analysis and Decisions. Harvard University Press, 2013.
152. Caitlin Knox, Christian Hampp, Mary Willy et al. Patient understanding of drug risks: An evaluation of medication guide assessments. *Pharmacoepidemiol. Drug. Saf.* 2015;24:518–525.
153. Gregory W. Daniel, Alexis Caze, Morgan H. Romine et al. Improving pharmaceutical innovation by building a more comprehensive database on drug development and use. *Heath Aff.* 2014;34(2):319–327.
154. Topol EJ, Steinhubl, SR, Torkamani, A. Digital medical tools and sensors. *JAMA* 2015;313(4):353–4.
155. Mega JL, Sabatine MS, Antman EM. Population and personalized medicine in the modern era. *JAMA* 2014;312:1969–1970.

3

Benefit–Risk Determinations at the FDA Center for Devices and Radiological Health

Telba Irony and Martin Ho

CONTENTS

ABSTRACT In March 2012, the Center for Devices and Radiological Health at the Food and Drug Administration issued a guidance document describing the factors to be considered when the Center makes benefit–risk determinations for medical device premarket reviews. Decision analysis provided the foundations and motivation for this guidance to industry and staff who have to weigh these factors when making benefit–risk determinations for medical device approval. In this chapter, we will discuss these factors and briefly provide examples to illustrate how to weigh these factors in order to reach regulatory decisions for approval of medical devices. A groundbreaking factor described in the guidance is "patient tolerance for risk and perspective on benefit." Until now, this factor has not been formally considered in the regulatory setting. Through an example, we will demonstrate how to obtain quantitative evidence on how patients weigh benefits against risks and how this evidence could be used in the regulatory setting.

3.1 Introduction

The Center for Devices and Radiological Health (CDRH) at the FDA has regulatory responsibility for medical devices and often faces difficult decisions when making a benefit–risk assessment for medical device premarket approval, in case of higher-risk medical devices, and de novo classifications, for lower- to moderate-risk devices.

In March 2012, CDRH issued a guidance document for industry and Food and Drug Administration (FDA) staff describing the factors to be considered when the Center makes benefit–risk determinations for certain premarket reviews for medical devices.[1]

We will discuss the roles of qualitative and quantitative methods for benefit–risk assessment and explain the factors for benefit–risk determination that are listed in the guidance document. We also present examples to illustrate how to weigh these factors in order to reach regulatory decisions for approval of medical devices. A groundbreaking factor described in the guidance is "patient tolerance for risk and perspective on benefit." Until recently, this factor has not been usually considered in the regulatory setting. We will describe a study that demonstrates how to obtain quantitative evidence on patient preferences and how regulators can use this evidence to inform benefit–risk determinations. This study has served as a proof of concept for the draft guidance document on how to collect, analyze, and submit patient preference information for medical device approval, which was released in May 2015.[2]

3.2 Decision Making at the CDRH

Decision making is essential to the FDA's role and it is often a challenge since each decision the agency makes involves different and special difficulties. A regulatory decision may involve the interests of various stakeholders such as patients, physicians, and caregivers. In addition, regulatory decisions often need to be made with limited information and in an efficient manner. Although every regulatory decision is unique, they usually involve the following challenges:

First, a regulatory decision may involve multiple objectives such as timely approving a medical product that is safe and effective and will promote and protect the public health. Frequently, however, effectiveness and safety progress in opposite directions. For example, a medical device that delivers a larger weight loss requires a riskier surgery for implantation and a more stringent diet than a nonimplantable weight-loss treatment does. In such cases, the decisions involve trading off effectiveness against safety. Second, more often than not, regulatory decisions involve uncertainty and acquiring information to reduce uncertainty may be a costly and time-consuming course of action that needs to be taken into account. Third, different perspectives and values may lead to different decisions. This issue arises when different stakeholders are affected by the consequences of the decision. They may see the problem from different angles and may disagree on the uncertainty or on the value of the various outcomes. As an example, patients may be willing to take high surgical risks to receive a breast implant whereas regulators and some physicians may be more conservative. Finally, an agency's decision may involve complex mathematical analysis and enumerating all realistic courses of action may require creativity and deep knowledge of the subject matter.

Keeping all objectives, factors, degree of uncertainty, courses of action, and consequences in mind at once is challenging, and a systematic approach to decision making can be very useful. A mathematical decision analysis framework can help organize the problem and confront the challenges even when the decisions involve a diverse group of stakeholders with different values.

Mathematical decision analysis is a set of tools to describe, inform and analyze decision making in the presence of uncertainty. It is a process of communication that provides insight and increases transparency by making objectives and preferences (i.e., values) that drive decisions explicit. The decision analysis approach provides a way to combine values and data, accounting for differences in values and uncertain information. Moreover, the approach allows for the determination of where resources could be allocated to obtain the information that has the highest value for decision making. The process also allows for identification of the points where stakeholders disagree (i.e., values, uncertainty, mathematical model) and thereby facilitates consensus building.

In the United States, high-risk medical devices are subject to approval applications (premarket applications or PMAs). Decisions for PMAs translate into determinations of whether there is reasonable assurance that the medical device under review is safe and effective. These determinations are made by "weighing any probable benefit to health from the use of the device against any probable risk of injury or illness from such use."[3] In addition, effectiveness can be reasonably assured when "it can be determined, based upon valid scientific evidence, that in a significant portion of the target population, the use of the device for its intended uses and conditions of use, when accompanied by adequate directions for use and warnings against unsafe use, will provide clinically significant results."[4] To support this process, PMA applicants submit valid scientific information that can include nonclinical and clinical study results, which CDRH reviews to determine whether the benefits of the device outweigh its risks under the intended conditions of use in the labeling of the device.

Similarly, devices that pose low to moderate risk and that have been determined to be not substantially equivalent to a device already in the market may submit a de novo request. CDRH will carefully consider the benefit–risk profile of such devices in the determination of whether or not there is reasonable assurance of safety and effectiveness for the de novo request to be granted.

In these two cases, the PMA approval and the de novo classification, the possible decisions available to the Center are to allow the device to be legally marketed in the United States, not to allow the device to be legally marketed in the United States, or to request more information.

These decisions involve assessments of safety and effectiveness of the medical device and the assessments depend on the context or additional factors to be described in Section 3.3. As an example, a risk posed by an implantable device may be acceptable to treat a chronic or life-threatening disease but may be unacceptable to treat an acute and mild disease. The idea is that under different scenarios, the weights placed on the benefits and the risks may be different. As a consequence, the relative degree of benefit and risk that could support approval of a PMA or to grant a de novo request could vary depending on the condition being treated, availability of alternative treatments, patient preferences, or other factors.

The idea that benefit–risk determinations depend on the context and should take into account additional factors raises several issues to be considered. How should values of benefits and risks be assessed in a way that they can be weighed in the same scale? Since patients, physicians, caregivers, and the public are all stakeholders in the benefit–risk determinations, who should assess the values on the benefits and risks for weighing? Is it conceivable that different stakeholders will place different weights on the benefits and risks? How should the Center assess the value of obtaining additional information about the safety and effectiveness of a device given that delaying a decision will incur a risk to the patients who need treatment and cannot get it until the treatment is on the market? In other words, the benefits and risks of allowing a medical product on the market can be considered in the context of the benefits and risks of not allowing a medical device on the market. Related to this issue is the assessment of the optimal amount of information needed before making a regulatory decision.

3.3 The Role of Qualitative and Quantitative Methods in Benefit–Risk Assessments

Making qualitative benefit–risk assessments of medical devices is needed to enumerate and elicit the benefits and risks that are important to patients and care providers and to explain and define the scope of benefits and risks. In addition, qualitative assessments are essential to characterize the benefits and risks of a treatment in order to select outcomes and the endpoints to be studied in clinical trials. However, qualitative methods cannot describe variability and cannot represent a full spectrum of values or preferences. Consequently, qualitative assessments will most likely lack representativeness. Furthermore, it is very difficult to weigh benefits against risks when they are not placed in the same scale.

Despite being a nascent field in need of research and advancement, quantitative benefit–risk assessments can be very important for regulatory decision making of medical products. Benefit–risk assessments are all about trade-offs. It is obvious that the desired outcome of any medical treatment is to experience all benefits with no risk. Since, unfortunately in most cases, this is not possible, there is a need to compare benefits to risks and decide which one wins. For comparisons, risks and benefits can be placed in the same scale of values, which may be an advantage for quantitative benefit–risk assessment for decision making.

Quantitative benefit–risk assessments can describe variability and represent the values of a full spectrum of stakeholders. They are conducive to validity and consistency checks whereby biases can be identified and mitigated. Quantitative methods are also very important when stakeholders have different values because they may help identify the source of the differences and hopefully lead to consensus. Quantitative methods also allow for sensitivity analyses to test assumptions and, when there is uncertainty or difference in values, to determine the best decision and its robustness under several scenarios.

Patients who have preferences for benefits and risks need to make them explicit in order to engage in shared decision making with their care providers. Each patient has a unique tolerance for risk and perspective on benefit. Therefore, there is a need to describe a whole spectrum of preferences in order to address the needs of a population of patients. This spectrum follows a distribution where the tails are important and the average, used for qualitative assessments, may not describe any individual very well. Quantitative assessments can represent a diverse patient population and help give a voice to most.

Industry, another stakeholder, would be interested in assessing qualitative and quantitative patient preferences in order to design their medical products to satisfy their customers and make the best business decisions.

It is important for CDRH to consider the whole spectrum of patient preferences to make decisions that are patient centric and that can address the needs of most including those that are not typical.

In conclusion, both qualitative and quantitative benefit–risk assessments are important for regulatory decision making, but quantitative assessments can address a diverse population and are conducive to validity checks and sensitivity analysis. Moreover, decision making becomes transparent and straightforward when benefits and risks can be weighed in the same scale.

3.4 Factors for Benefit–Risk Determination

The additional factors considered when CDRH makes benefit–risk determinations reflect the context in which a treatment is evaluated and could be thought of as reasons for either an increase or a decrease in the weights that are given to the benefits and to the risks of the device. For example, a treatment for a life-threatening disease will have a very high weight on its benefit of increasing survival, particularly if there are no alternative treatments available because the risk of not being treated would be very high. If several alternatives that increase survival are available, the survival increase of the new treatment will be less impactful, especially if the treatment poses more risks than the alternatives.

It is also important to highlight that the weights on the benefits and risks for a type of device may change over time because of changes in the context. New alternative treatments may become available and, consequently, the weight placed on benefits may decrease or the weight placed on risks may increase.

The main factors in the benefit–risk determinations made by CDRH at the FDA are described in Sections 3.4.1 through 3.4.3.

3.4.1 Benefits

3.4.1.1 Type of Benefit

Examples include improvement of patient health, relief of symptoms, patient satisfaction, improvement on quality of life, reduction of the probability of death, and so on. For diagnostic devices, the type of benefit can be measured by the device's ability to identify a specific disease or condition and thus to treat or manage it. It is important to take into account whether the primary endpoint used for effectiveness evaluation was well defined and reliably measured. Objective endpoints are more reliable than subjective endpoints that could be influenced by a placebo effect and less consistent measurements. Secondary effectiveness endpoints are also very important and again the reliability of measurements is an important aspect in the assessment of the overall type of benefit. If a surrogate endpoint is used to define the type of benefit, it is very important to validate it by verifying how well it correlates to the actual benefit.

3.4.1.2 Magnitude of the Benefit

When evaluating the magnitude of the effect, it is important to assess if the effect size is clinically meaningful and if it is estimated using valid statistical methods to avoid biases and statistical pitfalls.

3.4.1.3 Probability That the Patient Will Experience the Benefit

Sometimes, it is possible to predict which patients will experience the benefit whereas other times this is not possible. In addition, some patients may not be counted as responders but may still experience some benefits. Yet, in other situations, the patients who do not experience the benefits are the ones that incur the risks and those cannot be identified before the treatment is provided. Another point to consider is that sometimes a small proportion of patients experience a large benefit, whereas in other cases, a large proportion of patients experience small benefits. All these situations need to be considered when the Center makes benefit–risk determinations.

3.4.1.4 Duration of the Effect

Treatments that need to be repeated frequently may introduce greater risk or the benefit may diminish at each time the treatment is repeated. The duration of the effect may have great influence on the weight given to the benefit.

3.4.2 Risks

3.4.2.1 Severity, Types, Number, and Rates of Harmful Events Associated with the Use of the Device

These are considered in its risk assessment including device-related serious and nonserious adverse events and adverse events related to the procedure used in conjunction with the device.

3.4.2.2 Probability That the Patient Will Experience a Harmful Event

As in the case of benefit, the chance that a patient will experience an adverse event is an important consideration on the benefit–risk assessment.

3.4.2.3 Duration of the Harmful Events

Some harmful events are temporary while others can be permanent and irreversible. Temporary and reversible harms will have a lower weight than permanent and irreversible harms.

3.4.2.4 Risk of False Negative and False Positive from a Diagnostic Device

If a diagnostic device gives a false-positive result, the patient might receive additional testing or an unnecessary treatment and incur adverse events that accompany those interventions. A false-negative result may prevent a patient from receiving a necessary treatment and consequently the patient may incur the risks of the disease and miss out on the benefits from a treatment. Again, these risks will be carefully included as benefit–risk determinations are made.

3.4.3 Additional Factors

Benefits and risks are not considered in a vacuum. The context in which the device is evaluated will inform how much weight should be placed on the benefits and risks posed by the device. The context is described by the additional factors discussed in Sections 3.4.3.1 through 3.4.3.7 that are also considered when CDRH makes benefit–risk determinations.

3.4.3.1 Uncertainty

The degree of uncertainty of the benefits and harms of a device is an important factor considered in benefit–risk determinations. The higher uncertainty on the benefit, the lower will be its weight. On the other hand, if there is low assurance that the device will pose no harms, there will be a higher weight placed on its risks.

Poor design or conduct of clinical trials, missing data, or inadequate analyses of the outcomes can generate results that may not be reliable and thus have greater uncertainty than expected. In situations where the study design does not blind investigators and subjects, it may be difficult to tease out the placebo effect from the real treatment effect, and these studies may be subject to operational biases such as investigator bias, selection bias, or patient bias. Again, the uncertainty surrounding such study results may be higher than expected. It is also important that the analytical approach used in the evaluation of the endpoints is appropriate and validated to reduce uncertainty. Other factors that may contribute to reduction in the uncertainty of the results are repeatability, biological plausibility, and comparable results obtained from similar studies.

The generalizability of the trial results to the intended population is also a factor that contributes to uncertainty or lack thereof. Alternatively, it may be useful to treat or test a subgroup rather than the general population.

In summary, less uncertainty on the benefits will increase their value. More uncertainty on risks may also increase the weight placed on them. Readers could reference Chapter 4 for discussions on uncertainty considerations in benefit–risk assessment.

3.4.3.2 Characterization of the Disease

The clinical manifestation of the treated or diagnosed condition and how it affects patients who have it is an important additional factor considered by the FDA and will play an important role on the weights placed on the benefits and risks of a medical device treatment.

3.4.3.3 Patient Tolerance for Risk and Perspective on Benefit

CDRH recognizes that perspectives on benefits and tolerance for risk may vary across the patient population and that some patients may tolerate more risk than others to achieve the same benefit. Section 3.6 will elaborate on this factor and describe a proof-of-concept study for a method to elicit and incorporate patient preference in benefit–risk determinations. Patients can provide a unique perspective on benefits and risks of a medical device because patients live with their condition and the consequences of the decisions they make for their treatment.

CDRH will consider evidence relating to patient's perspectives of what constitutes meaningful benefits and risks and use this evidence to provide information about the weights that are given to benefits and risks. However, in the case where the probable risks outweigh the benefits for all reasonable patients, the Center will determine that the risks outweigh the benefits and not approve the PMA or not grant the de novo request.

Disease severity and disease chronicity may influence patient's risk tolerance. Patients suffering from severe diseases may tolerate more risks whereas patients suffering from chronic diseases may adapt over time, minimize the impact of the disease in their lives, and become less tolerant of treatment risks. If no alternative treatments are available, patients may be willing to accept more risks from a treatment.

It may be appropriate to approve a device when only a minority of the intended population would accept the risks in exchange for the benefits provided the information necessary for patients and health care providers to make well-informed decision is available and well understood. In that case, the subgroup that values the device will have access to it whereas the remaining population can choose not to use the device.

In summary, patient-centric assessments can be very helpful to inform the benefit–risk determination of a medical device.

3.4.3.4 Availability of Alternative Treatments and Diagnostics

If alternative therapies are available, the Center takes into account their effectiveness, safety, and benefit–risk profile. If no alternatives are available, the Center will also take into account the risk of not being treated for lack of alternatives.

3.4.3.5 Use of Risk Mitigation

The possibility of mitigating the risks and minimizing the probability of harmful events can improve the benefit–risk profile of a medical device and reduce the weight on its risks. Common forms of risk mitigation are restrictions on the indication for use and inclusion of warnings and precautions in the labeling. Some risks can be mitigated by providing special training to physicians and health care providers.

3.4.3.6 Possibility of Collecting or Using Postmarket Data

The possibility of collecting postmarket data on the use of the device in the real world can reduce the uncertainty on its benefits and risks and change the weights that are given to both. Postmarket studies or other information that becomes known after the device is in use in the real world may alter the benefit–risk profile of certain devices, particularly if new risks are identified or known risks are mitigated.

3.4.3.7 Novel Technology for Unmet Medical Need

FDA's assessment of the weights placed on the benefits and risks of medical devices takes into account breakthrough technologies particularly when they address unmet medical needs. Moreover, a new technology may improve with subsequent iterations and the benefit–risk profile of a breakthrough device tends to improve as the technology matures. In these cases, the Center may tolerate greater uncertainty on the benefits or risks in order to facilitate patient access to new devices and to encourage innovation that promotes the public health.

3.5 CDRH Benefit–Risk Guidance Document

In March 2012, the CDRH issued a guidance document for industry and FDA staff describing the factors to consider when making benefit–risk determinations for medical devices submitted to premarket approvals or de novo classifications.[1] The objective of the guidance document is to increase transparency, consistency, and predictability of the premarket review process.

The following two examples illustrate the role these factors play in CDRH's benefit–risk assessments:

1. A novel implantable device is designed to treat a severe chronic condition and improve mobility for patients who have failed all other existing treatment options. The pivotal trial to study the safety and effectiveness of the device shows that there is a 75% chance that a patient implanted with the device will experience a benefit and improvement in mobility. Since patient follow-up in the trial was 1 year, there is high uncertainty on the duration of the benefit beyond 1 year. In addition, missing data increases the uncertainty about the trial results. On the other hand, patients with this condition tend to have a longer life expectancy if they can maintain good mobility. The study also shows that patients have a 1% chance of death from the implant surgery and a 3% chance of harmful complications after the surgery, but these risks are not higher than those for similar treatments. Because of the uncertainty about the length of benefit and the rare but serious risks posed by this implant device, the benefit–risk determination for this device's premarket approval decision is challenging.

   Benefits: Patients who experience the benefits have an improvement in mobility and may have a longer life expectancy.

   Risks: Implantation procedure carries a 1% chance of death and there is a 3% chance of complications and adverse events.

   Additional Factors

   Uncertainty: The probability that a patient will experience a benefit is 75%; duration of the benefit is not known beyond 1 year. Missing data at the clinical trial was an issue but sensitivity analysis supports the primary analysis, suggesting that the results are robust.

Characterization of the disease: The disease is chronic and serious, especially because it affects patient mobility and ultimately survival.

Patient preference: Patient preference information shows that patients value the benefit provided by the device because it greatly improves quality of life and are willing to take the risk of having the device implanted for a 75% probability of benefit because of the lack of alternative treatment options.

Availability of alternative treatments: This treatment is indicated for patients who have failed all other existing treatments and consequently the benefits of this treatment are very important and the risk of not being treated is very high.

Risk mitigation: Risks from implantation surgery can be mitigated by limiting use to surgeons who have completed special training.

Possibility of collecting postmarket data: Postmarket data can be collected to reduce the uncertainty about the duration of the benefit beyond 1 year.

Novel technology for unmet medical need: The size of this device can be reduced at subsequent iterations, making the implantation procedure safer and further improving mobility.

Conclusion: The FDA is likely to approve this device because it is intended to treat a severe condition for which no alternatives are available. Patients are willing to take the risks even though it is uncertain they will experience the benefits because if they experience the benefit, there is an improvement in mobility and possibly in life expectancy. Patients have failed other alternatives and are not foregoing an effective treatment for an uncertain benefit. Surgery risk can be mitigated and the overall risk, although serious, is not higher than the risks of similar treatments. Finally, subsequent iterations may reduce the device's risk.

2. A device that uses a new technology to treat a rare cancer is compared to the standard of care, that is, chemotherapy, in a randomized clinical trial. The results show that the device performs as well as standard of care but not better. There is uncertainty on the effectiveness of chemotherapy but no alternatives are available. Neither the device nor the standard of care are curative and the cancer progresses rapidly and is terminal. The device treatment poses less harmful adverse events than chemotherapy and the technology can be improved at subsequent iterations.

   Conclusion: Despite the uncertainty about the benefits of the treatment and standard of care (chemotherapy), the FDA will probably approve the device in order to provide patients access to a treatment that does not cause the same severe adverse events as chemotherapy.

3.6 Groundbreaking Factor: Patient Benefit–Risk Trade-Off Preference

The FDA recognizes the unique role of patients to inform benefit–risk determinations for medical devices since patients, their caregivers, physicians, and regulators can differ in how benefits are weighed against the risks. In the opening statements of the draft guidance document on patient preference information[2] jointly released by CDRH and the

Center for Biologics Evaluation and Research in May 2015, the FDA states: "The U.S. Food and Drug Administration (FDA or the Agency) values the experience and perspectives of patients with devices. The Agency understands that patients and caregivers who live with a disease or condition on a daily basis and utilize devices in their care may have developed their own insights and perspectives on the benefits and risks of devices under PMA, HDE, or de novo review."

Patient preference information should be taken into account in conjunction with the values of the medical community and regulatory reviewers when benefit–risk determinations are conducted for regulatory approval of a medical device. Therefore, the FDA has released the draft guidance document to provide guidelines on how to collect and use patient preference information that may be considered in assessments of benefit–risk trade-offs.

On July 10, 2015, the US House of Representatives approved the 21st Century Cures Act[5] with a rare bipartisan vote of 344–77. The bill not only acknowledges the importance of a structured framework to assess the benefits and risks of medical treatments but also highlights the importance of patient preferences as a catalyst of innovations in medicine, asking the FDA to consider patient perspectives in its benefit–risk assessments.

Patient perspective information on benefit–risk trade-offs of medical treatments has also attracted the attention of public–private partnerships involving major stakeholders in the medical product ecosystem of the United States and Europe. The Medical Device Innovation Consortium (MDIC) is a public–private partnership created in the United States to advance medical device regulatory science whose members include a wide range of major stakeholders, from government (FDA, Centers for Medicare and Medicaid Services, National Institutes of Health, and Patient-Centered Outcomes Research Institute), patient groups (FasterCures and National Health Council), and the medical device industry.

Although the benefit–risk guidance document released by CDRH[1] in 2012 identifies patient perspectives as an important factor to consider in benefit–risk determinations, it does not advise on how to collect and use evidence on patient preferences for regulatory decisions. In absence of widely accepted practices to incorporate patient preferences information into the regulatory process, the MDIC initiated the Patient Centered Benefit–Risk Project (PCBR) to help major stakeholders such as patient groups, medical device industry, and the FDA to address this regulatory science gap. In May 2015, CDRH released the draft guidance on patient preference information and the MDIC released its PCBR Framework report, a catalog of patient preference elicitation methods.[6]

The PCBR Framework report explains how patient preference information can be used in all phases of medical device life cycle, from ideation and invention to prototyping, from preclinical testing, clinical trials, and premarket approval application to marketing and postmarket surveillance. First, the report defines important terms (e.g., *benefit*, *harm*, *risk*, and *preferences*) and introduces critical concepts (e.g., *minimum acceptable benefit*, *maximum acceptable benefit*, and *preference-sensitive decisions*). Next, it explains the potential value of patient preference information in regulatory benefit–risk assessments of medical technology and in the medical product life cycle. Then, it discusses some factors to consider when determining whether to conduct a patient preference study and how to select an appropriate method to answer the research question in hand. The report also describes the roles that patient preference data can play in various steps of the regulatory process and beyond and is concluded with suggestions of future research topics for better collection and considerations of patient preferences information among the major stakeholders. The process for developing the MDIC PCBR Framework report and the catalog of elicitation methods were supported by the FDA, reflecting the significance of patient preference information in benefit–risk determinations for premarket approval of medical devices.

Outside the United States, there is wide interest to consider patient preferences in benefit–risk assessment of medical products. The Innovative Medicines Initiative, also a public–private partnership including major stakeholders in the European pharmaceutical ecosystem, is sponsoring the Pharmacoepidemiological Research on Outcomes of Therapeutics project, which lists elicitation of preferences of patients and care providers as one of their four research components.

3.6.1 Preference-Sensitive Decisions

Preference-sensitive decisions refer to those decisions for which no option is clearly superior to others. For instance, some patients may prefer a treatment that prolongs life but decreases the quality of life whereas others may prefer a treatment that improves quality of life despite reducing life expectancy. The MDIC Framework report defines preference-sensitive decisions as those decisions for which no option is clearly superior to others either because the best option depends on patient values and preferences or because the evidence supporting one option over others is considerably uncertain (The MDIC Framework Report, Section II).[6] Patient preference information is crucial in benefit–risk assessments involving preference-sensitive decisions because there is a need to estimate the size and importance of the subgroup of patients who would chose a treatment option that is not clearly superior to others in order to determine if that option is worth approving.

3.6.2 The FDA CDRH Obesity Survey

In 2015, CDRH published a first-of-its-kind study designed to obtain quantitative evidence of patient preferences to inform regulatory benefit–risk determination for premarket approval decisions.[7] This work resulted from the collaboration between CDRH and RTI Health Solutions, which jointly designed a survey to serve as a proof of concept on how to elicit patient preferences for attributes of weight-loss medical devices and to explore ways to use the results in regulatory decision making.

The study demonstrated how to apply a well-established patient preference elicitation method to quantify the relative importance of benefits, risks, and other attributes of weight-loss devices. On the basis of the resulting evidence, the Center developed a decision-aid tool to incorporate quantitative patient preferences into its regulatory decision making. In particular, the quantitative nature of the study allows the FDA to estimate the distribution of patient preferences including patients that will tolerate higher risks and those that are risk averse. As a consequence, the size of the subgroup of patients who would tolerate the risks of a weight-loss device in exchange for its benefits can be estimated and can be taken into account for a regulatory decision. As highlighted by the study authors,[7] CDRH "will consider approving a medical device that demonstrates meaningful benefits even though its benefit-risk profile would be acceptable only to a subset of patients who are risk-tolerant. Such a device's *Indication for Use* will explain that the benefit-risk profile may be only suitable to those patients that are more risk-tolerant, who should consult with their care providers in a context of shared medical decision making."

CDRH selected weight-loss devices as the focus of its study because it acknowledges the preference-sensitive decisions that obese patients are facing: The available treatment options range from the relatively safe diet and exercise to the riskier gastric bypass surgery. The safe options typically deliver small benefits whereas the risky ones typically deliver larger benefits. No option is curative, and options strongly depend on the preference and risk tolerance of each obese patient. In other words, there is no single treatment option superior to other options in terms of low risks and high benefits. Therefore, preferences of obese patients play an important role in evaluating the benefit–risk profiles of weight-loss devices under review at CDRH.

The study used a representative sample of the US obese population and its results reflect preferences from a broad spectrum of respondents, including risk-tolerant and risk-averse obese patients. A discrete-choice experiment was used to elicit patient preferences as they compared hypothetical weight-loss device profiles. Each device profile was defined by eight attributes and each respondent was asked to compare eight pairs of different device profiles.

Regulatory reviewers at CDRH and health assessment experts from RTI Health Solutions collaborated closely to select attributes on the basis of clinical research, regulatory knowledge, and in-person interviews with obese patients. The chosen attributes are important to patients, physicians, and regulators and reflect the profiles of weight-loss devices that were under review by CDRH or in the pipeline. The following eight attributes were chosen for the survey: (1) total body weight loss, (2) duration of weight loss, (3) duration of mild-to-moderate side effects, (4) mortality risk, (5) chance of a side effect requiring hospitalization, (6) recommended dietary restrictions, (7) reduction in chance of comorbidity or reduction in prescription dosage for existing comorbidity, and (8) type of surgery to implant the weight-loss device. Each attribute had three to five levels.

The study results showed that the most important benefits of weight-loss devices are the amount and duration of weight loss. The most important risk is mortality risk. A very important attribute is diet restriction, whereas a side effect that requires hospitalization is the least important attribute.

The authors developed a decision-aid tool that can estimate the minimum acceptable benefit (i.e., weight loss) respondents would expect from a device to tolerate a specific level of risk. The tool also estimates the maximum acceptable risk (i.e., device-related mortality) respondents are willing to tolerate for a given weight loss and other device attributes. These values can be provided for risk-averse, for average, and for risk-tolerant patients and are critical to inform the FDA when determining the "minimum clinically meaningful effectiveness" that offsets the risks and inconveniences caused by devices under review. The minimum clinically meaningful effectiveness drives the sample size of pivotal studies designed to assess safety and effectiveness of medical devices and is crucial for the interpretation of clinical trial results as they become available.

The decision-aid tool can estimate the proportion of respondents who would prefer receiving a certain device profile over a no-device alternative. Table 3.1 shows the estimated proportions of patients accepting two different device profiles, Devices A and B.

TABLE 3.1

Estimated Percentages of Respondents Who Would Accept the Hypothetical Devices A or B Instead of Their Status Quo

Attributes of Hypothetical Devices	Device A	Device B
% Total body weight loss	9.2%	7.6%
Type of surgery	Laparoscopic	Endoscopic
Chance of dying from getting the device	0%	0%
Recommended diet restrictions	Eat ¼ cup at a time	Eat ¼ cup at a time
How long the weight loss lasts	12 months	6 months
How long minor side effect lasts	1 month	6 months
% Patients who would accept the device	9.0%	3.2%

3.6.3 Example

An implantable weight-loss device is under review. The existing treatment options are at the opposite ends of the benefit–risk spectrum: at one end, there is diet and exercise, which is noninvasive and safe but delivers limited weight loss, while at the other end, there is gastroplasty, which requires an invasive and irreversible surgery but delivers a substantial weight loss with high probability. The risk level of the device under consideration is in the middle between the risks of the safe and the aggressive therapy. A pivotal study submitted to the FDA shows that the device under review delivers a statistically significant but smaller-than-expected weight loss. However, the device is safer than the existing invasive option and the technology used by the device has an acceptable safety track record to treat other conditions. Making an approval decision for this device is a challenge because it delivers less benefit than expected. However, a valid patient preference study estimated that a meaningful portion of obese patients would be willing to receive the device and accept its risks in exchange for the weight loss it delivers. Therefore, the FDA is likely to approve this medical device.

3.7 Conclusion

The mission of the CDRH depends heavily on decision making and benefit–risk determinations. Often, benefit–risk determinations are very challenging and additional factors such as presence of uncertainty, patient preferences, availability of alternative treatments, characterization of the disease, the possibility of risk mitigation, the possibility of using postmarket data to reduce uncertainty on benefits and risks, and the possibility of improving a novel technology for an unmet medical need should be taken into account. These factors can be used as weights to help the assessment of benefits and risks.

It is very helpful to compare benefits against risks for decision making when the benefits and risks are weighed in the same scale. Quantitative methods can facilitate the elicitation of preferences and weights for benefits and risks of medical devices and enable the incorporation these weights into regulatory decisions that reflect the needs of a wide variety of stakeholders. In addition, quantitative methods can be validated and checked for robustness via sensitivity analysis.

Quantitative benefit–risk assessment is a nascent field that needs research and development to advance regulatory science so that regulatory decisions will reflect the values of a variety of stakeholders and be, at the same time, transparent, consistent, predictable, and rational.

References

1. U.S. Food and Drug Administration. 2012. Guidance for industry and Food and Drug Administration staff: Factors to consider when making benefit–risk determinations in medical device premarket approval and *de novo* classifications. http://www.fda.gov/downloads/MedicalDevices/DeviceRegulationandGuidance/GuidanceDocuments/UCM296379.pdf.

2. U.S. Food and Drug Administration. 2015. Draft guidance for industry, Food and Drug Administration staff, and other stakeholders: Patient preference information—Submission, review in PMAs, HDE applications, and de novo requests, and inclusion in device labeling. http://www.fda.gov/downloads/MedicalDevices/DeviceRegulationandGuidance/GuidanceDocuments/UCM446680.pdf.
3. Section 513(a) of the Federal Food, Drug & Cosmetic Act (21 CFR 860.7).
4. 21 CFR 860.7(e)(1).
5. U.S. House of Representatives. 2015. HR6, The 21st Century Cures Act. http://docs.house.gov/billsthisweek/20150706/CPRT-114-HPRT-RU00-HR6.pdf.
6. Medical Device Innovation Consortium. 2015. Medical Device Innovation Consortium (MDIC) patient centered benefit–risk framework report: A framework for incorporating information on patient preferences regarding benefit and risk into regulatory assessments of new medical technology. http://mdic.org/wp-content/uploads/2015/05/MDIC_PCBR_Framework_Web.pdf.
7. Ho, M. P., J. M. Gonzalez, H. P. Lerner, C. Y. Neuland, J. M. Whang, M. McMurry-Heath, A. B. Hauber, and T. Irony. 2015. Incorporating patient-preference evidence into regulatory decision making. *Surgical Endoscopy*, 1–10. http://link.springer.com/article/10.1007/s00464-014-4044-2.

Section III

Considerations of Benefit–Risk Assessment Development in Products' Life Cycle Management

4

Understanding and Evaluating Uncertainties in the Assessment of Benefit–Risk in Pharmaceutical Drug Development

Qi Jiang, Haijun Ma, Christy Chuang-Stein, Scott Evans, Weili He, George Quartey, John Scott, Shihua Wen, and Ramin B. Arani

CONTENTS

ABSTRACT Uncertainty has been recognized as a key issue in B–R assessment due to the challenges it adds to the decision-making process. In this chapter, the authors describe sources of uncertainties and discuss how uncertainties in B–R assessment are perceived by the community, and current positions of FDA and EMA in terms of handling of uncertainties in B–R assessment. The authors identified three major sources of uncertainty: uncertainties associated with the level of evidence, uncertainties associated with how to weigh benefit relative to risk, and uncertainties associated with premarketing to postmarketing translation. The authors also discussed approaches to quantify some of the uncertainties identified, and provided examples for illustration. Uncertainty is present throughout B-R assessment. Some uncertainties can be handled quantitatively. Others will require additional data to reduce uncertainty. Statistical tools are helpful to understand the impact of uncertainty, and clinical judgment is critical when a decision is to be made in presence of uncertainty.

4.1 Introduction

As Voltaire said, "Doubt is not a pleasant condition, but certainty is an absurd one." Dealing with uncertainties is an important aspect of the decision making of a product's benefit–risk (B–R) assessment. Although we will use the word *drug* in this article, the issues we discuss are generally common to all medical products, including drugs, devices, and biologics.

The Quantitative Sciences in the Pharmaceutical Industry Benefit:Risk Working Group (QSPI BRWG) was established in early 2013. Its main objectives are to educate the broader statistical community on this important area, to increase the role of statistical leadership in B–R assessment through cross-functional collaboration, and to foster communication between industry and regulatory agencies as use of structured B–R assessments increases. The BRWG is a diverse group, with members from pharmaceutical companies and the US Food and Drug Administration (FDA). The working group has three workstreams that focus on recommending appropriate methods to use (workstream 1), defining and promoting best practices (workstream 2), and addressing emerging topics including data sources, graphical representation, uncertainty evaluation and weight determination, and subgroup analysis (workstream 3). In this chapter, we discuss the issues on uncertainty evaluations. We will describe sources of uncertainties and share our thoughts on how to illustrate and assess uncertainties in B–R assessment.

4.2 Sources of the BRA Uncertainty

B–R assessment is dynamic. There are clear imbalances in the sources, timing, and nature of information available throughout a drug's life cycle (Hammad et al. 2013), which could cause uncertainties in B–R assessment. While some uncertainties are known and can sometimes be quantified and addressed, others may not be known. Stakeholders including regulatory agencies and governance bodies recognize the importance of uncertainties and the difficulties they present. Efficacy estimates and associated variability from clinical trials are often robust and can be considered as known knowns; adverse events (AEs) with low frequency may not be well understood in clinical trials and can be considered as known unknowns; unknown unknowns could include a very rare drug-induced safety issue that may only be observed in postmarketing after wide usage and large patient exposure.

We group the main uncertainties pertinent to B–R assessment into three categories: the uncertainties that are associated with the level of evidence for benefits and risks in clinical development, those associated with the relative importance of benefits versus risks, and those associated with translation of B–R assessment from a premarket to a postmarket setting. Below, we expand on this categorization and offer some guidance and thoughts on how to address and quantify uncertainties in B–R assessment.

4.2.1 Levels of Evidence for Benefit and Risk in Clinical Development

Evidence of benefits and risks obtained from clinical trials forms the primary basis for the B–R assessment of a drug. It is important to understand uncertainties of the evidence related to each key benefit or risk, respectively, and the implications of such information (ICH 2015). Uncertainties can arise because clinical trials evaluate efficacy in tightly controlled participant populations that cannot fully represent a drug's effectiveness or harm in more heterogeneous real-world populations. For example, the relatively short duration of a clinical trial leads to uncertainty about long-term effects for a drug that will be used chronically in its intended patient population. This entails uncertainty both about potentially diminishing efficacy over time and incidence of AEs with long latency periods, such as neoplasms. Recruitment to trials may underrepresent or exclude some vulnerable patient groups (e.g., the elderly, patients with multiple comorbidities, children, and women of childbearing age). The design of clinical trials often excludes those with a known high risk of the event of interest, particularly a previous history of that event, but in clinical practice, such patients are likely to be treated unless the treatment is contraindicated. This means that the absolute rate of the event of interest observed in clinical trials may not fully represent that inpatients who will likely take the drug once the drug is commercially available.

It is important to note that uncertainties between benefits and risks are usually asymmetrical. Clinical trials are designed to control Type I and Type II error rates for key efficacy endpoints, but seldom for safety endpoints. At the milestone of marketing authorization, the evaluation of efficacy is generally more robust than evaluation of safety data. Certain risks are particularly difficult to evaluate during premarket drug development, including serious AEs with low incidence, events that occur with low probability to the clinical trial population but may pose a greater risk to older patients, for example, or events that only occur after extended exposure or with a long latency period. In many cases, a drug's safety profile needs to be further evaluated during postmarketing.

In addition, estimated drug effects from clinical trials are associated with statistical uncertainties. In particular, safety endpoints often have low power and therefore greater uncertainty associated with the estimated rates.

Uncertainty about B–R profiles also arises when there are inconsistencies or conflicting findings across different subgroups, patient characteristics, geographic region, and studies. The FDA Draft Prescription Drug User Fee Act (PDUFA) Implementation Plan includes such conflicting findings among its examples of sources of uncertainty (FDA 2013b).

Post hoc findings are another source of uncertainty. While we generally pre-specify hypotheses for key efficacy endpoints, safety findings may be unexpected. Except for identified or known potential risks based on mechanism of action or previous experience, many safety issues are unexpected or were not well known before study data unblinding, and therefore there were no pre-specified hypotheses. For such post hoc observations, it is particularly difficult to distinguish real from chance findings. As the number of potential safety endpoints can be large, multiplicity may lead to false claims of safety issues.

Uncertainties can also be caused by issues such as possible biases in the data owing to study conduct, data quality, and so on. Missing data can introduce unknown bias. This occurs when data are missing not at random. It can also occur when data are missing at random but an inappropriate method is used to handle the missing data (Little et al. 2012).

4.2.2 Relative Importance of Benefits versus Risks

Uncertainty evaluation plays a critical role in B–R assessment, weight determination, and interpretation of the evidence and the conclusion (ICH 2015). B–R assessment involves synthesizing heterogeneous information, often for the purposes of a binary decision on a drug's approvability. This requires some way of making data of different nature comparable. Furthermore, we need to make a judgment on the relative importance of the benefit and risk elements and document the so-called weighting factors, to reflect this ranking exercise. The trade-offs between benefits and risks will depend on many considerations including the clinical importance of the endpoints, unmet medical need, the severity of the condition treated, and the current treatment options available for the given disease. Different stakeholders (e.g., sponsors, regulatory agencies, patients, and prescribers) may have different perspectives on these issues. For example, what is the acceptable increase in risk of severe bleeding for the benefit of reducing major adverse cardiac events? This may depend on the opinions of the assessors, as different stakeholders may weigh benefits and risks somewhat differently, especially when the results are marginal (FDA 2013b). This, of course, increases uncertainty in the final B–R assessment. Moreover, B–R assessments often do not include discussions to establish a "threshold of risk tolerance" that could differ among stakeholders with varying interests (e.g., regulators vs. payers vs. health care providers vs. patients). A patient's willingness to accept risk is likely to change over time depending on stage of life and severity of disease, which adds to the complexity of B–R decisions.

4.2.3 B–R Assessment in Postmarketing

Translation of clinical trial information into the postmarketing setting is challenging. Clinical trials are conducted in a somewhat artificial setting and are aimed at delineating the pure treatment effect from other confounding issues and risk factors. In general, patients in the real world are more heterogeneous, their adherence to the treatment regimen may not be as good (e.g., off-label use), and the clinical monitoring for them is often less rigorous than that in clinical trials. Consequently, the treatment efficacy could be diminished and safety signals could be complicated. For example, severity of AEs can be greater in the postmarket setting because in clinical trials, owing to frequent evaluation, AEs may be identified early and managed before they become severe. In contrast, AEs won't necessarily be identified until they become symptomatic in the postmarketing setting. One significant uncertainty in B–R balance when moving from premarketing to postmarketing is the potential of observing unexpected safety issues. The B–R balance observed in premarket may be subject to changes when generalized to the wider postmarket setting and these uncertainties make it difficult to predict the real-world treatment B–R profile at the time of approval.

Because of the uncertainty associated with premarket information, B–R assessments often need to be updated with emerging postmarket information. The updating of B–R assessment for marketed products has been formalized by regulatory agencies as the core of the periodic benefit–risk evaluation report. The update is more frequent shortly after market authorization and the frequency reduces over time (European Medicines Agency [EMA] 2013).

However, postmarket data have their own limitations. For example, risks often receive more attention than benefits in the postmarket setting, and postmarket data sources are usually less robust than clinical trial data. Observational studies can be susceptible to various sources of bias that might lead to overestimation or underestimation of adverse effects. Effectively synthesizing information from different sources with different levels of rigor is challenging; more research is needed in this area. Readers could refer to Chapter 7 for discussions on data source considerations in B–R assessment.

4.3 Current Status of Uncertainties in B–R Assessment

The uncertainties in B–R assessment described above are widely recognized. There have been many efforts to date devoted to improving the biopharmaceutical community's understanding of uncertainty and approaches to addressing them. However, considerable discrepancies remain in awareness of and approach to uncertainties between different stakeholders, attributed in part to different priorities.

Drug manufacturers are concerned about the impact of uncertainty in product development and have been working on ways to minimize it (Hughes et al. 2013). Regulators and payers recognize the importance of understanding uncertainty and are seeking more robust tools to articulate how it affects regulatory decision making (EMA 2012; FDA 2013b). Physicians recognize that each patient is different, but their understanding of the uncertainty and variability quantified in statistical terms remains limited (Ghosh and Ghosh 2005). Patients vary in their level of understanding uncertainty. While few people expect guarantees, many may have overoptimistic expectations of risks and benefits (Lloyd 2001). Regulatory agencies have long relied on B–R evaluations for new product approvals. However, past B–R assessments were generally informal, which may have led to a perception of lack of transparency. In recent years, regulatory agencies have moved toward a more structured B–R assessment process. This move has been accompanied by the issuance of regulatory guidelines, which outline approaches to B–R assessment and identify areas for further research (EMA 2012; FDA 2013b). Both FDA and EMA have noted the importance of and difficulty in handling uncertainty in B–R evaluations. FDA has developed a structured review framework for drugs and biologics, which includes the identification and evaluation of sources of uncertainty. The following two areas of focus were also identified for uncertainty characterization: how to translate premarket B–R assessment on the basis of clinical trial data to the postmarket setting and how to evaluate postmarket findings from sources of varying levels of rigor (FDA 2013b).

EMA has acknowledged that there are uncertainties associated with favorable and unfavorable effects. For example, there are uncertainties because of possible biases in the data, soundness and representativeness of clinical trials, and the potential for unobserved adverse effects. EMA has also acknowledged that the balance between favorable and unfavorable effects is affected by uncertainty. While judgment plays a key role in B–R assessment, a quantitative model could be useful to explore the impact of uncertainty on the overall B–R balance (EMA 2012).

The new initiatives described above place increased emphasis on the role of structured B–R assessment in the regulatory review process. The importance of incorporating patient opinions has been recognized as well. FDA has committed to a new initiative called Patient-Focused Drug Development with the goal of obtaining the patient perspective on certain disease areas for drugs and biologics during the 5-year period (2013–2018) of PDUFA V. In the medical devices arena, FDA has developed a Patient Preference Initiative and has begun to apply quantitative patient preference evidence to inform regulatory approval decisions (Ho et al. 2015).

4.4 Approaches to Address Different Sources of Uncertainty in B–R Assessment

In Section 4.2, we discussed three major sources of uncertainty: uncertainties associated with the level of evidence, uncertainties associated with how to weigh benefit relative to risk, and uncertainties associated with premarketing to postmarketing translation. In this section, we turn our attention to approaches that can be used to address some of these uncertainties.

4.4.1 Approaches to Address Uncertainties Associated with the Level of Evidence for Benefits and Risks in Clinical Development

The most common way to describe uncertainties in treatment effect estimates is to provide a quantitative measure of sampling variability associated with these estimates. This is often done in the form of confidence intervals. Confidence intervals could be constructed from a single trial or from meta-analyses of relevant trials. Confidence intervals could be provided in tabular or graphical format. Figure 4.1 is extracted from the Briefing Document prepared by the sponsor of rivaroxaban for a Cardiovascular and Renal Drugs Advisory Committee meeting on September 8, 2011. The Advisory Committee reviewed rivaroxaban for the prevention of stroke and systemic embolism in patients with nonvalvular atrial fibrillation. Data used to support the indication came from a single study ROCKET AF, in which rivaroxaban was compared with warfarin (Johnson and Johnson 2011).

The primary efficacy endpoint in ROCKET AF is a composite endpoint of stroke or non–central nervous system systemic embolism. The sponsor also specified two major secondary efficacy endpoints, both of which are also composite. The first major secondary efficacy endpoint is stroke, embolism, or vascular death. The other major secondary efficacy endpoint is stroke, embolism, myocardial infarction, or vascular death. Another important secondary efficacy endpoint is all-cause mortality.

The principal safety endpoints are major and non–major clinically relevant (NMCR) bleeding events. Major bleeding events include fatal bleeding, critical organ bleeding (intracranial and other sites), bleeding that required blood transfusion, and bleeding causing a >2 g/dl decrease in hemoglobin concentration (Hgb).

All efficacy and safety endpoints are binary. One can estimate the treatment effect on each endpoint by the difference in the incidence (proportion) of the endpoint in the two treatment groups (rivaroxaban—warfarin) or the difference in the incidence rate (e.g., events

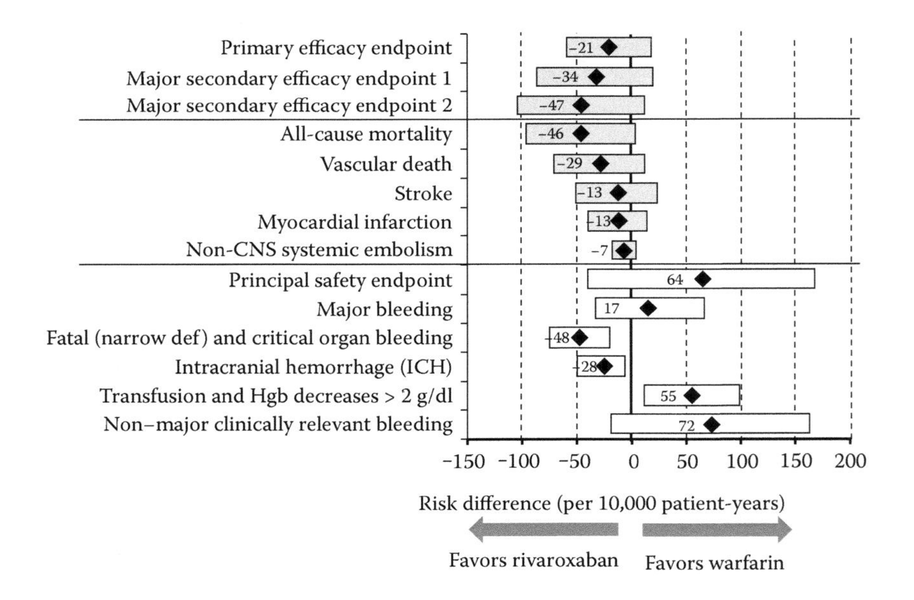

FIGURE 4.1
Forest plot of point estimates and 95% confidence intervals of treatment comparisons of main efficacy and safety endpoints. (From Johnson and Johnson Briefing Document, 2011. Rocket AF: ITT Analysis Set up to follow-up visit, Figure 9.2.)

per 10,000 patient years). Since all events (both efficacy and safety) are undesirable, low incidences (incidence rates) are desirable. A negative difference favors rivaroxaban while a positive difference favors warfarin. Figure 4.1 displays the point estimate and a 95% confidence interval, constructed by the sponsor, for the effect of rivaroxaban compared to warfarin on the main efficacy and safety endpoints discussed above. Here, 95% confidence intervals could be constructed by applying normal approximation (or exact methods) to data for individual endpoints separately. Alternatively, they could be constructed by applying the bootstrap method to account for correlation between endpoints.

In Figure 4.1, statistics for individual components of the composite endpoints are also displayed to examine the consistency of the results. The results pertain to the Intent-to-Treat (ITT) Analysis Set with data up to the follow-up visit. (The sponsor also considered other analysis data sets.) On the basis of the graphical display, the sponsor claimed that rivaroxaban has better efficacy results on all efficacy endpoints in Figure 4.1. The pattern is consistent across all components of the efficacy endpoints. Figure 4.1 also includes major and NMCR bleeding events, where the excessive events observed in the rivaroxaban group were mainly NMCR bleeding events and major bleeding events that required transfusions and caused a >2 g/dl decrease in Hgb.

Another way to express uncertainties is to describe the limitations of the data in a qualitative fashion. For example, in an effects table where important information of benefit and risk endpoints relevant to the B–R assessment is displayed in one table, weakness of the source data for these endpoints can be described in the "uncertainties" column (EMA 2012). One can add treatment effect estimates as well as sampling variability associated with the estimates to the effects table, thus combining the qualitative and quantitative discussions.

In the FDA-conducted B–R assessment for riociguat (Adempas), a first-in-class pulmonary arterial hypertension drug, uncertainties (or certainties) of clinical benefit were described qualitatively by pointing out the appropriateness of endpoints and the robustness of benefit evidence across endpoints and studies (FDA 2013a).

It is important to note that uncertainties associated with study design, conduct, and quality (e.g., missing data, confidentiality breach of interim results, improper means of measurement) are best addressed by good planning and careful execution (Little et al. 2012). Issues associated with design may be hard to remediate, although analytical remedies and adjustments are sometimes possible. For example, one may use analytical approaches such as multiple imputations to estimate treatment effects in the presence of missing data. Approaches of this kind, however, rely on assumptions about missing data processes that are generally not verifiable.

4.4.2 Approaches to Address Uncertainties Associated with the Relative Importance of Benefits versus Risks

The most common approach to address uncertainties associated with the importance of endpoints relative to each other is to repeat B–R assessment with different choices of weights, that is, conduct a sensitivity analysis by varying weights. We discuss a couple of approaches in this section.

We consider a hypothetical case of two important efficacy endpoints and two important safety endpoints. For simplicity, we assume that all the endpoints are binary and that treatment effect on each endpoint is estimated by the difference in the incidence of events in the two groups (new treatment − control). For convenience, we assume (1) the efficacy endpoints represent desirable outcomes, so a positive difference favors the new treatment;

and (2) the safety endpoints represent undesirable outcomes, so a positive difference favors the control. We use d_1 and d_2 to denote the difference in the incidence of the first and the second efficacy endpoints and d_3 and d_4 to denote the difference in the incidence of the first and the second safety endpoint. We use $\{w_i, i = 1, \ldots, 4\}$ to denote the weights assigned to the four endpoints such that $w_i \geq 0$ and $\sum_{i=1}^{4} w_i = 1$. These weights may reflect importance given to the four endpoints by clinical experts, by members of a data monitoring committee (DMC), or by patients (e.g., via conjoint analyses) (Freedman et al. 1996).

Using the weights w_i, we can construct a linear B–R score as

$$\text{Linear score} = \sum_{i=1}^{2} w_i\, d_i - \sum_{i=3}^{4} w_i\, d_i.$$

A positive linear score favors the new treatment. A critical question is how to choose $\{w_i\}$. One approach is to first decide how to weigh the safety endpoints relative to the efficacy endpoints, that is, $(w_3 + w_4)/(w_1 + w_2)$. We can then decide how to weigh the two endpoints within each category, that is, w_1/w_2 and w_3/w_4. In our hypothetical example, we assume that $w_1/w_2 = 0.8$ and $w_3/w_4 = 1$. In other words, the first efficacy endpoint weighs 80% of the second efficacy endpoint and the two safety endpoints weigh the same. We next focus on $(w_3 + w_4)/(w_1 + w_2)$, which reflects the importance of risk relative to benefit. From these three ratios, one can construct $\{w_i, i = 1, \ldots, 4\}$ with different scenarios. For example, if $(w_3 + w_4)/(w_1 + w_2) = 0.4$, then the four weights are $w_1 = \{100/(100 + 40)\} \times \{80/(80 + 100)\}$, $w_2 = \{100/(100 + 40)\} \times \{100/(80 + 100)\}$, $w_3 = w_4 = \{40/(100 + 40)\} \times 0.5$. Instead of focusing on only one choice of $(w_3 + w_4)/(w_1 + w_2)$, one can examine a range of this ratio and see how B–R comparison varies as a function of the ratio. This is shown in Figure 4.2 where $(w_3 + w_4)/(w_1 + w_2)$ varies between 0.05 and 2, that is, risk weighing between 5% and 200% of the benefit. In the hypothetical

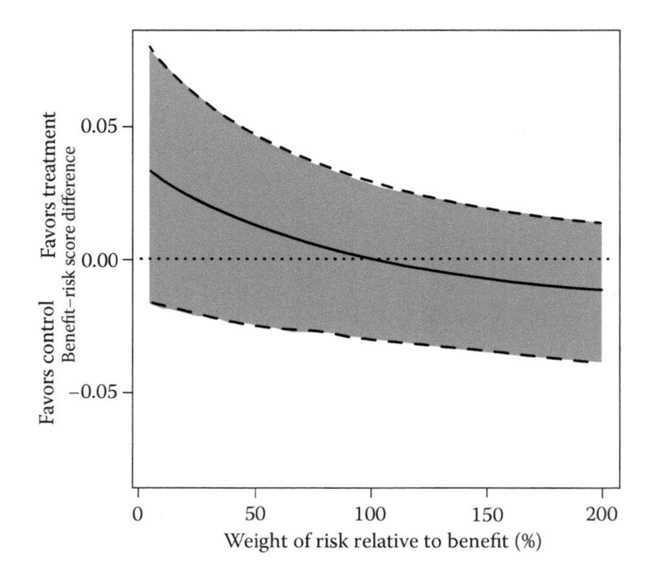

FIGURE 4.2
Linear B–R score with point-wise confidence interval as a function of the relative weight of risk to benefit.

example displayed in Figure 4.2, the two treatment groups have the same linear score when risk weighs the same as the benefit. As more weight is placed on risk (i.e., $(w_3 + w_4)/(w_1 + w_2) > 1$), the comparison favors control. This pattern is common in situations where a new treatment offers more benefit but also causes more treatment-related side effect. Figure 4.2 includes a 95% confidence interval for each choice of the relative weight. No adjustment is made for the numerous choices of $(w_3 + w_4)/(w_1 + w_2)$ displayed in the figure.

In Figure 4.2, we assess B–R at a particular point in time. In many clinical trials involving chronic administration of medications over a long period (e.g., longer than 2 years), it is often desirable to assess B–R over time with benefit and risk measured cumulatively over time. Results of the assessment can be displayed as a function of time as in Figure 4.3. Figure 4.3 assumes, again, four endpoints, two being efficacy endpoints and two being safety endpoints. Four types of weights are considered in Figure 4.3, Equal Weight, Weighted by Rank, Swing Weight (B–R = 100:40), and Ranged Swing Weight (B–R = 100:10 to 100:200).

Under the "Equal Weight" approach, the same weight was assigned to the four endpoints (i.e., $w_i = 0.25$, $i = 1, \ldots, 4$). For the "Weighted by Rank" approach, the four endpoints were first ranked by their relative importance with more important ones having higher ranks. Then, weights were assigned on the basis of their ranks so that the most important endpoint has a weight of 4/10 while the least important endpoint has a weight of 1/10. For the "Swing Weight" approach, the weights were assigned using the two-level approach employed in Figure 4.2 with $(w_3 + w_4)/(w_1 + w_2) = 0.4$. For the "Ranged Swing Weight" approach, we let $(w_3 + w_4)/(w_1 + w_2)$ vary between 0.10 and 2. The resulting linear B–R scores over time were plotted in gray. Confidence intervals are not included in Figure 4.3. However, they could be added for any choice of weights to address uncertainty associated with data. Bootstrap method could be used to construct confidence intervals. The advantage of bootstrap is that it preserves the correlation between different endpoints.

For the simulated example, Figure 4.3 suggests that for most choices of weights, the new treatment has a more favorable B–R score than control. The B–R score using swing weight was negative, favoring control after treatment initiation but became positive at approximately month 3 and remained positive during the study period. Figure 4.3 allows one to

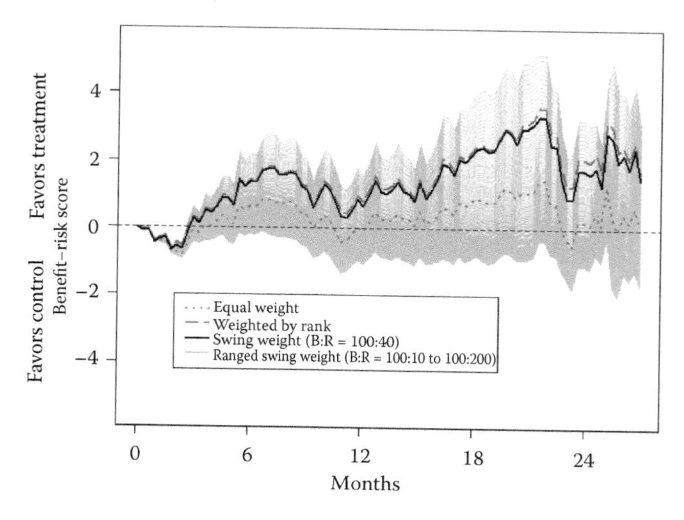

FIGURE 4.3
Display of B–R score over time with four different choices of weights.

assess the B–R profile over time as well as how this profile varies under different choices of weights.

In the examples above, all endpoints are measured in terms of proportion. There are many situations when endpoints important to B–R assessment are measured on different scales. For example, percentage HbA1c reduction from baseline is often a primary endpoint to assess the efficacy of a new treatment for diabetes. When endpoints have different units, it is often desirable to transform them to be on the same scale so that they can be meaningfully combined. One way to do this is to define a value function for each endpoint that maps the admissible range for that endpoint to [0,1]. The function can be chosen in such a way that a more favorable efficacy outcome and a more detrimental safety outcome all map to a higher value within [0,1]. Once endpoints are standardized, they can be combined using weights assigned to them. The process to assess uncertainty associated with weight choice in the context of the scale-free endpoints could proceed as described in this section.

In the above examples, weights are fixed. Their values are varied to assess the impact on B–R conclusion. Weights could be considered as random and based on data, and the B–R decision can be based on criteria incorporating the uncertainty of weighting, such as in the stochastic multicriteria acceptability analysis (Tervonen et al. 2011).

There are a few other approaches to address uncertainty. The construction of a "benefit–risk" cloud was proposed to incorporate uncertainty surrounding data (Sashegyi 2011). The proposal originated from a desire to facilitate DMC–sponsor communication and to help a DMC make B–R decisions on the basis of interim data. The idea is simple. For each endpoint, one can construct a 95% confidence interval reflecting the uncertainty around the population mean for the endpoint and for each treatment group. One can simulate an endpoint by making a random draw from the confidence interval. The draw should reflect the "likelihood" of values within the confidence interval (i.e., values closer to the middle are more likely than those near the boundaries of the confidence interval). With simulated data for each important endpoint, one could recalculate the benefit and risk measure. Sashegyi proposed separate weightings for benefit and risk endpoints. Plotting the weighted benefit result versus the weighted risk result for each treatment group on a two-dimensional plane creates a B–R cloud for each treatment. The relative position of the two clouds as well as the spread of the clouds can help a DMC decide if there is a clear separation of the clouds and, if so, in what manner they separate. Sashegyi's idea could be extended in multiple ways. First, the idea could be applied to differences between treatment groups instead of to each treatment group individually. Next, a B–R cloud for the difference between two groups could be displayed for each of multiple studies in the same graph to examine the consistency of additional benefit and additional risk across studies. Furthermore, one could construct confidence interval for each endpoint based on a meta-analysis of comparable studies and develop a single B–R cloud based on the meta-analysis results. In all of the cases above, different clouds under different weightings (for benefit and risk separately) could be displayed, although one needs to be careful not to overload the graph. Overloading a graph could diminish the usefulness of the visualizations.

Another approach is the B–R plane (Lynd and O'Brien 2004). The plane is a two-dimensional plot where the average difference in the probability of achieving a benefit with a new therapy relative to a comparator is plotted against the average difference in the probability of an AE between the two treatments. Lynd and O'Brien applied this approach to assess the use of low-dose unfractionated heparin versus enoxaparin for preventing venous thrombosis after a major trauma. This approach is covered in detail in Chapter 10 of this book and will therefore not be further discussed here.

4.4.3 Approaches to Address Uncertainties Associated with Premarketing to Postmarketing Translation of B–R Assessment

Clinical trials have many known limitations. The most important ones include short treatment duration, highly selected populations, and intensive monitoring of patient safety and compliance to minimize untoward outcome. Once a product is approved and available for public use, the product may be used by many patients not represented in clinical trials and in a way not consistent with the product label. It is often impossible to anticipate in advance how these patients may respond to the product. While one may attempt to build a prediction model based on an estimated pharmacokinetics and pharmacodynamics relationship, the success of the attempt is based largely on the existence of a useful biomarker and the availability of data. Absence of either makes it impossible to build a prediction model with a reasonable prediction capability. This is why it is critical to continue B–R assessment in the postmarketing phase.

Besides the above, another factor that affects B–R postmarketing assessment is the impact attributed to the regression to mean (RTM) effect. Products are selected on the basis of observed benefit and safety results that are favorable. This selection means that the actual benefit and safety may not be as favorable as observed in clinical trials. This is known as the RTM effect. The effect works in the opposite directions for benefit and risk and could lead to a less favorable B–R profile because of this statistical phenomenon.

Regulators have various options for marketed products whose B–R balance has become less favorable based on postmarketing data. The most common one is to include a box warning to the product label. The most severe one is to withdraw the product from the market. Options in between include requiring patients/prescribers to register for product use or restricted access through a managed access program.

4.5 Concluding Remarks

There is much increased emphasis from regulatory agencies, industry, and the medical community on the efforts on further enhancing structured B–R assessments and improving transparency, consistency, and communication. Uncertainty has been recognized as a key issue in B–R assessment, owing to the challenges it adds to the decision-making process.

In this chapter, we discussed the potential sources of uncertainty in B–R assessment and classified them into three categories: those related to the level of evidence from clinical trials, those related to the relative importance of benefits and risks, and those related to translation from premarketing to postmarketing. We reviewed regulatory agencies' reports and literature about B–R methodology and frameworks. We also summarized the current positions of FDA and EMA in terms of handling of uncertainties in B–R assessment. In addition, we discussed potential approaches to quantify some of the uncertainties identified and provided examples for illustration.

There are other sources of uncertainties in addition to those discussed in this section. Some could relate to endpoint definitions. For example, in the rivaroxaban example, hemorrhagic strokes were included in both the primary efficacy and principal safety endpoints, which could lead to these events being counted twice in the linear B–R score analysis when scores are constructed based on the composite endpoints. Double counting could also occur if serious adverse reaction is identified as an important safety endpoint and malignancy is cited as a separate safety endpoint for B–R assessment. One option in this case is to conduct sensitivity analysis using endpoints that do not overlap.

It is important to address uncertainty in B–R assessment considering a few aspects including the complexity of the decision-making process with consideration of both quantitative and qualitative dimensions, while recognizing that not all drugs are created equal—context matters, sources of uncertainties (clinical, methodological, and statistical) matters, and operational challenges may compound the picture (Hammad 2014).

B–R assessment is a continuous and dynamic process and is conducted by sponsors during clinical development and during drug life cycle management. Uncertainty is present throughout B–R assessment. Some uncertainties can be handled quantitatively with the use of confidence intervals and sensitivity analysis. Others will require additional data to reduce uncertainty. Statistical tools are helpful to understand the impact of uncertainty and clinical judgment is critical when a decision is to be made in the presence of uncertainty. For this reason, B–R assessment requires cross-functional efforts and close collaboration is critical.

References

EMA. "The Benefit–risk methodology project documents: Work Packages (WP) 4," (2012), currently available on EMA website at: http://www.ema.europa.eu/ema/index.jsp?curl=pages/special_topics/document_listing/document_listing_000314.jsp&mid=WC0b01ac0580223ed6.

EMA. "ICH guideline E2C (R2) on periodic benefit–risk evaluation report (PBRER)," (2013).

FDA. "Briefing Document on Adempas (riociguat) for the Cardiovascular and Renal Drugs Advisory Committee," (2013a), currently available at: http://www.fda.gov/downloads/AdvisoryCommittees/CommitteesMeetingMaterials/Drugs/CardiovascularandRenalDrugsAdvisoryCommittee/UCM363541.pdf.

FDA. "Draft PDUFA V Implementation Plan: Structured Approach to Benefit–Risk Assessment in Drug Regulatory Decision-Making," (2013b).

Freedman L, Anderson G and Kipnis V. "Approaches to monitor the results of long-term disease prevention trials: Examples from the Women's Health Initiative." *Control Clin Trials*, (1996), 17, pp. 509–525.

Ghosh AK and Ghosh K. "Translating evidence-based information into effective risk communication: Current challenges and opportunities." *Journal of Laboratory and Clinical Medicine*, (2005), 145(4), pp. 171–180.

Hammad TA. "Key Sources of Uncertainty in the Assessment of Benefits and Risks of Pharmaceuticals and Associated Challenges," (2014), Institute of Medicine Workshop: Characterizing and Communicating Uncertainty in the Assessment of Benefits and Risks of Pharmaceutical Products, available at: http://iom.nationalacademies.org/~/media/Files/Activity%20Files/Research/DrugForum/2014-Feb-13/February%2012%20-%20Session%20I%20-%20Hammad.pdf.

Hammad TA, Neyarapally GA, Iyasu S, Staffa JA, Dal Pan G. "The future of population-based postmarket drug risk assessment: A regulator's perspective." *Clinical Pharmacology and Therapeutics*, (2013), 94(3), pp. 349–358.

Ho MP, Gonzalez JM, Lerner HP et al. "Incorporating patient-preference evidence into regulatory decision making." *Surg Endosc.*, (2015), 29(10), pp. 2984–2993.

Hughes D, Waddingham EAJ, Mt-Isa S et al. "IMI-PROTECT Recommendations for the methodology and visualisation techniques to be used in the assessment of benefit and risk of medicines," (2013), available at: http://protectbenefitrisk.eu/documents/HughesetalRecommendationsforthemethodologyandvisualisationtechniquestobeusedintheassessmento.pdf.

ICH. "Final Concept Paper M4E(R2): Enhancing the Format and Structure of Benefit–Risk Information in ICH M4E(R1) Guideline," (2015), available at: http://www.ich.org/fileadmin/Public_Web_Site/ICH_Products/CTD/M4E_R2_Efficacy/M4E_R2__Final_Concept_Paper_27_March_2015.pdf.

Johnson and Johnson. "Advisory Committee Briefing Document Rivaroxaban for the Prevention of Stroke and Non-Central Nervous System (CNS)," (2011), available at: http://www.fda.gov/downloads/AdvisoryCommittees/CommitteesMeetingMaterials/Drugs/CardiovascularandRenalDrugsAdvisoryCommittee/UCM270797.pdf.

Little RJ, D'Agostino R, Cohen ML et al. "The Prevention and Treatment of Missing Data in Clinical Trials." *N Engl J Med*. (2012), 367, pp. 1355–1360.

Lloyd AJ, 2001. "The extent of patients' understanding of the risk of treatments." *Quality in Health Care*, p. 10 (suppl. 1): i14–i18.

Lynd L and O'Brien B. "Advances in risk-benefit evaluation using probabilistic simulation methods: An application to the prophylaxis of deep vein thrombosis." *J Clin Epidemiol.*, (2004), 57(8), pp. 795–803.

Sashegyi A. "A benefit–risk model to facilitate DMC-sponsor communication and decision making." *Drug Information Journal*, (2011), 45, pp. 747–757.

Tervonen T, van Valkenhoef G, Buskens E, Hillege HL, Postmus D. "A stochastic multicriteria model for evidence-based decision making in drug benefit–risk analysis." *Stat Med*. (2011), 30(12), pp. 1419–428.

5

Quantifying Patient Preferences for Regulatory Benefit–Risk Assessments

F. Reed Johnson and Mo Zhou

CONTENTS

ABSTRACT In 2006, a preference study of patients' risk tolerance was submitted to the US Food and Drug Administration (FDA) Tysabri Advisory Committee as part of the drug's reapproval application. This submission marked the first time such evidence was included in support of drug licensing. The Center for Drug Evaluation and Research (CDER) currently is developing a benefit–risk evaluation framework to better communicate which benefits and risks are considered, how the available evidence is interpreted, and how the benefits and risks are weighed. FDA's Center for Devices and Radiological Health (CDRH) issued guidance in 2012 and 2015 for conducting benefit–risk assessments which explicitly includes consideration of patients' tolerance for risks and perspectives on benefits. A decision tool using patient-preference weights is being used to evaluate benefits and risks of new devices. This chapter provides a conceptual framework for quantifying patient benefit–risk tradeoff preferences, outlines procedures for eliciting valid preference weights for therapeutic benefits and harms, and reviews applications of these methods in two recent regulatory case studies for Duchenne's muscular dystrophy and weight-loss devices. It concludes with an evaluation of prospects for integrating quantitative evidence on patients' willingness to accept therapeutic risks in return for improved efficacy in regulatory decision making.

5.1 Introduction

5.1.1 Benefit–Risk Evidence and the Weighting Problem

Pharmaceutical benefit–risk (B–R) evaluations pose many measurement challenges, including multiple potential efficacy and safety endpoints; large uncertainty about the likelihood, causality, reversibility, and latency of low-frequency adverse events; and heterogeneity of effects among patient subgroups. These problems are the focus of lively debate and continuing research. However, even if all the difficulties related to measuring benefits and harms could be resolved, it still would be impossible to determine whether the benefits exceed the harms of a particular treatment on the basis of accurate outcome measures. B–R assessment requires value judgments to compare dissimilar beneficial and harmful outcomes. Although balancing benefits and risks inevitably involves societal value judgments, B–R evaluations typically are informed by advisory bodies composed of scientists and clinicians.

The fundamental question for drug development and regulatory decision making is how much risk of adverse outcomes, including mortality, is acceptable for a treatment that offers improvements in efficacy relative to the current standard of care. For some decision makers, a relatively small benefit in a sufficiently large population could offset a given adverse event risk, while for others, any risk of a fatal side effect would make a treatment unacceptable.

In Figure 5.1, a comparison of enoxaparin and unfractionated heparin indicates an incremental benefit of 0.12 and an incremental risk of 0.03 (Lynd and O'Brien 2004). Decision maker 1 subjectively assigns equal weights to major bleed and deep vein thrombosis (DVT) events, so the willingness to accept one major bleed to prevent one DVT is $\mu_A = 1$. Decision maker 2, however, requires four times more benefit to accept one major bleed, so $\mu_B = 1/4$.

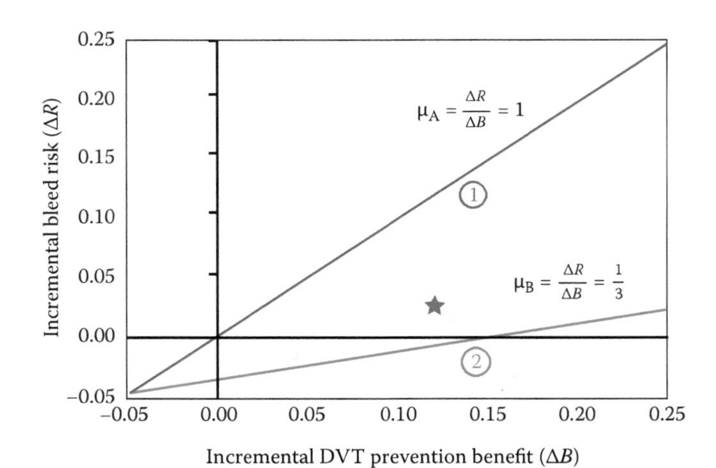

FIGURE 5.1
Willingness to accept one major bleed to prevent one DVT. (Adapted from Lynd, L.D. and O'Brien, J. 2004. Advances in risk–benefit evaluation using probabilistic simulation methods: An application to the prophylaxis of deep vein thrombosis. *J Clin Epidemiol* 57 (8):795–803.)

The red star indicates the actual B–R ratio, which is approximately 1/3. Decision maker 1 would favor approving enoxaparin, while decision maker 2 would not favor approval.

The disagreement between 1 and 2 is not related to the quality of the evidence. Decision maker 1 simply is more risk-tolerant and decision maker 2 is more risk-averse. Medical experts have personal risk attitudes but are asked to make societal evaluations. The practice of delegating such societal value judgments entirely to medical experts is being challenged.

5.1.2 Whose Preferences Should Count?

Patients are the potential beneficiaries of more effective treatments and also bear the risks associated with those treatments. Their subjective judgments arguably warrant consideration as well. However, current evaluation practices do not require quantification or even formal consideration of the values of patients in the treatment review and approval process. The values and risk tolerance of patients typically are presented qualitatively to advisory panels and policy makers either individually or through advocacy organizations. However, such anecdotal testimony does not constitute evidence of the willingness of well-informed patients to accept risks to obtain therapeutic benefits. In addition, it is unclear whether those who advocate for less restrictive or more restrictive access to treatments actually represent the affected patient population.

The principle of informed consent requires that patients play a meaningful role in therapeutic decisions. The American Medical Association's official statement on informed consent states that informed consent is a process involving disclosure and discussion of specific potential benefits and risks of treatment so that patients can make an informed decision to proceed or to refuse a particular treatment (Chilton and Collett 2008). Informed consent and shared decision making shift the focus of decision making from physicians determining what is best for patients to physicians helping patients choose what is best for them.

An early trade-off study compared cancer patients' and hospital caregivers' acceptance of radiotherapy toxicity in return for survival benefits (Brundage et al. 1998). Figure 5.2

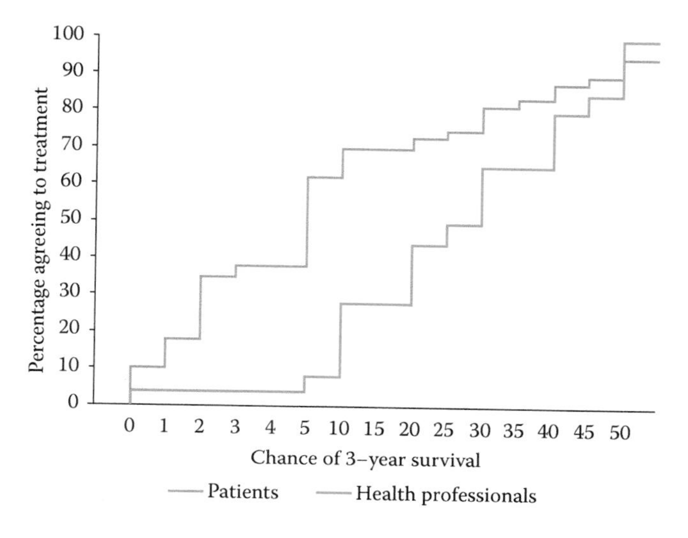

FIGURE 5.2
Trade-off survival thresholds for cancer patients and health professionals. (Adapted from Brundage, M.D. et al. 1998. Using a treatment-tradeoff method to elicit preferences for the treatment of locally advanced non-small-cell lung cancer. *Med Decis Making* 18 (3):256–67.)

indicates that larger percentages of patients were willing to accept treatment toxicities than healthcare professionals for each likelihood of survival to 3 years. At the plausible benefit level of 5%, 60% of patients would accept high-dose radiotherapy toxicities compared to only 10% of hospital caregivers.

Despite well-established principles of informed consent and increasing support for shared decision making, patient concerns are unlikely to play a meaningful role in regulatory B–R evaluations in the absence of valid, quantitative evidence on patients' tolerance for treatment-related risks. Fortunately, more than 40 years of development of stated-preference methods in market research, transportation, environmental policy, and health have produced a robust set of tools for quantifying the value that patients place on the potential benefits of a treatment and their willingness to accept risk in return for treatment benefits. A leading stated-preference researcher, Daniel McFadden, received the Nobel Prize in Economics in 2000 for his development of the theoretical and statistical foundations for these stated-preference methods (McFadden 1974). Various terms are used to describe identical or closely related stated-preference approaches, including conjoint analysis, stated-preference surveys, best–worst scaling (BWS), and discrete-choice experiments (DCEs). In this chapter, we focus on obtaining preference weights and B–R acceptance thresholds using DCEs, or simply choice experiments. Choice experiments have scientific credibility and are compatible with widely accepted standards for evidence. Using choice experiments to understand and quantify how much side effect risk patients will tolerate in return for better efficacy can help inform consistent, principled regulatory decisions.

5.1.3 Patient Preferences and Recent Regulatory Developments

B–R assessments are included in regulatory evaluations of premarket and postmarket reviews process of human drugs, biological products, and devices. These evaluations take into account evidence of safety and effectiveness of a product, the severity of the condition the product intends to prevent or treat, the benefits and risks of other available treatments, and potential risk management tools that may reduce the risks of the product. Both the US Food and Drug Administration (FDA) and the European Medicines Agency (EMA) are developing institutional arrangements to provide more involvement for individual patients and patient organizations in regulatory decision making (EMA 2013; FDA 2012).

The FDA's Center for Drug Evaluation and Research (CDER) conducts evaluations of new pharmaceutical products. These assessments involve both quantitative analyses and qualitative weighting of the evidence. Improving transparency and formalization of CDER's regulatory B–R assessments were significant concerns in reauthorizing the Prescription Drug User Fee Act (PDUFA) in 2010. The Food and Drug Administration Safety and Innovation Act (FDASIA) (Public Law 112–144) requires CDER to "implement a structured risk–benefit assessment framework in the new drug approval process to facilitate the balanced consideration of benefits and risks, a consistent and systematic approach to the discussion and regulatory decision-making, and the communication of the benefits and risks of new drugs." To fulfill this requirement, CDER published a 5-year plan that describes the approaches the Agency will take to develop and implement structured B–R assessments in the drug review and approval process.

On the basis of an analysis of prior regulatory decisions, CDER has developed a basic B–R framework. The key decision factors in the framework include analysis of the severity of the condition, current treatment options, benefits defined by results from clinical trials, risks defined by observed or expected adverse events, and risk management options to mitigate potential safety concerns. Within each factor, the regulatory decision is informed by two considerations—evidence and uncertainties based on facts, and conclusions and reasons that explain the bases for decisions. The Benefit–Risk Summary Assessment in the final row of the framework explains how the FDA integrated these evidences on benefits and risks and reached the regulatory decision. It also includes the rationale to support labeling and postmarketing requirements. While acknowledging the importance of quantifying certain components of the B–R assessment to support decision making, the framework describes a structured qualitative approach to identify and communicate key considerations in the FDA's B–R assessments and explains how that leads to a regulatory decision.

In addition to developing a B–R assessment framework, CDER also established a new Patient-Focused Drug Development initiative. Although patients' unique perspective would benefit the drug development and review process, there have been few opportunities for patients to contribute insights from their experience. CDER is soliciting patients' perspectives for various disease areas over a 5-year period. Twenty conditions were identified for the first 3 years. A public meeting is to be conducted for each disease area with participants from CDER review divisions, the patient-advocacy community, individual patients, and other interested stakeholders. The information obtained from these meetings will be used to improve drug development and the review process. Recently, CDER issued draft guidance on patient engagement for rare conditions such as Duchenne muscular dystrophy (US FDA CDER 2015a).

The Center for Devices and Radiological Health (CDRH) is the branch within the FDA that approves, regulates, and monitors medical devices. In contrast to CDER's qualitative approach to B–R assessments, CDRH is developing a quantitative approach to patients' tolerance for treatment-related risks. The Center issued preliminary guidance in 2012 (US FDA CDRH and Center for Biologics Evaluation and Research 2012) and more extensive draft guidance in May 2015 (US FDA CDRH and Center for Biologics Evaluation and Research 2015).

This chapter suggests that valid measures of patients' B–R trade-off preferences could provide evidence on societal values to assist decision makers in evaluating such treatments. We first outline a conceptual framework for accounting for probabilistic treatment outcomes and the utility theoretic basis for quantifying B–R trade-off preferences. We then summarize the steps necessary to elicit patient preferences using a DCE and provide examples from previous studies. Finally, we summarize two recent patient-preference studies that have had significant impacts on FDA draft guidance. A CDRH-sponsored case study on obese individuals' willingness to accept risks of weight-loss devices is being used in reviews of such devices and recently was the basis for approving a device that failed to achieve its clinical-trial primary endpoint and helped inform draft guidance. CDER invited a Duchenne muscular dystrophy patient-advocacy group to propose guidance on patient engagement. The resulting report formed the basis of recent draft guidance on regulatory reviews involving rare conditions.

5.2 Conceptual Framework for Measuring B–R Trade-Off Weights

5.2.1 Preferences for Probabilistic Outcomes

At the individual-patient level, all outcomes are probabilistic to some degree. Some patients could be more sensitive to gastrointestinal side effects than others. Some patients could have a genetic mutation that increases their chance of achieving beneficial outcomes from a particular therapy. In the absence of prior information about a patient's likely response to therapy, mean outcomes from clinical-trial and postmarketing data can be used to assess the likelihood a given patient will experience beneficial or harmful outcomes.

Of course, some risks are more consequential than others. Harms that take the form of life-threatening or seriously disabling conditions are irreversible, are mutagenic or teratogenic, or for which there are no effective treatments are far more serious than short-term, self-limiting or treatable, mild-to-moderate side effects such as transitory vomiting and nausea, fatigue, sleeplessness, headache, and other common conditions. Patients generally can decide whether such side effects are tolerable or whether to avoid the associated discomfort by discontinuing treatment.

As a practical matter, risk tolerance relates primarily to the more serious category of side effects. It is tempting to employ the simplifying assumption used in cost–utility analysis that the expected value of a harmful outcome is just the value of that outcome times the probability of its occurrence. This assumption requires that people be risk-neutral. Conventional economic utility theory assumes that people are risk averse. Risk neutrality generally is inconsistent with observed behavior (Gafni and Torrance 1984; Bala et al. 1998). When faced with a choice between two uncertain outcomes with the same expected value, people prefer the more certain alternative. Insurance markets exist because people are risk-averse. Because they are averse to both the harmful outcome itself and having to live with the uncertainty of the harm occurring, people are willing to pay an insurance premium that is significantly larger than the expected monetary value of the harm.

The fact that different people carry different amounts of insurance that covers different kinds of hazards indicates that people's tolerance for risk varies and that risk tolerance can be quantified. In the case of insurance, we can observe the value of avoiding monetary damages. In the case of healthcare, such markets often do not exist. When they do exist, they usually are uninformative about patients' preferences because of reimbursement rules and the role of physician intermediaries. In the absence of clinical data on risk tolerance, we need to design controlled experiments to provide evidence on patients' B–R trade-off preferences.

5.2.2 B–R Thresholds

Figure 5.1 shows patients' B–R acceptability threshold (Johnson et al. 2013a). It indicates that patients on average will accept therapeutic risks only if they are sufficiently compensated with better efficacy, which requires that the B–R acceptability threshold slope upward. Combinations of benefits and risks that lie above the line indicate outcomes for which the perceived (negative) value of additional risks relative to a comparator are greater than the corresponding perceived value of the additional benefits. Conversely, outcomes that lie below the line indicate outcomes for which the subjective value of the marginal risks are less than the corresponding subjective value of the marginal benefits. Holding efficacy constant at a given level, the threshold indicates the subjective risk value at which benefits are exactly offset by risks for that level of efficacy.

To construct the B–R acceptability threshold, it is necessary to obtain estimates of the relative importance of benefits and risks. We discuss an empirical approach to obtaining such estimates.

5.2.3 Using the B–R Threshold to Compare Benefits and Risks

Many discussions about B–R comparisons focus on the need to convert benefits and harms into a common metric to facilitate direct calculation of net benefits. Finding such a metric

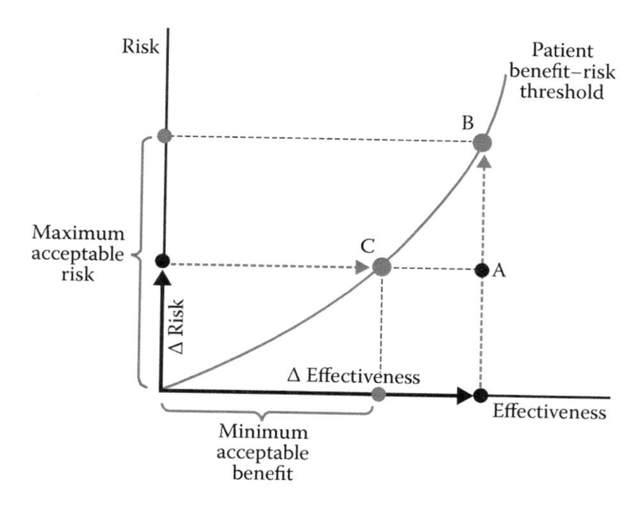

FIGURE 5.3
Minimum acceptable benefit and maximum acceptable risk from a B–R acceptability threshold. The shape of the B–R threshold depends on the shapes of the underlying preference utility functions for benefit and risk.

requires the quantitative evaluation of relative importance across benefits and harms. In contrast, the B–R acceptability threshold offers a framework for directly comparing quantitative measures of benefits and risks. Suppose Figure 5.3 shows the B–R threshold for a specific patient population in a given therapeutic area. Suppose also that the benefits and risks associated with a treatment in that therapeutic area correspond to point A. Because A is located below the threshold, the improved efficacy more than compensates for the increased risk. At the given risk increase, the minimum acceptable efficacy improvement is shown by C, which is less than the actual efficacy indicated by A. Similarly, for the actual efficacy indicated by A, the maximum acceptable risk is shown by B, which is more than the actual risk.

B–R acceptability thresholds are likely to be nonlinear and to differ across risk types and among individuals. Some patients may be more tolerant than others of side-effect risks as a result of inherent differences in their aversion to bearing risk, severity of their health condition, or other factors.

5.3 Steps for Quantifying Patient B–R Trade-Off Preferences*

Properly designed and implemented choice experiments can yield valid and reliable estimates of patient-preference weights for beneficial and harmful treatment outcomes following the steps shown in Figure 5.4. Additional details for implementing these steps can be found in Johnson et al. (2013a).

5.3.1 Identify Treatment Attributes and Levels

Attributes are beneficial and harmful treatment outcomes or trial endpoints that will be used to construct trade-off questions. They can be defined using a value tree as shown in

* This section was adapted from material in Johnson et al. (2013a).

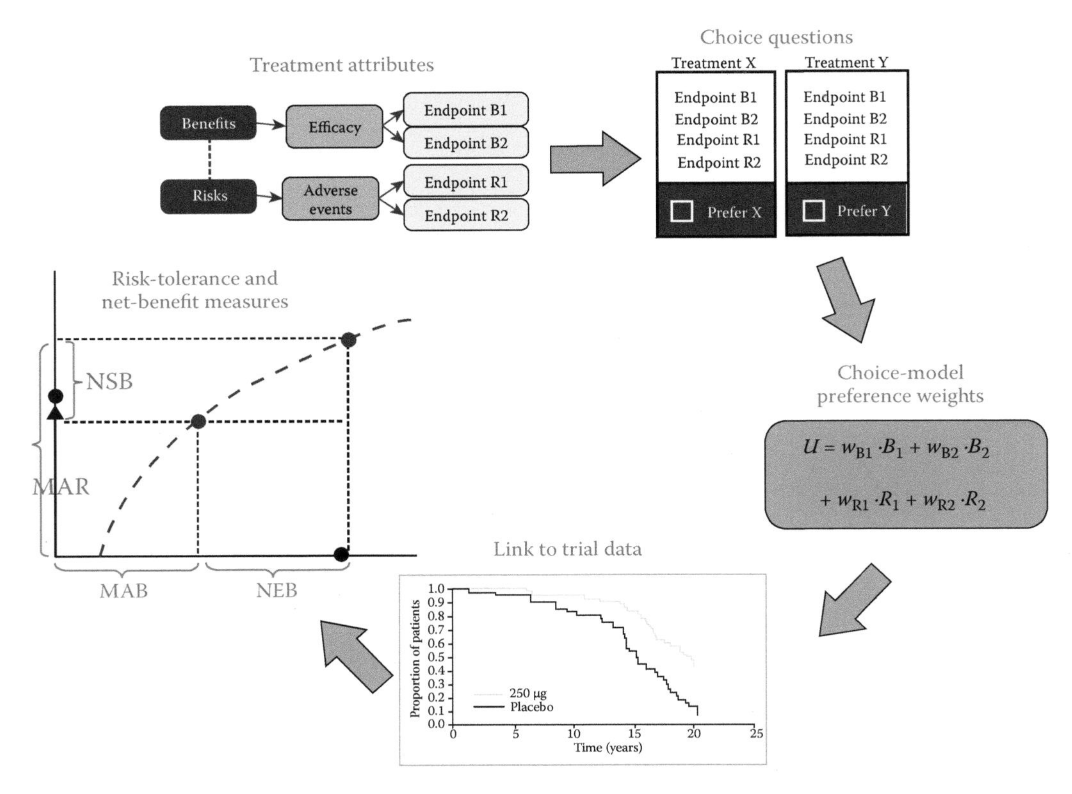

FIGURE 5.4
Steps in a B–R DCE study. (Adapted from Muehlbacher, private correspondence.)

Figure 5.4. The content of the value tree can come from published literature, professional judgment, trial data, qualitative data on patient concerns, or some combination of these. In B–R preference assessments designed to provide evidence for regulatory decision making, efficacy endpoints are typically endpoints measured in clinical trials. Adverse event attributes should include those adverse events of concern to regulators. Each attribute can have two or more levels. For example, a lymphoma risk attribute could have risk levels of 0.005, 0.010, and 0.02. A time-to-progression cancer-treatment attribute could have levels of 6, 12, and 18 months. Table 5.1 shows an attribute table for a B–R study of biologic treatments for multiple sclerosis.

5.3.2 Construct Trade-Off Questions

The most common choice-question format uses two or three hypothetical treatment alternatives. An example choice question from a renal cell carcinoma study is shown in Figure 5.5, including risk grids to minimize numeracy requirements for comparing probabilistic outcomes (Mohamed et al. 2011). In a choice-experiment survey, each treatment profile specifies benefit and risk endpoints corresponding to ranges observed in the clinical data. Combinations of endpoints are varied according to an experimental design with known statistical properties. Each respondent evaluates several questions to obtain enough data to ensure feasible statistical estimation of all the desired preference weights. Marshall et al. (2010) found that most published choice-experiment studies have used between 7 and

TABLE 5.1

Attribute Table for Multiple Sclerosis (MS) B–R Choice Experiment

Treatment Attribute	Levels
Number of relapses during the next 5 years	• No relapse • 1 relapse • 3 relapses • 4 relapses
Time (from today) until your MS gets worse	• 8 years • 5 years • 3 years • 1 year
Chance of dying from liver failure within 10 years	• None would die • 5 patients out of 1000 (0.5%) would die • 20 patients out of 1000 (2%) would die • 50 patients out of 1000 (5%) would die
Chance of dying or severe disability from PML within 10 years	• None would die or have disability • 5 patients out of 1000 (0.5%) would die or have disability • 20 patients out of 1000 (2%) would die or have disability • 50 patients out of 1000 (5%) would die or have disability
Chance of dying from leukemia within 10 years	• None would die • 5 patients out of 1000 (0.5%) would die • 20 patients out of 1000 (2%) would die • 50 patients out of 1000 (5%) would die

Source: From Johnson, F.R. et al. 2009. Multiple sclerosis patients' benefit–risk preferences: Serious adverse event risks versus treatment efficacy. *J Neurol* 256 (4):554–562.

15 questions per respondent. The resulting survey instrument must be carefully pretested with patients from the target sample population to ensure that the information provided in preparation for the choice questions is adequate and understandable, that patients are willing to accept trade-offs among the ranges of treatment attributes shown, and that the overall burden of taking the survey is acceptable.

5.3.3 Estimate Preference Weights

Statistical analysis of the pattern of choices observed from appropriately designed study reveals the implicit preference weights employed by respondents in evaluating the hypothetical treatments. Choice questions generate data that require analysis using advanced statistical techniques (Train 2002; Train and Sonnier 2005). The observed choices contain information on the implicit weights respondents used to evaluate the relative importance of the outcomes. These weights are estimated using an appropriate statistical model that accounts for the particular characteristics of the choice data.

Subgroup analysis and other statistical techniques help identify how risk tolerance varies by individual characteristics such as age, health history, current symptom severity, treatment experience, and time since diagnosis. Unfortunately, it is rarely possible to obtain a strictly random sample from the full population of patients with a particular condition. Furthermore, the sample must be sufficiently large and diverse to enable statistical weighting of estimates to approximate those of a more representative sample or identify preferences for groups of patients with particular characteristics of clinical interest.

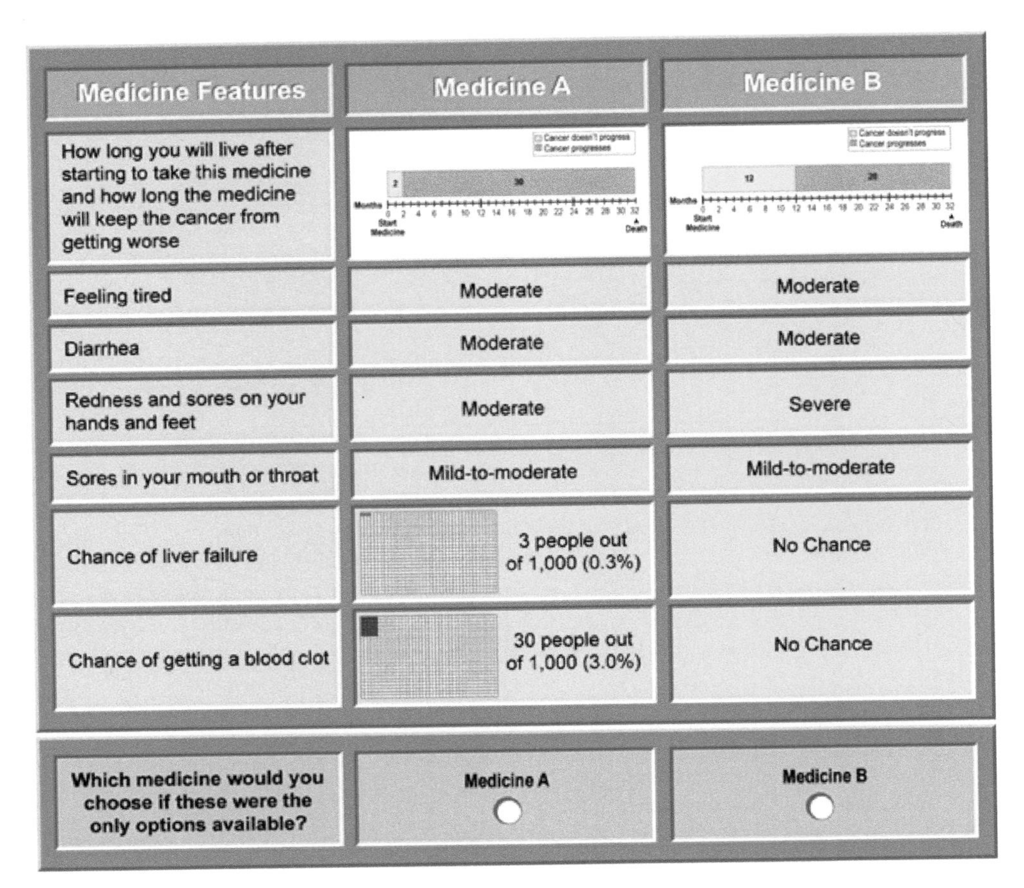

FIGURE 5.5
Example choice–experiment trade-off question. (From Mohamed, A.F. et al. 2011. Patient benefit–risk preferences for targeted agents in the treatment of renal cell carcinoma. *Pharmacoeconomics* 29 (11):977–988.)

Figure 5.6 contains estimated preference weights for Crohn's disease treatments that offer improvements in beneficial outcomes but have potential risks of serious infection, progressive multifocal leukoencephalopathy (PML), and lymphoma (Johnson et al. 2007). The study was submitted to the FDA Tysabri Advisory Committee in 2008. The efficacy attributes and steroids are categorical severity levels, while the risk attributes are continuous probabilities. The height of the plots indicates the relative importance of the attributes over the ranges evaluated. Hence, a symptom improvement from severe to remission is most important, followed by 0.5% risk of PML, while 0.5% risk of serious infection and lymphoma are about equally important, as are preventing complications and avoiding steroid use.

5.3.4 Calculate Risk Tolerance and Net Benefit Metrics for Trial Data

To evaluate the preference-weighted benefits and adverse event outcomes of one or more drugs, the preference weights must be combined with results from clinical or observational studies (Manjunath et al. 2012). Because no relative preference weights exist for outcomes that are not included in the stated choice survey, nothing can be said about the relative importance of nonincluded outcomes. This requires the implicit assumption that

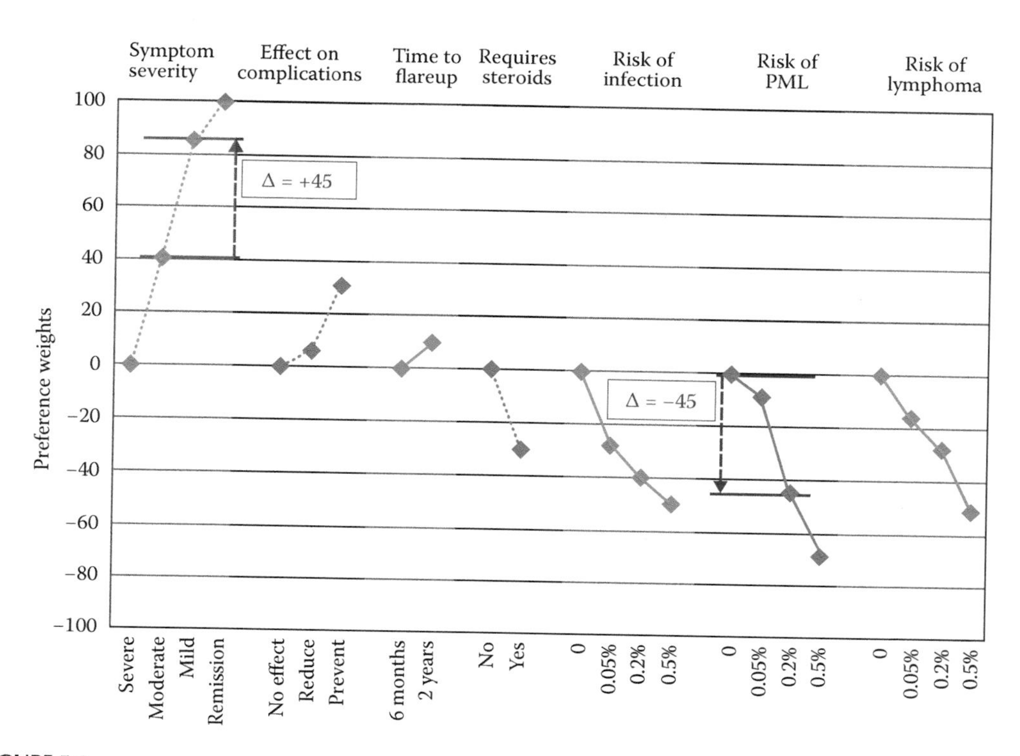

FIGURE 5.6
Estimated B–R preference weights, Crohn's disease. (Adapted from Johnson, F.R. et al. 2007. Crohn's disease patients' risk–benefit preferences: Serious adverse event risks versus treatment efficacy. *Gastroenterology* 133 (3):769–779.)

outcomes not included in the stated choice survey are not relevant to the decision that the B–R assessment is designed to inform.

Preference weights are measured on an ordinal scale; hence, individual weights cannot be compared directly; an outcome with a preference weight of 80 is not twice as important as an outcome with a preference weight of 40. However, we can compare relative differences in weights. Thus, we can say a *difference* in preference weights of 0.8 is twice as important as a *difference* in preference weights of 0.4. In Figure 5.6, on average, an improvement in symptoms had a difference in weights of 45 (85–40). In return for that benefit, patients would tolerate a weighted equivalent increase in PML risks of 0.2%.

5.4 Potential Bias and Measurement Error

While the choice-experiment approach described here is a promising method for quantifying patient preferences for beneficial and harmful outcomes, developing valid and reliable evidence using this approach can be challenging. The most serious threat to validity is that the data consist of choices among hypothetical alternatives. Hypothetical choices do not involve the same clinical, emotional, and financial consequences as actual choices. Potential hypothetical bias can be limited by constructing choice questions that mimic realistic clinical choices as closely as possible, subjecting the data to tests of logic and consistency, and mapping attribute levels clearly to clinical evidence.

Successful elicitation of patient preference data requires that all members of the patient sample share a common, clear understanding of the treatment features they are evaluating. In the case of eliciting preferences, including probabilistic outcomes, researchers must cope with the generally low level of numeracy in the general population. Some well-established findings include the following (Slovic 1987):

- People have difficulty evaluating small probabilities (smaller than approximately 1 in 1000) accurately.
- People care as much about such risk characteristics as voluntariness, familiarity, catastrophe, dreadfulness, and timing as they do about probability.
- People evaluate risk information from different sources differently.
- People evaluate decisions framed as gains differently from decisions framed as losses.
- People translate population risks to personal risks using a variety of heuristics.

Attitudes toward bearing risk and related behavior depend strongly on the decision context, sources of risk, and content of available information, as well as specific characteristics of the risks in question. When choice experiments replicate the same context, information, and outcomes encountered in a treatment setting, they are a legitimate expression of preferences as defined in that setting.

While the literature of stated-choice applications in healthcare generally is significant, there are less than 100 published studies specifically related to B–R trade-off preferences. Many clinicians, regulators, and other potential users of B–R assessments therefore are unlikely to be familiar with these methods and may be skeptical of their validity and reliability. While obtaining valid and reliable measures of patient preferences is challenging, it is possible to quantify patient preferences and subject the results to the same rigorous standards as those applied to clinical, epidemiological, and patient-reported outcomes data.

5.5 Applications to Pharmaceuticals and Devices

5.5.1 Case Study: FDA Center for Drugs—Duchenne's Muscular Dystrophy

Duchenne muscular disorder (DMD) is a rare and inherited neuromuscular disorder caused by a defective gene for dystrophin. The main sign of the condition is progressive muscular weakness, which usually leads to loss of ambulation during the teenage years and premature death caused by respiratory failure or cardiac disease in the 20s. The condition is associated with significant care-related and financial burden to the families (Bushby et al. 2010).

Despite the severity of the disease, currently there are no FDA-approved therapies for DMD. Similar to other conditions, patients and caregivers managing DMD seek to accelerate approvals of new therapies to save lives. Because of the serious and progressive nature of the condition and limited treatment options, patients and caregivers have expressed the willingness to accept potential risks in the absence of conclusive efficacy and safety data.

Patients and patient advocates want regulators to consider the nature of the disease and be more flexible in applying approval criteria (Mullard 2013).

CDER's Patient-Focused Drug Development Initiative intends to engage patients to understand the impact of disease and integrate patient perspective in the drug review and approval process, but the initiative is limited to patient and caregiver engagement activities to 20 disease areas (Mullard 2013). Patients with other conditions, including DMD, have received little guidance on how to provide information that may be useful to the FDA's regulatory decision making. The only existing mechanism is providing testimony to FDA advisory committees. However, the small number of participants who provide such anecdotal testimony may not represent the views of the general DMD patient population and caregivers (Vogt et al. 2006).

To help inform regulatory review of the therapies under investigation, Parent Project Muscular Dystrophy (PPMD), an advocacy organization focusing on improving treatment for DMD, conducted a study to quantify caregiver preferences for benefits and risks using stated-preference methods (Hollin et al. 2015). Such quantitative methods can elicit perspectives from a large group of stakeholders and generate more formal evidence that may inform regulatory decision making. On the basis of a replicable and community-engaged approach, the study from PPMD demonstrated how an advocacy organization could develop scientific evidence on patient treatment preferences to inform regulatory decision making.

The study was conducted as a collaboration among PPMD staff, academic researchers, and an advocacy oversight team (a clinician, a scientist experienced in drug development, and two DMD caregivers). The study began by identifying the treatment-preference research question that met the expressed requirements of the DMD community, the caregiver study population, and respondent recruitment strategies.

This study employed a variant of stated-preference methods called BWS. Instead of eliciting preferences using treatment-profile pairs as is done in DCEs, BWS elicits preferences by asking respondents to identify the best and worst features of single profiles (Flynn et al. 2007; Gallego et al. 2012; Louviere and Flynn 2010). The authors combined each BWS question with a DCE question comparing the single profile with the respondent's status quo. Figure 5.7 is an example question from the PPMD survey.

Identifying relevant and comprehensible attributes and levels is an important step to generate meaningful study outcomes. As indicated above, when the study is intended to provide relative importance weights for clinical-trial endpoints, the attributes and levels must map into those outcomes. In this case, the study is intended to provide regulators with information about patients' concerns, which may not correspond to trial endpoints determined by clinicians and regulators without patient involvement. The study used a community-engaged approach to identify attributes and levels that were clinically relevant, meaningful, and understandable to caregivers. PPMD identified and invited stakeholder informants to participate through the advocacy-facilitated industry roundtable, PPMD's grassroots family networks, PPMD's clinician database, and self-nomination after the notification of program launch in the community.

The initial discussions yielded more than 20 potential benefit and risk attributes. The advocacy oversight team ultimately selected six treatment attributes with three levels each, including effect on muscle function, life span, available evidence on the drug, nausea, risk of bleeding, and risk of heart arrhythmia. The study used a 3^6 main-effects orthogonal design to accommodate the six attributes and three levels each. The design consisted of 18 profiles, the minimum number to ensure no structural correlation among the attributes (Johnson et al. 2013b). All profiles included the six attributes but had different combination

Choose the best thing by clicking the circle under "best" and choose the worst thing by clicking the circle under "worst." You have to choose a best thing and a worst thing to move on. Remember that a computer chose combinations to make the experiment work, and some of them seem bad. Even so, please pick the best and worst thing.

Best	Treatment	Worst
o	Slows the progression of weakness	o
o	2 year gain in expected lifespan	o
o	1 year of post-approval drug information available	o
o	Causes loss of appetite	o
o	Increased risk of bleeding gums and increased bruising	o
o	Increased risk of harmless heart arrhythmia	o

	If this treatment were real, would you use it for your child?
o	Yes
o	No
o	I don't know

FIGURE 5.7
Preference-elicitation question from the Duchenne Muscular Dystrophy Survey. (From Hollin, I.L. et al. 2015. Caregiver preferences for emerging Duchenne muscular dystrophy treatments: A comparison of best–worst scaling and conjoint analysis. *Patient* 8 (1):19–27.)

of levels. In each profile, caregivers were asked to choose the best and worst aspects of the profile. Before completing the tasks, caregivers were provided with detailed description of the attributes and levels, detailed instruction, and an example task. They were also told that the treatments did not currently exist, but to assume that the treatments were approved by the FDA, provided by their doctor, and the costs were covered by health insurance.

A convenience sample of 119 caregivers who self-identified as a parent or guardian of an individual with DMD completed the Web-enabled survey. The respondents were predominantly white, married, and biological mothers. Respondents' age ranged from 28 to 66 years old with an average of 44 years. The age of the affected patient ranged from 2 to 38 years old, with an average of 12 years.

A relative importance score was calculated for each level within each attribute by subtracting the number of times a level was chosen as worst from the number of times the level was chosen as best, dividing by the total number of time it was available, and rescaling the resulting weights between 0 and 100. "Stops progression of weakness" (0.877) and "slows progression of weakness" (0.800) had the highest relative importance scores among all attributes and levels. The importance of these outcomes was almost twice as large as the next-highest scores assigned to "5-year gain in expected life span" (0.464) and "2-year gain in expected life span" (0.408). "Increased risk of dangerous heart arrhythmia and sudden death" (−0.786) and "increased risk of hemorrhagic stroke and lifelong disability" (−0.720) had the largest negative importance scores, followed by "causes loss of appetite with occasional vomiting" (−0.280). Effects on muscle function were the most important overall attribute (28.7%), while evidence about the drug was the least important attribute (2.3%). In terms of B–R trade-offs, caregivers in this study were willing to accept an increased risk (magnitude not quantified) of disabling stroke or arrhythmia-induced cardiac arrest in return for stopping progression of muscle weakness. Conversely, they would require that a treatment stopped progression of muscle weakness if the treatment also had an increased risk of a severe side effect.

This study documented the value that caregivers place on even moderate function benefits and their considerable tolerance for side-effect risks as well as for evidence uncertainty. Following the completion of the study, PPMD reported the results to CDER and the DMD community. They also submitted a patient-initiated FDA draft guidance for DMD in June 2014 that included an engagement framework and guidance on the use of stated-preference methods to inform drug development and regulatory review (Parent Project Muscular Dystrophy 2014). On the basis of this document, the FDA issued a draft guidance in June 2015 (US FDA 2015a). In addition to informing FDA regulatory decision making about DMD therapies, this study described a successful community-engagement process to understand treatment preferences among a large group of stakeholders. It also demonstrated how a patient-advocacy group could use quantitative methods to systematically quantify caregiver experience and concerns.

5.5.2 Case Study: FDA's Center for Devices—Weight-Loss Devices

Since the release of its guidance on B–R assessment in 2012, the CDRH has emphasized the importance of incorporating patient preference in the evaluation and approval of medical devices. The regulatory agencies had made numerous efforts to reach out to patients with different conditions and listen to their opinions before 2012 to obtain patient perspectives on benefits and risks, but similar to the process with drug development and review, the approaches used in patient engagement had been qualitative.

To enhance the strength of evidence on patient preferences and improve patient engagement, CDRH, in collaboration with researchers from RTI Health Solutions, conducted a study to quantify the relative importance of safety and effectiveness of weight-loss devices to patients (Ho et al. 2015). It quantified the minimum benefit patients expected from a weight-loss device to tolerate a given level of risk and the maximum risk patients were willing to tolerate for a given level of expected weight loss. This study is the first patient preference study that was sponsored by a regulatory agency and used to inform regulatory decision making.

Using a DCE approach, researchers developed a survey instrument based on clinical research on obesity, regulatory knowledge about weight-loss devices, and interviews with obese individuals. Eight attributes were selected on the basis of the primary concerns expressed by physicians, regulators, and obese individuals during survey development and the knowledge of devices that were likely to be reviewed in the near future. They included the percentage of total body weight loss compared to current weight, duration of weight loss, duration of mild-to-moderate side effects, risk of mortality, chance of a side effect that requires hospitalization, recommended dietary restrictions, reduction in chance of comorbidity or in prescription dosage for current comorbidity, and type of surgery. Each attribute had three to five levels. The levels for clinical-outcome attributes were described as average effects or average risks to people who used the device.

Each choice question elicited a judgment about which of two hypothetical device profiles was better for individuals like them. In a separate follow-up question after each choice task, the respondents were also asked whether they would accept the better device if it was available in the market or whether they would prefer no device. Respondents were told to answer the questions assuming that all costs were covered by insurance. Figure 5.8 is an example DCE question.

An experimental-design algorithm yielded 120 choice questions on the basis of the eight attributes (Kuhfeld et al., 1994; Kuhfeld 2010). The design was used to construct 15 survey versions with 8 questions each. Respondents were randomly assigned to one of the survey versions. The study design included several internal validity tests to verify that respondents understood the basic risk concepts. Additionally, each respondent was given a risk tutorial and asked to answer a question to verify their understanding of risks before starting to answer the choice questions.

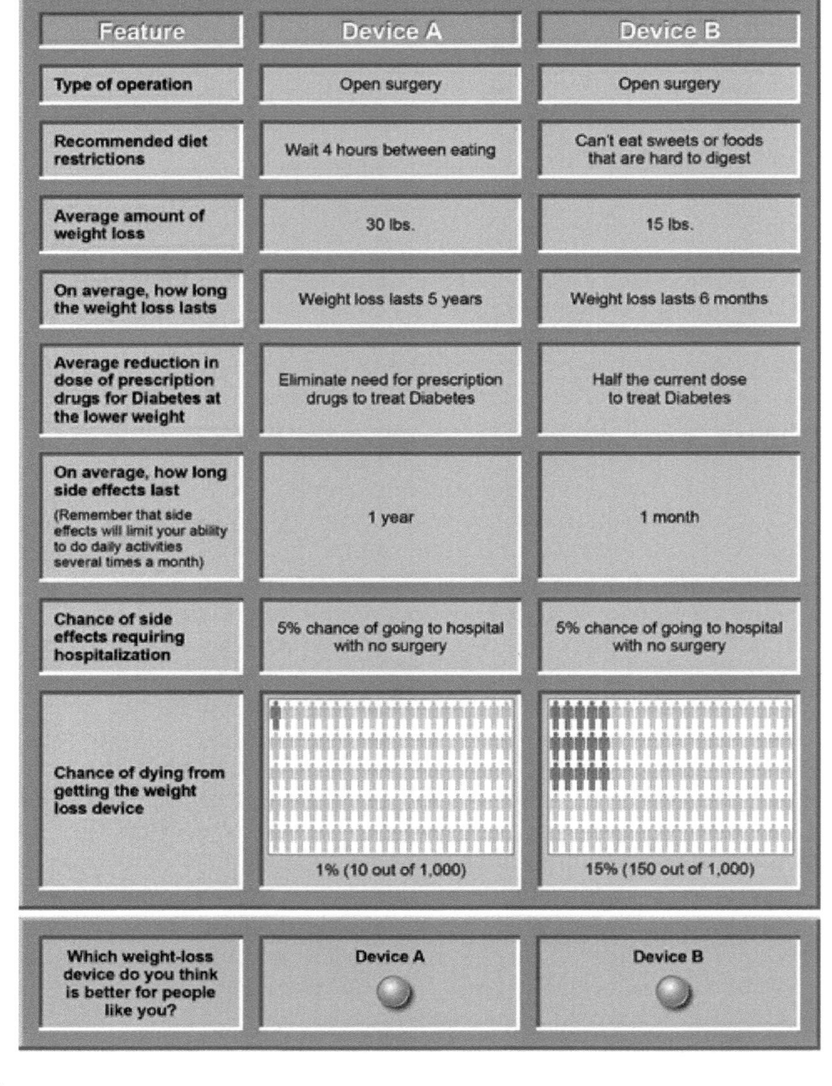

Feature	Device A	Device B
Type of operation	Open surgery	Open surgery
Recommended diet restrictions	Wait 4 hours between eating	Can't eat sweets or foods that are hard to digest
Average amount of weight loss	30 lbs.	15 lbs.
On average, how long the weight loss lasts	Weight loss lasts 5 years	Weight loss lasts 6 months
Average reduction in dose of prescription drugs for Diabetes at the lower weight	Eliminate need for prescription drugs to treat Diabetes	Half the current dose to treat Diabetes
On average, how long side effects last (Remember that side effects will limit your ability to do daily activities several times a month)	1 year	1 month
Chance of side effects requiring hospitalization	5% chance of going to hospital with no surgery	5% chance of going to hospital with no surgery
Chance of dying from getting the weight loss device	1% (10 out of 1,000)	15% (150 out of 1,000)
Which weight-loss device do you think is better for people like you?	Device A	Device B

FIGURE 5.8
Preference-elicitation question from the Weight-Loss Device Survey. (From Ho, M.P. et al. 2015. Incorporating patient-preference evidence into regulatory decision making. *Surg Endosc.* doi: 10.1007/s00464-014-4044-2.)

After pretesting in face-to-face interviews, the Web-enabled survey was administered between September and November 2012 to the GfK KnowledgePanel, a large Web panel that matches the demographics of the general US population. A total of 1057 English-speaking respondents with a previous or current body mass index (BMI) of at least 30 kg/m^2 and an intention to lose weight were randomly drawn from the panel. The sample was stratified by BMI and was equally divided among the 30–35, 35–40, and ≥40 BMI groups. After deleting respondents who failed data-quality checks, 540 of 710 responses were included in the final analysis. Overall, the analysis sample was approximately 2 years older and 8.5% heavier than the general obese population in the United States. Internal validity tests indicated that the data met high quality standards.

Figure 5.9 shows the estimated preference weights from the study. The overall importance of each attribute in explaining device choices is indicated by the difference between the best and worst preference weights for each attribute. Mortality risk was the most important attribute, followed by percentage of total body weight loss, duration of weight loss, and duration of mild-to-moderate side effects.

In addition to relative importance, the study used the estimated preference scores to calculate the minimum acceptable benefits for specific levels of risk and the maximum acceptable risks for given levels of weight loss. Obese respondents were segmented on the basis of their risk tolerance. For example, the gastric band, which is implanted by laparoscopic surgery, offers 13% total body weight loss that lasts for an average of 5 years. It is

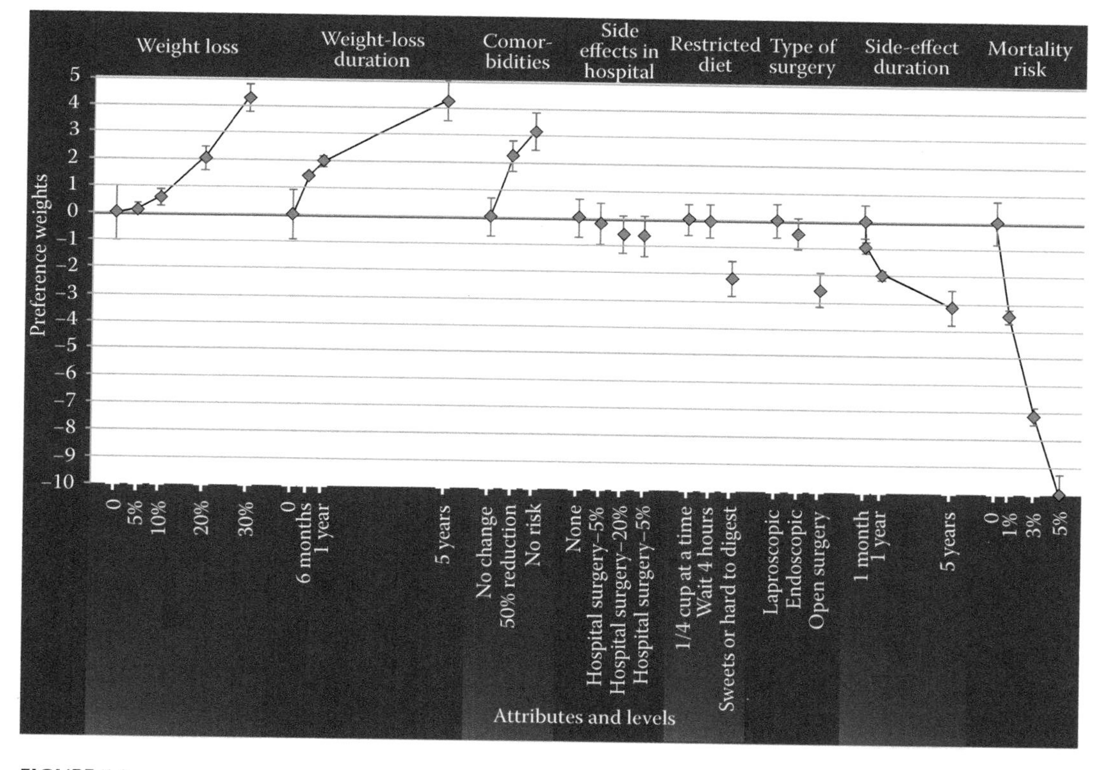

FIGURE 5.9
Weight-loss device preference—weight estimates. (From Ho, M.P. et al. 2015. Incorporating patient-preference evidence into regulatory decision making. *Surg Endosc*. doi: 10.1007/s00464-014-4044-2.)

associated with 1% mortality rate, 5% chance of hospitalization for side effects requiring surgery, and some minor side effects that can last for 5 years. It requires patients to limit their diet to 1/4 cup of food at a time after surgery and does not improve comorbidities. On the basis of the study estimates, respondents in the middle 50% of the distribution had a minimum acceptable weight-loss benefit of more than 30% given other attributes of the gastric band or a maximum acceptable mortality risk of 0.16% and therefore would prefer no device. However, risk-tolerant individuals in the upper 25% of the distribution had a minimum acceptable weight-loss benefit of only 13.0% and a maximum acceptable risk of 7.1%. Since the benefits and risks associated with gastric band met their threshold, they would prefer gastric band to no device. Overall, the study predicted that only 11.6% of respondents would choose gastric band over no device on the basis of the estimates, which is consistent with market data (Nguyen et al. 2011).

One of the main issues that regulatory reviewers consider in the B–R assessments is what level of "minimum clinical effectiveness" is sufficient to offset the risks and inconveniences associated with the treatment under review. This study built a calculator using the preference-score estimates to quantitatively assist CDRH reviewers in identifying the minimum effectiveness threshold. The tool can estimate the maximum acceptable risk for average or risk-tolerant patients for a given effectiveness benefit, the minimum acceptable benefit for a given risk for the same patients, and the predicted percentage of patients who would choose the treatment if available. Regulatory reviewers can use the minimum effectiveness threshold set by the tool to determine the size of clinical studies or use it as a reference to evaluate the treatment for premarket approval.

Using results from the weight-loss study, CDRH approved EnteroMedics's Maestro Rechargeable System in January 2015 (US FDA 2015b). Although the device failed to meet its co-primary clinical-trial endpoints, the agency took into consideration patients' B–R trade-off preferences. It is the first approval to result from CDRH's pilot program to formally incorporate patient preference into risk–benefit determinations for obesity devices, and it is the first new obesity device approved by the FDA since 2007. The study informed the draft guidance issued in May 2015 (US FDA CDRH and Center for Biologics Evaluation and Research 2015a).

5.6 Conclusions

B–R evaluations inevitably require assessments of both data quality and the relative importance of endpoints measured in clinical data. Relative importance requires value judgments about which both experts and nonexperts could reasonably disagree. Incorporating quantitative patient perspectives on these value judgments is consistent with the growing interest in greater patient involvement in healthcare decision making. While public outreach efforts may give voice to patient concerns about regulatory decisions, it is not obvious how such outreach efforts could influence regulatory policy and decision making. This chapter suggests that, to be relevant and useful in an evidence-based regulatory process, preferences should be quantified and evaluated in the same way as other forms of evidence in evaluating the benefits and risks of new and existing therapies. Eliciting and quantifying the preferences of patients will allow for more formal, evidence-based consideration of patient perspectives that is currently lacking in regulatory decision making.

References

Bala, M. V., L. L. Wood, G. A. Zarkin, E. C. Norton, A. Gafni, and B. O'Brien. 1998. "Valuing outcomes in health care: A comparison of willingness to pay and quality-adjusted life-years." *J Clin Epidemiol* 51 (8):667–676. doi: S0895-4356(98)00036-5 [pii].

Brundage, M. D., J. R. Davidson, W. J. Mackillop, D. Feldman-Stewart, and P. Groome. 1998. "Using a treatment-tradeoff method to elicit preferences for the treatment of locally advanced non-small-cell lung cancer." *Med Decis Making* 18 (3):256–267.

Bushby, K., R. Finkel, D. J. Birnkrant, L. E. Case, P. R. Clemens, L. Cripe, A. Kaul, K. Kinnett, C. McDonald, S. Pandya, J. Poysky, F. Shapiro, J. Tomezsko, C. Constantin, and D. M. D. Care Considerations Working Group. 2010. "Diagnosis and management of Duchenne muscular dystrophy, part 1: Diagnosis, and pharmacological and psychosocial management." *Lancet Neurol* 9 (1):77–93. doi: 10.1016/S1474-4422(09)70271-6.

Chilton, F., and R. A. Collett. 2008. "Treatment choices, preferences and decision-making by patients with rheumatoid arthritis." *Musculoskeletal Care* 6 (1):1–14. doi: 10.1002/msc.110.

European Medicines Agency (EMA). 2013. Guidance document on the content of the Rapporteur day 80 critical assessment report.

Flynn, T. N., J. J. Louviere, T. J. Peters, and J. Coast. 2007. "Best–worst scaling: What it can do for health care research and how to do it." *J Health Econ* 26 (1):171–189. doi: 10.1016/j.jhealeco.2006.04.002.

Gafni, A., and G. W. Torrance. 1984. "Risk Attitude and Time Preference in Health." *Management Science* 30 (4):440–451. doi:10.1287/mnsc.30.4.440.

Gallego, G., J. F. Bridges, T. Flynn, B. M. Blauvelt, and L. W. Niessen. 2012. "Using best–worst scaling in horizon scanning for hepatocellular carcinoma technologies." *Int J Technol Assess Health Care* 28 (3):339–346. doi: 10.1017/S026646231200027X.

Ho, M. P., J. M. Gonzalez, H. P. Lerner, C. Y. Neuland, J. M. Whang, M. McMurry-Heath, A. B. Hauber, and T. Irony. 2015. "Incorporating patient-preference evidence into regulatory decision making." *Surg Endosc*. doi: 10.1007/s00464-014-4044-2.

Hollin, I. L., H. L. Peay, and J. F. Bridges. 2015. "Caregiver preferences for emerging duchenne muscular dystrophy treatments: A comparison of best–worst scaling and conjoint analysis." *Patient* 8 (1):19–27. doi: 10.1007/s40271-014-0104-x.

Johnson, F. R., A. B. Hauber, and J. Zhang. 2013a. "Quantifying Patient Preferences to Inform Benefit–Risk Evaluations. " In *Benefit–Risk Analysis in Pharmaceutical Research and Development*, edited by A. Sashegyi, J. Felli and B. Noel. New York: Chapman & Hall.

Johnson, F. R., E. Lancsar, D. Marshall, V. Kilambi, A. Muhlbacher, D. A. Regier, B. W. Bresnahan, B. Kanninen, and J. F. Bridges. 2013b. "Constructing experimental designs for discrete-choice experiments: Report of the ISPOR Conjoint Analysis Experimental Design Good Research Practices Task Force." *Value Health* 16 (1):3–13. doi: 10.1016/j.jval.2012.08.2223.

Johnson, F. R., S. Ozdemir, C. Mansfield, S. Hass, D. W. Miller, C. A. Siegel, and B. E. Sands. 2007. "Crohn's disease patients' risk–benefit preferences: Serious adverse event risks versus treatment efficacy." *Gastroenterology* 133 (3):769–779. doi: 10.1053/j.gastro.2007.04.075.

Johnson, F. R., G. Van Houtven, S. Ozdemir, S. Hass, J. White, G. Francis, D. W. Miller, and J. T. Phillips. 2009. "Multiple sclerosis patients' benefit–risk preferences: Serious adverse event risks versus treatment efficacy." *J Neurol* 256 (4):554–562. doi: 10.1007/s00415-009-0084-2.

Kuhfeld, W. F. 2010. *Marketing Research Methods in SAS: Experimental Design, Choice, Conjoint, and Graphical Techniques*. Cary, NC: SAS Institute Inc.

Kuhfeld, W. F., R. D. Tobias, and M. Garratt. 1994. "Efficient experimental design with marketing research applications." *Journal of Marketing Research (JMR)* 31 (4):545–557.

Louviere, J. J., and T. N. Flynn. 2010. "Using best–worst scaling choice experiments to measure public perceptions and preferences for healthcare reform in australia." *Patient* 3 (4):275–283. doi: 10.2165/11539660-000000000-00000.

Lynd, L. D., and J. B. O'Brien. 2004. "Advances in risk–benefit evaluation using probabilistic simulation methods: An application to the prophylaxis of deep vein thrombosis." *J Clin Epidemiol* 57 (8):795–803. doi: 10.1016/j.jclinepi.2003.12.012.

Manjunath, R., J. C. Yang, and A. B. Ettinger. 2012. "Patients' preferences for treatment outcomes of add-on antiepileptic drugs: A conjoint analysis." *Epilepsy Behav* 24 (4):474–479. doi: 10.1016/j.yebeh.2012.05.020.

Marshall, D., J. F. Bridges, B. Hauber, R. Cameron, L. Donnalley, K. Fyie, and F. R. Johnson. 2010. "Conjoint Analysis Applications in Health—How are Studies being Designed and Reported?: An Update on Current Practice in the Published Literature between 2005 and 2008." *Patient* 3 (4):249–256. doi: 10.2165/11539650-000000000-00000.

McFadden, D. 1974. "Conditional logit analysis of qualitative choice behavior." In *Frontiers in Econometrics*. New York: Academic Press.

Mohamed, A. F., A. B. Hauber, and M. P. Neary. 2011. "Patient Benefit–Risk Preferences for Targeted Agents in the Treatment of Renal Cell Carcinoma." *Pharmacoeconomics* 29 (11):977–988. doi: 10.2165/11593370-000000000-00000.

Mullard, A. 2013. "Patient-focused drug development programme takes first steps." *Nat Rev Drug Discov* 12 (9):651–652. doi: 10.1038/nrd4104.

Nguyen, N. T., H. Masoomi, C. P. Magno, X. M. Nguyen, K. Laugenour, and J. Lane. 2011. "Trends in use of bariatric surgery, 2003–2008." *J Am Coll Surg* 213 (2):261–266. doi: 10.1016/j.jamcollsurg.2011.04.030.

Parent Project Muscular Dystrophy. 2014. Guidance for Industry: Duchenne Muscular Dystrophy Developing Drugs for Treatment over the Spectrum of Disease. Hackensack, NJ. http://www.parentprojectmd.org/site/DocServer/Guidance_Document_Submission_-_Duchenne_Muscular_Dystrop.pdf?docID=15283.

Slovic, P. 1987. "Perception of risk." *Science* 236 (4799):280–285.

Train, K. E. 2002. *Discrete Choice Methods with Simulation*. Cambridge: Cambridge University Press.

Train, K., and G. Sonnier. 2005. "Mixed Logit with Bounded Distributions of Correlated Partworths." In *Applications of Simulation Methods in Environmental and Resource Economics*, edited by Riccardo Scarpa and Anna Alberini, 117–134. Springer-Verlag.

U.S. Food and Drug Administration (FDA). 2012. Factors to Consider When Making Benefit–Risk Determinations in Medical Device Premarket Approval and De Novo Classifications: Guidance for Industry and Food and Drug Administration Staff. Center for Devices & Radiological Health and Center for Biologics Evaluation & Research.

U.S. Food and Drug Administration (FDA). 2015. Patient Preference Information–Submission, Review in PMAs, HDE Applications, and De Novo Requests, and Inclusion in Device Labeling: Draft Guidance for Industry, Food and Drug Administration Staff, and Other Stakeholders. Center for Devices and Radiological Health and Center for Biologics Evaluation and Research.

U.S. Food and Drug Administration (FDA). 2015a. Duchenne Muscular Dystrophy and Related Dystrophinopathies—Developing Drugs for Treatment Guidance for Industry: Draft Guidance. edited by Center for Drug Evaluation and Research (CDER).

U.S. Food and Drug Administration (FDA). 2015b. "FDA approves first-of-kind device to treat obesity." Last Modified 02/04/2015. http://www.fda.gov/NewsEvents/Newsroom/PressAnnouncements/ucm430223.htm.

Vogt, F., D. L. Schwappach, and J. F. Bridges. 2006. "Accounting for tastes: A German perspective on the inclusion of patient preferences in healthcare." *Pharmacoeconomics* 24 (5):419–423.

6

Choice of Metrics and Other Considerations for Benefit–Risk Analysis in Subgroups

Steven Snapinn and Qi Jiang

CONTENTS

ABSTRACT Evaluation of subgroups is a routine part of the analysis of nearly every large clinical trial. The purpose is to determine whether the effects of the treatment are consistent across the study population or whether there are patient characteristics that can be used to predict which patients will experience a particularly large benefit or a particularly large harm (i.e., treatment-by-factor interactions). Unfortunately, the power to detect interactions is typically low, and there is a belief that subgroup analyses are far more likely to lead to false-positive findings than to identify true interactions. However, it is important to note that the presence of an interaction depends on the scale on which the treatment effect is measured, and this has important implications for the assessment of benefit–risk in subgroups. Notably, when there is reason to believe that the relative effects of a treatment (e.g., the hazard ratio for a time-to-event endpoint) are consistent across subgroups, the absolute effects (e.g., the absolute risk reductions) are often highly variable. This is because there are often subgroups with greater and lesser disease severity, where event rates vary considerably; in this case, a constant hazard ratio across subgroups will lead to highly variable absolute risk reductions. In this chapter, we argue that benefit–risk conclusions should be based on the absolute effects for benefits and harms and, therefore, that subgroup analyses play a particularly important role.

6.1 Introduction to Subgroup Analyses

Clinical trials are conducted in a population of subjects defined by a set of inclusion and exclusion criteria. Regardless of the restrictions imposed by these criteria, the population is always somewhat heterogeneous, including subjects with different demographics, different disease severity and treatment history, different genetic profiles, and so on. While the primary analysis will typically involve all enrolled subjects, there is often interest in how the effects of the treatment under study vary across the various subject characteristics. For this reason, a set of subgroup analyses is often performed.

A subgroup analysis is one conducted on a subset of the enrolled subjects; for example, an analysis including just the men or just the women, or an analysis including just the patients whose ages fall in a defined range. Randomized clinical trials often employ a technique called stratification, which ensures that the treatment groups have roughly similar numbers of subjects in the subgroups that are levels of the stratification factors. For example, if sex is a stratification factor, the treatment groups will contain similar proportions of men and similar proportions of women. For all other subgroups, the proportions in the treatment groups may be similar or not, depending on the play of chance. However, all subgroup analyses, whether the subgroup is part of a stratification factor or not, are valid in the sense that they are protected by randomization. For example, if sex were not a stratification factor, the proportions of men could differ in the various treatment arms, but randomization would ensure that the men in all treatment arms were similar with respect to all measured and unmeasured confounding factors.

Note that, throughout this chapter, we assume that all subgroups can be defined by information available at the time of randomization. Analyses based on subgroups that involve postrandomization information, such as change in a laboratory parameter during follow-up, or the initial response to treatment, may provide misleading results.

While there is often considerable interest in how the effects of the treatment vary across subgroups, subgroup analyses have serious limitations. The main limitation has to do with sample size: The study's sample size is generally chosen to ensure adequate power to detect a reasonable effect size in the overall population, leaving inadequate power in subgroups that necessarily have smaller sample size. In addition, there are often many subgroup analyses performed, with many opportunities for false-positive findings. Therefore, subgroup analyses suffer from increased rates of both type I and type II errors. This issue has been discussed frequently in the literature (Alosh et al. 2015; Cui et al. 2002; Julian 2000; Pocock et al. 2002; Sleight 2000; Wang et al. 2007).

One common approach for interpretation of subgroup analyses is to assume a priori that the treatment's effects are consistent across subgroups unless there is strong evidence to the contrary. This leads to testing for treatment-by-factor interaction (Lagakos 2006), or evidence that the apparent heterogeneity in the treatment effect across the subgroups within a factor (e.g., for men and women) differs more than would be expected by chance alone. The results of this test, perhaps along with an understanding of the biological mechanisms of the treatment (Yusuf et al. 1991), are then used to draw conclusions.

Regulatory agencies around the world have an important stake in the correct interpretation of subgroup analyses and have written relevant guidance documents, most recently "Guideline on the Investigation of Subgroups in Confirmatory Clinical Trials" by the European Medicines Agency (EMA) (2014). Clearly, one of the greatest concerns of regulatory agencies is approval of a drug for a subpopulation on the basis of a false-positive subgroup analysis; as discussed above, because of the large number of subgroup analyses typically conducted, the probability of such a false-positive finding can be extremely high. The EMA document attempts to find the right balance between dismissing subgroup analysis in order to avoid such inappropriate drug approvals and appropriately identifying subpopulations with enhanced benefits. Discussing various regulatory guidance documents, Grouin et al. (2005) provided guidance on when subgroup analyses can and should be done, and on their interpretation.

Various authors have attempted to improve the statistical analysis of subgroups. Alosh and Huque (2009) describe a flexible strategy for testing a prespecified sequence of hypotheses for both the overall population and a subgroup. Foster et al. (2011) present a method to find subgroups with an enhanced treatment effect that involves predicting response probabilities for treatment and control "twins" for each subject. Moyé and Deswal (2001) discuss a new approach, distinct from the use of a treatment-by-subgroup interaction term, which provides an evaluation of the effect of an intervention within a particular subgroup stratum prospectively declared to be of interest to the investigators. Song and Chi (2007) propose a general statistical methodology for testing both the overall and subgroup hypotheses, which has optimal power and strongly controls the familywise type I error rate. White et al. (2005) describe a Bayesian approach with informative priors to interpret subgroup results in a specific clinical setting.

One notable example of the debate regarding subgroup analysis (DeMets 2004) involves a clinical trial known as MERIT-HF, which evaluated the effects of metoprolol relative to placebo in the treatment of congestive heart failure (MERIT-HF Study Group 1999). Overall, the results were quite favorable for metoprolol, with highly significant risk reductions of 34% for mortality and 19% for a composite endpoint of mortality and all-cause hospitalization. The results were relatively consistent across nearly all prespecified and post hoc subgroups evaluated; however, one notable exception was that there was a nonsignificant 5% increase in risk of mortality in the subgroup enrolled in the United States. Note that 14 countries participated in this trial, and 1071 of the total of 3991 randomized subjects were from the United States. In a paper discussing the challenges of subgroup analyses, Wedel et al. (2001) concluded that the inconsistent finding was likely attributed to the play of chance. They went further to state that "Thus the best estimate of the treatment effect on total mortality for any subgroup is the estimate of the hazard ratio for the overall trial."

The general advice to dismiss heterogeneity of effect across subgroups as likely due to the play of chance is widespread in the clinical trial community, and, because of the high likelihood of false-positive findings, seems sensible. However, it is important to note that the presence or absence of heterogeneity often depends strongly on the scale on which the treatment effect is measured. Let X represent the summary measure of a clinical variable, such as the mean posttreatment blood pressure across subjects in a treatment arm, or the percentage of subjects in that arm who experience a clinical event. Now, let the subscripts 0 and 1 represent the control and treatment groups, and the subscripts A and B represent two subgroups. On a difference scale, the treatment effects in the two subgroups are $D_A = X_{A1} - X_{A0}$ and $D_B = X_{B1} - X_{B0}$, while on a ratio scale, the treatment effects are $R_A = X_{A1}/X_{A0}$ and $R_B = X_{B1}/X_{B0}$. In this case, $D_A = D_B$ only implies $R_A = R_B$ when $X_{A0} = X_{B0}$.

Subgroup analyses can be conducted for efficacy variables and for safety variables, and this issue of scales is important in both cases. However, the issue of scales is of particular importance for subgroup analyses evaluating the benefit–risk ratio, as will be discussed in the subsequent sections of this chapter.

6.2 Metrics for Assessing Benefits and Harms

Various metrics for assessing a treatment effect are in common use, depending on the type of measurement. The treatment effect for continuous variables is typically measured by the difference in mean values between groups, or the difference in mean within-group changes from baseline. Continuous variables are also sometimes converted into binary or ordinal data using a set of prespecified cut-points in the continuous scale, although this practice is somewhat controversial (Snapinn and Jiang 2007). The treatment effect for binary data can be assessed on an absolute scale, such as the risk difference, or a relative scale, such as the risk ratio or odds ratio. Let p_0 and p_1 represent the proportions of patients who experience the event in the control and treatment groups, respectively; in this case, the risk difference is $p_1 - p_0$, the risk ratio is p_1/p_0, and the odds ratio is $\{p_1/(1 - p_1)\}/\{p_0/(1 - p_0)\}$. As with binary data, the treatment effect for time-to-event variables can be assessed by absolute measures such as the risk difference or by relative measures such as the hazard ratio. The simplest model for analyzing a time-to-event variable is the exponential model, in which the risk or hazard of the event is constant over time. Let r_0 and r_1 represent the constant hazard rates in the control and treatment groups, respectively; in this case, the risk difference is $r_1 - r_0$, and the hazard ratio is r_1/r_0.

It is probably fair to say that there is more consistency in the metrics chosen for benefits than for harms, although the analysis of safety data has received increased attention recently (Snapinn and Jiang 2015; Zhou et al. 2015). Focusing specifically on a time-to-event endpoint, benefits are typically measured by the hazard ratio, often calculated using the Cox proportional hazards model, although such relative measures have been criticized as overstating the magnitude of the benefit (Kraemer et al. 2003; Replogle and Johnson 2007). With respect to harms, there is much more of a mixture of absolute and relative measures presented.

To illustrate the lack of consistency in measuring harms, consider the following four examples, all of which correspond to high-profile safety issues with marketed drugs:

- Natalizumab, marketed as Tysabri, is a treatment for multiple sclerosis. It was approved in the United States in 2004; it was withdrawn from the market because of a rare but extremely serious side effect, progressive multifocal leukoencephalopathy, or PML, but returned to the market in 2006 because the drug's benefit was felt to exceed this important risk. According to a newspaper report (Reuters 2011), the rate of PML with natalizumab was 1.16 cases per 1000 patients. If we assume that the rate of PML in untreated patients would essentially be zero, then this value can be interpreted as a risk difference; however, since it is based on the number of patients rather than patient-years, it appears to treat the occurrence of PML as a binary variable rather than as a time-to-event variable.
- Rofecoxib, which was marketed as Vioxx, was a treatment for pain due to osteoarthritis. It was approved in the United States in 1999 and withdrawn from the market in 2004 because of an unexpected increase in the risk of thrombotic events. As reported by the authors of the APPROVe study (Bresalier et al. 2005), there were 1.50 cases of thrombotic events per 100 patient-years with rofecoxib and 0.78 per 100 patient-years with placebo, for a relative risk of 1.92. The treatment effect metric used by the authors, the relative risk, is essentially equivalent to the hazard ratio; however, they also provide the risk estimates within each treatment group, which would allow the reader to calculate a risk difference.
- Cerivastatin, which was marketed as Baycol, was a statin used to treat hyperlipidemia. Although all statins, which are among the most commonly used prescription drugs in the world, are believed to have the potential to cause a condition known as rhabdomyolysis, the frequency of this adverse event appeared to be much greater with cerivastatin than with other statins. As reported by Furberg and Pitt (2001), there were 31 fatalities attributed to rhabdomyolysis among 700,000 users of cerivastatin in the United States, a figure 10 times higher with cerivastatin

than with other approved statins. The authors focused on the risk relative to that of other drugs in the class, but the figures they presented allow the calculation of an absolute risk difference with respect to other statins as well as to no treatment (assuming rhabdomyolysis occurs at a rate of zero in untreated patients).

- Rosiglitazone, which is marketed as Avandia, is a treatment for diabetes. While rosiglitazone remains on the market, concerns have been raised with respect to a potential increase in risk of cardiovascular events. As reported by Graham et al. (2010), the hazard ratio for a composite endpoint including acute myocardial infarction (MI), stroke, heart failure, and death relative to another drug (pioglitazone) in the same class was 1.18, and the risk difference was 1.68 excess events per 100 patient-years.

A quantitative assessment of benefits and harms requires some means of combining information on both endpoints. Again focusing on time-to-event endpoints, we argue here that both the benefits and harms should be measured as absolute risk differences.

First, consider the simplest case in which the benefit of the treatment is assessed by a single time-to-event efficacy variable, and similarly the harm is assessed by a single time-to-event safety variable. Further assume that the efficacy and safety variables are statistically independent and that the benefit and the harm are of equal importance. For example, suppose that the benefit of the treatment is a reduction in risk of cardiovascular death, and the harm is an increase in the risk of noncardiovascular death. Let the baseline hazard rates (i.e., the rates in the control group) of the efficacy and safety variables, respectively, be γ_e and γ_s, and let the treatment effects for these two variables, as measured by the hazard ratios, be λ_e and λ_s. Both the efficacy and safety variables are adverse, and the expectation is that the treatment will reduce the risk of the efficacy variable but increase the risk of the safety variable: that is, $\lambda_e < 1$ and $\lambda_s > 1$. Therefore, the overall rate of any adverse event (i.e., either the safety or the efficacy event) is $(\gamma_e + \gamma_s)$ in the control group and $(\lambda_e\gamma_e + \lambda_s\gamma_s)$ in the treatment group. The overall treatment effect is $(\lambda_e\gamma_e + \lambda_s\gamma_s) - (\gamma_e + \gamma_s)$ when measured as a risk difference, where values less than zero represent net benefit, and $(\lambda_e\gamma_e + \lambda_s\gamma_s)/(\gamma_e + \gamma_s)$ when measured as a hazard ratio, where values less than one represent net benefit. A key question, then, is which separate measures of effect for benefit and harm, when combined, will yield the appropriate conclusion about net benefit.

The absolute risk differences for efficacy and safety, respectively, are $(\lambda_e\gamma_e - \gamma_e)$ and $(\lambda_s\gamma_s - \gamma_s)$, and the hazard ratios are λ_e and λ_s. It is clear that the sum of the two risk differences equals the overall risk difference. While neither individual metrics can reproduce the overall hazard ratio, the individual risk differences determine whether there is net benefit as measured by the overall hazard ratio: the overall hazard ratio, $(\lambda_e\gamma_e + \lambda_s\gamma_s)/(\gamma_e + \gamma_s)$, is less than one if an only if $(\lambda_e\gamma_e - \gamma_e) + (\lambda_s\gamma_s - \gamma_s)$ is less than zero. The same is not true of the individual hazard ratios, since there can always be examples of net benefit and net harm regardless of the values of λ_e and λ_s. In other words, when assessing net benefit–risk, the individual risk differences for benefit and harm are far more meaningful than the individual hazard ratios.

Consider now a second case where the efficacy and safety variables are not of equal clinical importance: suppose that the consensus in the clinical community is that an efficacy event has clinical importance c times that of a safety event. Therefore, there is net benefit if $c * (\lambda_e\gamma_e - \gamma_e) + (\lambda_s\gamma_s - \gamma_s)$ is less than zero. Again, this is a combination of the individual risk differences for the efficacy and safety variables, and the individual hazard ratios are insufficient to determine whether or not there is net benefit.

6.3 Assessment of Benefit–Risk in Subgroups

Published results of clinical trials often present results of analyses evaluating the primary endpoint within subgroups, but it is less common to present safety analyses in subgroups, and less common still to present benefit–risk analyses in subgroups. This seems to reflect a belief that, while the benefits of a drug might be reasonably expected to vary among subgroups, there is less likelihood of variability in the safety profile of the treatment. In this case, if the benefits can be shown to be consistent across subgroups, then the benefit–risk profile is likely to be consistent as well.

We discuss the issue of the evaluation of benefit–risk in subgroups in the context of the Heart Outcomes Prevention Evaluation (HOPE) trial (Arnold et al. 2003), a study to determine whether the angiotensin-converting enzyme inhibitor, ramipril, could prevent the development of heart failure in high-risk patients without existing heart failure. The study randomized 9297 patients to ramipril or placebo, followed them for approximately 4.5 years, and found that ramipril significantly reduced the risk of the development of heart failure (relative risk, 0.77; 95% confidence interval, 0.68 to 0.87; $p < 0.0001$). (Note that the paper refers to relative risks, and we have followed that convention in this chapter; however, they are actually hazard ratios calculated using a Cox proportional hazards model.)

As is common in large outcomes trials, the HOPE publication included a forest plot of the primary endpoint results in selected subgroups. The key features of this forest plot have been recreated in Figure 6.1. In this figure, the relative risks are represented as dots and the confidence intervals are denoted by horizontal lines. The bold vertical line represents a relative risk of 1, or no difference between groups, and the thin vertical line represents a relative risk of 0.77, or the overall treatment effect. Note that the relative risks and confidence intervals were not tabulated in the publication, and interpolating them from the published figure would have been imprecise. Therefore, we have chosen to calculate them using the following approximations: the hazard ratio is approximately equal to $\ln(1 - p_R)/\ln(1 - p_P)$, where p_R and p_P are the event proportions in the ramipril and placebo groups, respectively, and the variance of the natural log of the hazard ratio is $4/(e_R + e_P)$, where e_R and e_P are the event counts in the two treatment groups.

The figure also contains relevant summary statistics for each subgroup (the number of subjects and percentage of subjects with an event for each treatment group) and a test for treatment-by-factor interaction. As shown, the estimates of the relative risk are less than one in all subgroups, and in only one case is the treatment-by-factor interaction nominally (i.e., without adjustment for multiplicity) statistically significant at the 5% level: the treatment effect in the subgroup with systolic blood pressure less than 139 mmHg was greater than that in the subgroup with systolic blood pressure of 139 mmHg or greater. The HOPE investigators considered the apparent interaction with respect to systolic blood pressure to be interesting enough to describe it in the abstract of their paper, but with respect to all other subgroups, they simply commented that "the benefits of ramipril in reducing all heart failure were consistent across major relevant subgroups."

The approach taken by the HOPE investigators is typical in our experience of trials with time-to-event endpoints: subgroup analyses for the primary efficacy endpoint are presented within subgroups, and conclusions regarding the consistency of the treatment effect are guided by an assessment of the relative treatment effect, typically as measured by the hazard ratio. However, as discussed above, it is the absolute risk differences that are of greater relevance to an assessment of benefit–risk, and there is often considerably greater evidence of differences across subgroups with respect to the absolute differences.

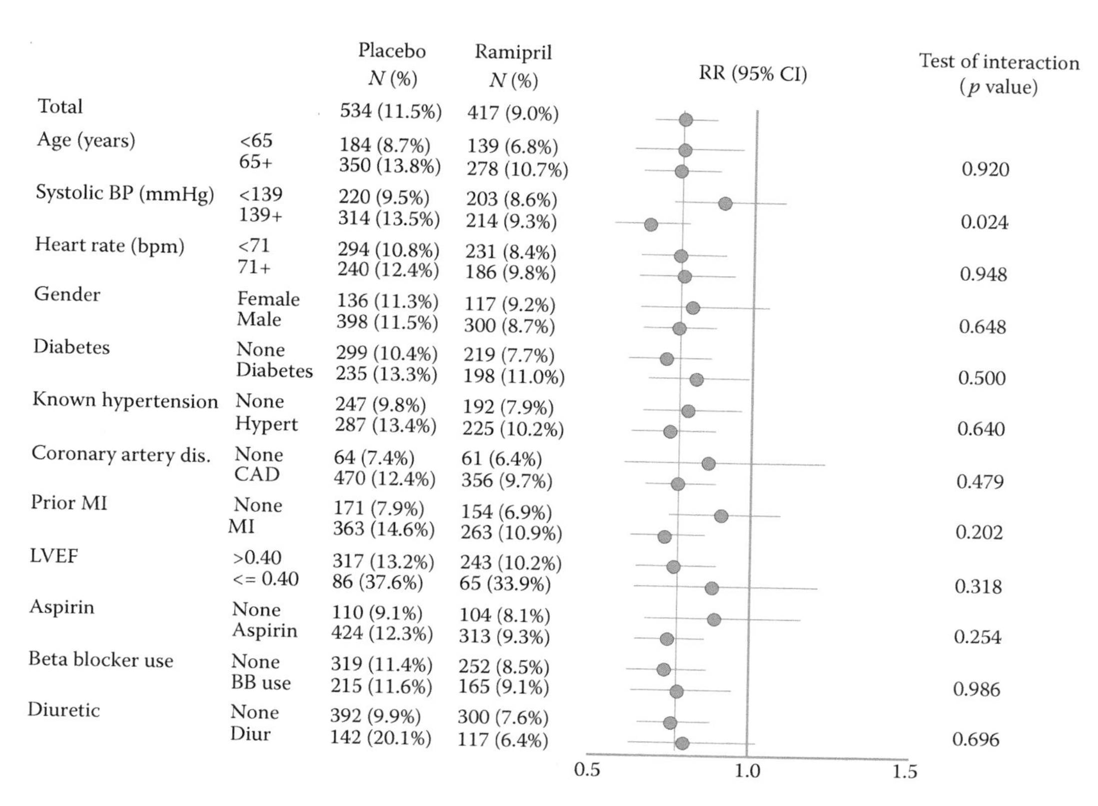

		Placebo N (%)	Ramipril N (%)	Test of interaction (p value)
Total		534 (11.5%)	417 (9.0%)	
Age (years)	<65	184 (8.7%)	139 (6.8%)	
	65+	350 (13.8%)	278 (10.7%)	0.920
Systolic BP (mmHg)	<139	220 (9.5%)	203 (8.6%)	
	139+	314 (13.5%)	214 (9.3%)	0.024
Heart rate (bpm)	<71	294 (10.8%)	231 (8.4%)	
	71+	240 (12.4%)	186 (9.8%)	0.948
Gender	Female	136 (11.3%)	117 (9.2%)	
	Male	398 (11.5%)	300 (8.7%)	0.648
Diabetes	None	299 (10.4%)	219 (7.7%)	
	Diabetes	235 (13.3%)	198 (11.0%)	0.500
Known hypertension	None	247 (9.8%)	192 (7.9%)	
	Hypert	287 (13.4%)	225 (10.2%)	0.640
Coronary artery dis.	None	64 (7.4%)	61 (6.4%)	
	CAD	470 (12.4%)	356 (9.7%)	0.479
Prior MI	None	171 (7.9%)	154 (6.9%)	
	MI	363 (14.6%)	263 (10.9%)	0.202
LVEF	>0.40	317 (13.2%)	243 (10.2%)	
	<= 0.40	86 (37.6%)	65 (33.9%)	0.318
Aspirin	None	110 (9.1%)	104 (8.1%)	
	Aspirin	424 (12.3%)	313 (9.3%)	0.254
Beta blocker use	None	319 (11.4%)	252 (8.5%)	
	BB use	215 (11.6%)	165 (9.1%)	0.986
Diuretic	None	392 (9.9%)	300 (7.6%)	
	Diur	142 (20.1%)	117 (6.4%)	0.696

FIGURE 6.1
Subgroup results for the HOPE Study.

Take, for example, the age subgroups in HOPE. The hazard ratios for subjects younger than 65 years (0.774) and for those 65 years or older (0.762) were virtually identical, and the interaction test ($p = 0.920$) provided little evidence of a true difference in relative risk by age. However, the percentage of placebo subjects with an event was considerably greater for older subjects (13.8%) than for younger subjects (8.7%). When measured as an absolute risk difference, the effect of ramipril was considerably greater among older subjects (3.1%) than among younger subjects (1.9%).

The HOPE investigators did not provide a test for interaction on the basis of absolute risk differences, and it is possible that the difference between 3.1% and 1.9% in the two age groups is within the bounds of chance. However, regardless of the results of the interaction test, it is not possible for the treatment effect to be the same in both age categories on both scales. If the relative risks are truly consistent between age categories, and the event rate is truly greater in older patients than in younger patients (which certainly appears to be the case, and would be expected a priori), then the observed difference in the absolute effect of ramipril between age groups is real, with important implications for the benefit–risk evaluation.

The term *prognostic factor* is used to describe a factor that is associated with the risk of an event, and there is typically a host of prognostic factors in every disease setting, some stronger than others. Age is a common prognostic factor for many adverse outcomes; other common prognostic factors include variables that measure the severity of the disease and genetic markers. In the presence of a prognostic factor, the effect of the treatment may be consistent across the levels of that factor on a relative scale, or on an absolute scale, but not on both.

There are good reasons to believe that treatment benefits are more typically consistent on a relative scale than on an absolute scale. First, empirically, forest plots like those for HOPE, where the relative risks appear consistent across subgroups, are extremely common across studies in multiple disease areas. Second, a constant absolute risk difference simply does not seem plausible in many settings and may be impossible in some. For example, the overall treatment effect of ramipril in HOPE on an absolute scale was 2.5%. If there are subgroups where the risk of the event in untreated subjects is less than 2.5%, then clearly a decrease of 2.5% is impossible. A treatment can only prevent an event in a subject who would have the event in the absence of the treatment; we refer to such a subject as "at risk." In order for a treatment to have a constant effect on an absolute scale, the probability that the treatment benefits a specific at-risk subject would have to depend somehow on the proportion of subjects in that subgroup who are not at risk, which does not seem plausible.

For safety endpoints, on the other hand, there is more reason to believe that the treatment effect could be relatively consistent across subgroups on an absolute scale. Note that with a safety event, the notion of an at-risk population is reversed: subjects who are at risk of being harmed by the treatment are those who would not have the event without the treatment. If the safety event is relatively rare, such that the at-risk population is approximately the same as the overall population, then the effect can be consistent on both a relative and absolute scale.

In other words, a very simple causal model, in which a constant percentage across subgroups of at-risk subjects experience the benefit, and a constant percentage across subgroups of at-risk subjects experience the harm, leads to a consistent benefit on a relative scale and a nearly consistent harm on an absolute scale. If we let r be the size of the at-risk population (i.e., for an efficacy event, the proportion of subjects who would experience the event in the absence of the treatment, or, for a safety event, the proportion who would not experience the event in the absence of treatment), and p be the proportion of this at-risk population, constant across subgroups, affected by the treatment, then the effect of the treatment is rp on an absolute scale. For efficacy endpoints, where there are often important prognostic variables, r will often vary across subgroups, leading to inconsistent effects on an absolute scale. For safety endpoints, on the other hand, r is often approximately equal to 1, in which case the effect will be consistent on both absolute and relative scales.

The HOPE results highlight a related issue. As with age, prior MI appeared to be an important prognostic factor, with a placebo event rate that was considerably higher among subjects with a prior MI (14.6%) than in other subjects (7.6%). In addition, the relative risk was somewhat better in the prior MI subjects (0.731) than in other subjects (0.905), although the test for interaction was not statistically significant (p = 0.202). These two factors together led to a considerably greater observed absolute risk difference in prior MI subjects (3.7%) than in other subjects (0.7%). However, it is not clear whether these observed results provide the best estimate of the magnitude of the difference in effect size between subgroups. Some might argue that the difference in relative risks between the subgroups was likely attributed to chance, in which case the best estimate of the relative risk in each subgroup is the overall relative risk of 0.77. Applying this relative risk estimate to the placebo event rates in each subgroup results in absolute risk differences of 3.3% among subjects with prior MI and 1.7% among other subjects. There is still a large difference in absolute benefit between these subgroups, but not as great as that based on the observed results.

6.4 Summary

While both subgroup analyses and benefit–risk evaluation have been the focus of considerable research and discussion in the scientific literature, the intersection of the two, the evaluation of benefit–risk in subgroups, has received less attention. In this chapter, we have argued that the traditional approach of evaluating the consistency of the treatment effect across subgroups on a relative scale is inadequate for benefit–risk analysis. While heterogeneity of the treatment effect on a relative scale is typically unexpected, and observed heterogeneity on this scale is often dismissed as likely being attributed to chance, heterogeneity on an absolute scale is expected and common. This implies that the benefit–risk profile of the treatment will often vary, sometimes considerably, across subgroups.

Sculpher (2008) discussed some of the concepts discussed here, though in the context of cost-effectiveness analysis rather than benefit–risk analysis. Differences in prognosis across subgroups, as well as differences in cost, can affect the cost-effectiveness analysis. He also argued that relative measures of effect are inadequate for cost-effectiveness analysis and that baseline event rates should be considered. In fact, if one considers an adverse event to be a kind of cost of the treatment, there is much in common between benefit–risk analysis and cost-effectiveness analysis.

While there is good reason to believe that the benefit–risk profile of treatment will vary across subgroups, many of the concerns of subgroup analyses remain in this setting. Observed differences in the benefit–risk profile across subgroups will reflect both true differences and the play of chance, and, with many subgroups being evaluated, the probability of a type I error can be considerably inflated. Regulators are likely to remain cautious about approving a drug based solely on a favorable benefit–risk analysis within a subgroup. However, there will likely be some cases where regulatory approval is warranted for a subgroup and others where patients and prescribers should be aware of clear differences in the benefit–risk profile for specific subgroups.

Much of this chapter has focused on a relatively simple situation where there is a single time-to-event benefit endpoint and a single time-to-event safety endpoint. Most real situations will be considerably more complex, with multiple benefit and risk endpoints on multiple scales. However, it will still be true that differences in the benefit–risk profile across subgroups can and often will exist and that a thorough analysis of a clinical trial should include an evaluation of the benefit–risk profile within subgroups.

References

Alosh, Mohamed, Kathleen Fritsch, Mohammad Huque et al. "Statistical Considerations on Subgroup Analysis in Clinical Trials." *Statistics in Biopharmaceutical Research* (2015): doi: 10.1080/19466315.2015.1077726.

Alosh, Mohamed, and Mohammad Huque. "A Flexible Strategy for Testing Subgroups and Overall Population." *Statistics in Medicine* 28 (2009): 3–23.

Arnold, J. Malcolm O., Salim Yusuf, James Young et al. "Prevention of Heart Failure in Patients in the Heart Outcomes Prevention Evaluation (HOPE) Study." *Circulation* 107 (2003): 1284–1290.

Bresalier, Robert S., Robert S. Sander, Hui Quan et al. "Cardiovascular Events Associated With Rofecoxib in a Colorectal Adenoma Chemoprevention Trial." *New England Journal of Medicine* 352 (2005): 1092–1102.

Cui, Lu, H. M. James Hung, Sue Jane Wang, and Yi Tsong. "Issues Related to Subgroup Analysis in Clinical Trials." *Journal of Biopharmaceutical Statistics* 12 no. 3 (2002): 347–358.

DeMets, D. L. "Statistical Issues in Interpreting Clinical Trials." *Journal of Internal Medicine* 255 (2004): 529–537.

European Medicines Agency. "Guideline on the Investigation of Subgroups in Confirmatory Clinical Trials." (2014) http://www.ema.europa.eu/docs/en_GB/document_library/Scientific_guideline/2014/02/WC500160523.pdf.

Foster, Jared C., Jeffrey M. G. Taylor, and Stephen J. Ruberg. "Subgroup Identification From Randomized Clinical Trial Data." *Statistics in Medicine* 30 no. 24 (2011): 2867–2880.

Furberg, Curt D., and Bertram Pitt. "Withdrawal of Cerivastatin From the World Market." *Current Controlled Trials in Cardiovascular Medicine* 2 (2001): 205–207.

Graham, David J., Rita Ouellet-Hellstrom, Thomas E. MaCurdy et al. "Risk of Acute Myocardial Infarction, Stroke, Heart Failure and Death in Elderly Medicare Patients Treated With Rosiglitazone or Pioglitazone." *Journal of the American Medical Association* 304 no. 4 (2010): 411–418.

Grouin, Jean-Marie, Maylis Costa, and John Lewis. "Subgroup Analysis in Randomized Clinical Trials: Statistical and Regulatory Issues." *Journal of Biopharmaceutical Statistics* 15 (2005): 869–882.

Julian, Desmond G. "Debate: A Subversive View of Subgroups – A Dissident Clinician's Opinion." *Current Controlled Trials in Cardiovascular Medicine* 1 (2000): 28–30.

Kraemer, Helena Chmura, George A. Morgan, Nancy L. Leech, Jeffrey A. Gliner, Jerry J. Vaske, and Robert J. Harmon. "Measures of Clinical Significance." *Journal of the American Academy of Childhood Adolescent Psychiatry* 42 no. 12 (2003): 1524–1529.

Lagakos, Stephen. "The Challenge of Subgroup Analyses – Reporting Without Distorting." *New England Journal of Medicine* 354 no. 16 (2006): 1667–1669.

MERIT-HF Study Group. "Effect of Metoprolol CR/XL in Chronic Heart Failure: Metoprolol CR/XL Randomised Intervention Trial in Congestive Heart Failure." *The Lancet* 353 (1999): 2001–2007.

Moyé, Lemuel A., and Anita Deswal. "Trials within Trials: Confirmatory Subgroup Analyses in Controlled Clinical Experiments." *Controlled Clinical Trials* 22 (2001): 605–619.

Pocock, Stuart J., Susan E. Assmann, Laura E. Enos, and Linda E. Kasten. "Subgroup Analysis, Covariate Adjustment and Baseline Comparisons in Clinical Trial Reporting: Current Practice and Problems." *Statistics in Medicine* 21 (2002): 2917–2930.

Replogle, William H., and William D. Johnson. "Interpretation of Absolute Measures of Disease Risk in Comparative Research." *Family Medicine* 39 vol. 6 (2007): 432–435.

Reuters. "Biogen Reports 10 More Tysabri PML Cases, 4 Deaths." February 18, 2011. http://www.reuters.com/article/2011/02/18/biogen-tysabri-idUSN1811430320110218#sthash.jznJf7Zw.dpuf.

Sculpher, Mark. "Subgroups and Heterogeneity in Cost-Effectiveness Analysis." *Pharmacoeconomics* 26 no. 9 (2008): 799–806.

Sleight, Peter. "Debate: Subgroup Analyses in Clinical Trials – Fun to Look at But Don't Believe Them!" *Current Controlled Trials in Cardiovascular Medicine* 1 (2000): 25–27.

Snapinn, Steven M., and Qi Jiang. "Responder Analysis and the Assessment of a Clinically Relevant Treatment Effect." *Trials* 8:31 (2007).

Snapinn, Steven, and Qi Jiang. "Analysis of Safety Data." In *Cancer Clinical Trials: Current and Controversial Issues in Design and Analysis*, chapter 4. Boca Raton: CRC Press, 2015.

Song, Yang, and George Y. H. Chi. "A Method for Testing a Prespecified Subgroup in Clinical Trials." *Statistics in Medicine* 26 (2007): 3535–3549.

Wang, Rui, Stephen W. Lagakos, James H. Ware, David J. Hunter, and Jeffrey M. Drazen. "Reporting of Subgroup Analyses in Clinical Trials." *New England Journal of Medicine* 357 no. 21 (2007): 2189–2194.

Wedel, Hans, David DeMets, Prakesh Deedwania et al. "Challenges of Subgroup Analyses in Multinational Clinical Trials: Experiences From the MERIT-HF Trial." *American Heart Journal* 142 (2001): 502–511.

White, Ian R., Stuart J. Pocock, and Duolao Wang. "Eliciting and Using Expert Opinions About Influence of Patient Characteristics on Treatment Effects: A Bayesian Analysis of the CHARM Trials." *Statistics in Medicine* 24 (2005): 3805–3821.

Yusuf, Salim, Janet Wittes, Jeffrey Probstfield, and Herman A. Tyroler. "Analysis and Interpretation of Treatment Effects in Subgroups of Patients in Randomized Clinical Trials." *Journal of the American Medical Association* 266 no. 1 (1991): 93–98.

Zhou, Ying, Chunlei Ke, Qi Jiang, Seta Shahin, and Steven Snapinn. "Choosing Appropriate Metrics to Evaluate Adverse Events in Safety Evaluation." *Therapeutic Innovation & Regulatory Science* 49 no. 3 (2015): 398–404.

7

Sources of Data to Enable Benefit–Risk Assessment

Christy Chuang-Stein, George Quartey, Weili He, Qi Jiang, Haijun Ma, Jonathan Norton, John Scott, and Jesse A. Berlin

CONTENTS

ABSTRACT Benefit–risk (B–R) assessment is required at the time a product is submitted for marketing authorization. Data for this assessment typically come from clinical trials (randomized and nonrandomized). However, B–R assessment is an ongoing process and assessment beyond the initial marketing application will require data from the broad use of the product in the real-world setting. Fortunately, such data have become increasingly available in recent years. Examples include spontaneous reports of adverse events and data registered in administrative and registry databases. Administrative databases describe the patient's usage of, as well as experience with, all kinds of pharmaceutical products. In this chapter, we will discuss these additional data sources and how the available data could be used to assist B–R assessment. We will also describe a set of principles on how data from these different sources could be examined together to provide an overall picture of the B–R profile of a product.

7.1 Introduction

Benefit–risk (B–R) assessment is a continuous process throughout the life cycle of a pharmaceutical product. During the development phase of a product, a manufacturer needs to determine, at various stages, whether the observed/potential risks are likely to outweigh the observed/anticipated benefits. For example, after single- and multiple-dose ascending studies in healthy volunteers, a manufacturer needs to decide if the observed adverse experience in the healthy volunteers together with preclinical animal testing findings supports continuing with the product development even if no evidence of benefit has been observed. A similar decision is necessary at the end of the dose-finding studies that offer early results on the product's benefit. A critical B–R decision point comes when results from confirmatory trials become available. With available data in a more diverse population (or populations), a manufacturer needs to decide if a marketing application is warranted, on the basis of a B–R assessment using all available information. Once a product is submitted for regulatory approval, regulators will make the marketing decision, based on their own B–R assessment of the product.

Clinical trials are the primary source of information on treatment effects for B–R assessment in the initial marketing authorization application of a new product. Most of the clinical trials are randomized, providing direct head-to-head comparisons between the new product and a comparator. The single-arm design, although not common in Phase III trials, could be considered when the target patient population is too small to make conducting a randomized trial practical. Another example of a nonrandomized trial is a long-term extension study, which enrolls patients from earlier randomized trials so that patients can receive the investigational product for an extended period. Because randomization removes bias attributed to treatment selection, it results in comparable patients between treatment groups and enables comparisons between them without bias owing to treatment confounding. This feature is lost for single-arm studies when historical information is used for comparison. Similarly, extension studies often allow control subjects to cross over to receiving the experimental therapy, thereby losing the benefits of randomization.

Randomized clinical trials (RCTs), however, have their limitations. Foremost is the restriction placed on patients through the inclusion/exclusion criteria. Patients in clinical trials generally have fewer medical conditions and receive fewer concomitant medications. For example, a clinical trial may exclude patients with preexisting psychological disorders or receiving certain medications. As a result, the trial population may not be completely representative of the target patients in the real-world setting. Second, except for a few situations, the duration of the exposure in a clinical trial is typically limited, ranging from a few weeks to a couple of years, even for medications intended for chronic use. This is because most clinical trials are designed from the efficacy perspective and benefit can often be realized over a shorter duration. This is especially true for products intended for symptomatic relief. On the other hand, risk can show up later in a user's life or adversely affect future generations. Examples of drugs with such risks are diethylstilbestrol (DES) and thalidomide.

DES is a potent synthetic estrogen. It was prescribed to millions of pregnant women from 1938 to 1971 (and to a small number of women for several years after 1971) in the United States to reduce morning sickness and to prevent miscarriages. Its use in other parts of the world continued into the mid-1980s. Unfortunately, DES was later found to be one of the most toxic carcinogens and developmental disrupters (see, e.g., Matter 2013). Currently established adverse effects of DES exposure include greater risk for breast cancer in women exposed during pregnancy, a rare vaginal cancer in daughters of exposed women, possible risk for testicular cancer in sons of exposed women, and abnormal reproductive organs for all DES offspring. The full effect of DES in multiple generations is still being researched.

Thalidomide was used as a sedative, hypnotic, and anti-inflammatory medication by pregnant women to combat morning sickness and as a sleep aid in nearly 50 countries outside of the United States from 1957 to 1961. The product was never approved in the United States. More than 10,000 children of women who took thalidomide during their pregnancies were born with a wide range of birth defects, including shortened arms and legs, blindness, deafness, heart problems, and brain damage (see, e.g., Kim and Scialli 2011).

There are recent examples of product withdrawals based on information emerging after product launch. Daggumalli and Martin (2012) reported 15 product withdrawals between 2001 and 2010. All of the cases involved new information on risk, tipping the B–R balance that was previously considered to be favorable. Major reasons for product withdrawals between 2001 and 2010 include increased risk of cardiac toxicity, hepatic toxicity, renal toxicity, bone toxicity, progressive multifocal leukoencephalopathy (PML), bronchospasm, and death.

The need to continue B–R assessment postmarketing in the real-world setting prompted the revision of the International Conference on Harmonization (ICH) E2C. The revision (i.e., E2C(R2)) recommends a manufacturer to submit a Periodic Benefit–Risk Evaluation Report (PBRER) to regulatory agencies (ICH E2C(R2) 2012). The revision, which reached Step 4 (implementation) by the ICH regions in November 2012, was implemented to ensure that the periodic reports for marketed drugs would include all cumulative knowledge of the product as well as an evaluation of the product's B–R profile. New information could come from many different sources including data associated with uses other than the approved indication(s), if the inclusion of the latter is judged to be relevant and appropriate.

Because of the limitations and expense of RCTs, postmarketing studies may take the form of observational studies using data from claims databases or electronic medical records. The studies could be postapproval safety studies or postapproval efficacy studies. The objectives of these studies are to gather additional safety or efficacy data about a product in patients who take the product and are being cared for in the regular clinical setting.

Other data sources for B–R assessment of marketed products include product registries or patient registries. Spontaneous reports have long been used as a major source for pharmacovigilance of marketed products. Recently, social media has emerged as another data source. Researchers have increasingly used text mining techniques to identify adverse experiences associated with product usage in social media. Because of the lack of structure and the inability to follow up on adverse experiences reported at the social media sites, data gleaned from this source should be viewed with great caution. As such, we do not plan to cover social media in the remainder of this chapter.

In this chapter, we focus on different data sources for B–R assessment. The need to use different data sources reinforces the fact that B–R assessment is a continuous process. While the initial decision to grant a marketing authorization is typically based on RCTs, findings from the continuous B–R assessment can lead regulators to revisit the initial marketing authorization decision or to take other regulatory actions. Section 7.2 of this chapter focuses on clinical trials; Section 7.3 focuses on spontaneous reports; Section 7.4 focuses on observational studies; and Section 7.5 focuses on patient registries. In Section 7.6, we offer principles outlining how data from these sources should be handled in the conduct of B–R assessment. These principles are applicable to the development of PBRER mentioned above. In Section 7.7, we include four examples of using information to assess B–R assessment and make informed decisions. We offer some additional comments in Section 7.8.

7.2 Clinical Trials as the Data Source for B–R Assessment

Most of the existing quantitative B–R methodologies focus on data from RCTs (Quartey et al. 2016). RCTs offer direct comparisons between treatments without the need to worry about confounding owing to treatment selection. In addition, RCTs are typically conducted under good clinical practice principles. Except for a few rare cases, information collected in RCTs is generally of good quality and integrity. Individual patient data in RCTs allow efficacy and safety to be assessed jointly at the individual patient level. Having individual patient data may also allow the identification of biologically defined subgroups that may experience a more favorable B–R experience than other subgroups.

When there are multiple randomized trials of the same product, it is common to combine results from these studies in a meta-analysis to obtain more precise estimates for treatment effects, if the studies are judged to be appropriate for combining. Meta-analysis is sometimes used to integrate efficacy data concerning an important clinical endpoint whose occurrence in individual studies is limited. More often, meta-analysis of clinical trials is used to integrate safety data in order to understand the risk for adverse events that are uncommon (incidence proportion between 1/1000 and 1/100) or rare (incidence proportion between 1/10,000 and 1/1000). Here, the classification of frequencies is based on the recommendations from the CIOMS (Council for International Organizations of Medical Sciences) Working Groups III and V (1999). Because of the low incidence of events and the limited duration of randomized trials, some trials may not even record any of the events of interest. For important adverse events that are of special interest, a manufacturer can convene a committee to adjudicate these events real-time throughout the development program so that a preplanned meta-analysis of these events will have the rigor expected of a confirmatory meta-analysis.

An example of the above is the assessment of cardiovascular (CV) toxicity of medications for type 2 diabetes mellitus (T2DM). In December 2008, the Food and Drug Administration (FDA) in the United States issued a guidance document on evaluating CV risk of new therapies for T2DM (US FDA 2008). The guidance states that if the premarketing clinical data rule out a relative risk >1.8 on a major adverse CV endpoint and the overall risk–benefit analysis is favorable, the product could be approved, provided that the sponsor also demonstrates that a relative risk >1.3 can be ruled out after the product is on the market. For a manufacturer who initiated the development program for a new T2DM product after December 2008, one strategy is for the manufacturer to arrange to have all reported CV events of interest evaluated by an Adjudication Committee during the trials. The adjudicated events will be analyzed in a prespecified meta-analysis of late-stage trials to satisfy the 1.8 requirement. Variations of this strategy have been used by manufacturers of T2DM medications since 2009 such as including in the meta-analysis interim results from an ongoing CV outcome trial (Marchenko et al. 2015).

Meta-analysis has been used to combine safety information of products approved for an indication to assess the risk of these products and better inform B–R decisions. For example, the FDA conducted and presented a meta-analysis on the effect of antiepileptic drugs (AEDs) on suicidality behavior and ideation at a joint meeting of the FDA Peripheral and Central Nervous System Drugs Advisory Committee and the Psychopharmacologic Drug Advisory Committee in July 2008. The meta-analysis included 11 commercially available AEDs. The meta-analysis led to the requirement that all labels for AEDs carry a warning about an increased risk in suicidality behavior and ideation associated with anticonvulsant use. Similarly, FDA conducted a meta-analysis to investigate the risk of serious but relatively infrequent occurrences of severe asthma exacerbations and asthma-related death of long-acting beta-agonists (LABAs). The analysis included four drugs and was reviewed at a joint meeting among three FDA Advisory Committees (Pediatric, Pulmonary–Allergy Drugs, Drug Safety and Risk Management) in December 2008. As a result of the meta-analysis and subsequent discussions, FDA required updates to the labels of LABAs for the asthma indication in June 2010.

New and emerging treatments are often compared to placebo or standard of care, but rarely to each other. Data from randomized controlled trials have been used as evidence to indirectly compare treatments of interest in the absence of head-to-head data, thus providing insights on the relative treatment benefit in terms of efficacy and safety across drug classes for the same indication. These comparisons can help guide internal decision making and select comparators for clinical trials. Indirect comparisons and, more broadly, mixed treatment comparisons require assumptions about the studies included in the analyses. Interested readers are referred to Lumley (2002), Lu and Ades (2004), and Ohlssen et al. (2013) for theories and applications of these approaches.

In order to obtain longer exposure data and to incentivize patients to enroll in trials, many manufacturers cross patients from randomized trials into an extension study at the end of the planned duration in the randomized trials. Since these extension studies are usually of longer duration, we are more likely to observe events that occur only after a prolonged exposure. For development programs that conduct placebo-controlled trials, extension trials often do not include a randomized control. When a small number of clinically meaningful adverse events that are not usually associated with the disease of interest or the patient population enrolled are reported in an extension study, it can be difficult to interpret the significance of these events in the absence of a control group. One could consider reporting incidence rates for these events to minimize the impact of exposure duration. However, other potential confounding factors such as patient population, geographic variation, severity of disease under study, and concomitant therapy, can make the interpretation of the incidence rates challenging.

Because of these concerns, we suggest that manufacturers consider the use of at least a contemporaneous control with data from sources external to the clinical program, for example, large, electronic health care data sets, ongoing cohort or registry studies, or other clinical programs to help interpret data observed in noncontrolled open-label extension studies. While a randomized control group provides the best comparison, it is not always realistic to demand the inclusion of a randomized control in an extension study. Another type of control, which may be slightly better, is a nonrandomized concurrent control in the form of a concurrent cohort. In essence, data from these uncontrolled studies should be treated similarly as data from observational studies. We will discuss observational studies in more detail in Section 7.4.

7.3 Spontaneous Reports as a Data Source for Risk

One mechanism to monitor the safety of a product once it is approved for marketing is through the voluntary reporting of adverse events by users, health care providers, family members, or the manufacturers to a system set up for this purpose. The events don't need to be serious or judged to have a clear causal relationship with the product. The reports are called "spontaneous" because they are not solicited or sought as in clinical trials.

Many countries have spontaneous reporting systems (SRSs). For example, the United Kingdom began the "Yellow Card" system in 1964 to collect spontaneous reports. In the United States, FDA established its SRS in 1969. SRS was replaced by the Adverse Event Reporting System (AERS) in November 1997. AERS allows users to encode and search reports as well as export data into spreadsheets and other software for more complex analyses. Data files from AERS were made available to the public on a quarterly basis.

In August 2012, FDA moved data from AERS to FDA Adverse Event Reporting System (FAERS). The remit of the system remains the same, that is, to support FDA's postmarketing safety surveillance program for drug and therapeutic biologic products. Entries in FAERS are coded in MedDRA. See http://www.fda.gov/Drugs/GuidanceComplianceRegulatoryInformation/Surveillance/AdverseDrugEffects/default.htm for additional information. In addition to FAERS, FDA also maintains Vaccine AERS (VAERS) to house spontaneous reports related to vaccines.

There are other databases for spontaneous reports. For example, manufacturers typically maintain spontaneous reports on their products (drugs, biologics, vaccines, and devices) in their in-house pharmacovigilance databases. In December 2001, the European Medicines Agency (EMA) launched a web-based information system designed to manage information on safety reports of suspected adverse reactions to medicines that are authorized or being studied in clinical trials in the European Economic Area. EudraVigilance Post-Authorisation Module in the EudraVigilance Database Management System is designed to receive individual case safety narratives related to spontaneous reports and reports from noninterventional studies.

Interpreting spontaneous reports properly and judging if the number of reports increased over time require information on drug use or exposure. For example, a twofold increase in the number of reports does not represent an increase if the usage is increased by fivefold. In addition, the number of certain adverse events reported to a system like FAERS can be affected by several factors. For example, it is well known that new products tend to receive a lot of attention, which often results in an initial spike in reports, a phenomenon called the Weber effect. When there is media coverage on the adverse reactions to a particular product, this will likely generate more attention to the product and produce more reports. In addition, the introduction of a risk minimization measure may raise more awareness and prompt more reporting. Still other factors that could lead to heightened reporting include pending lawsuits and the introduction of generic copies of the branded product. Above all, one needs to keep in mind inherent data issues such as duplicated reports, underreporting, coding errors, and variations in coding rules in a spontaneous report database. All these are recognized limitations of a passive surveillance system and have been discussed extensively by others (Gould et al. 2015; Hammad et al. 2013; Ishiguro et al. 2014).

As stated earlier, we need to have knowledge on the exposure to a product to assess the reporting rate of an event. Here, exposure could be measured in terms of exposure duration or the number of patients exposed to the product. In the remainder of this section, we will discuss two approaches that have been used to estimate exposure duration and the number of exposed patients, respectively. Both are approximations, because individual-level data on actual consumption are unavailable.

7.3.1 Estimating Postmarketing Exposure Duration

Postmarketing exposure can be estimated in a number of different ways. Telfair et al. (2006) used ex-factory distribution data to estimate postmarketing exposure to pharmaceutical products. The approach could be described briefly as below.

Assume that there are K different dosage strengths d_i ($i = 1, \ldots K$) in milligrams. Suppose U_i units of d_i were sold during a predefined time frame. Units can refer to tablets or capsules for a solid formulation or volume for a liquid formulation and should be clearly defined. The total drug sold in grams during the time frame is

$$TD = \frac{1}{1000}\sum_{i=1}^{K} U_i \times d_i.$$

Suppose there are I different indications, which may have different recommended daily doses. Let q_i denote the average daily dose in grams for subjects using the product for the ith indication. An example is when a higher daily dose is used to manage a more severe manifestation of a disorder. Telfair et al. suggested getting the estimate of the average daily dose from the manufacturer's internal core data sheet or using the recommended daily dose in the product label. If an average daily dose cannot be determined for a product, Telfair et al. suggested using a range of the minimum to maximum daily dose.

Assume that the proportion of the sales for the ith indication of the total sales for the product during the defined time frame is p_i ($0 < p_i < 1$). One can then estimate E_i, the total exposure (in days) for the ith indication and the total drug exposure TE (in days). If one divides TE by 30.4 (the average number of days in a month), one obtains the total exposure in months.

$$E_i = \frac{p_i \times TD}{q_i}$$

$$TE = \sum_{i=1}^{K} E_i$$

The approach proposed by Telfair et al. is a population-based approach. Although it is arguably simplistic, it provides a framework for estimating exposure to a drug with a fixed dose and relatively high dosing frequency. It relies on several assumptions: First, it assumes that patients took the medications as recommended. Second, it assumes that the administration schedule remains the same for all indications (e.g., QD, BID, or TID) and the only difference across indications is the recommended daily dose. Third, it implicitly assumes that the amount of drug given to health care providers as free starter samples is negligible. In addition, it should be remembered that distribution is not consumption. Further limitations include potential lag time (period between distribution and consumption) and stockpiling for small molecules.

Adaptations are necessary for many other situations. For example, for weight-based medications (e.g., many cancer drugs), one needs to take patient weight into consideration.

Alternatively, one may use the average weights within different geographic regions. When the average daily dose can only be given in a range, E_i can be expressed as a range (LE_i, UE_i). The total exposure TE could be expressed as a range of (LE, UE).

The estimated TE could be used to calculate a reporting rate for an event, defined as the number of reports of an event divided by TE, during a defined period. As Telfair et al. stated, the reporting rate is not the same as exposure-adjusted incidence rate calculated in clinical trials because of limitations of the SRS and the method used to estimate exposure. In addition, underreporting is a major issue with spontaneous reports (Alvarez-Requejo et al. 1998; Hazell and Shakir 2006). However, the reporting rate, calculated in a consistent manner, can be used to judge if the rate appears to have changed over time, recognizing that, as noted above, many factors other than a real drug effect could affect the rate. One can also compare reporting rates for different drugs for the same disorder. A manufacturer could include reporting rates in the PBRER of their product to support statements concerning risk over time.

7.3.2 Estimating the Number of Patients Exposed to a Medication in the Postmarketing Setting

Tramadol HCl was approved as a nonscheduled opioid pain medication in April 1995 in the United States, contingent upon the development of a proactive surveillance program, to be overseen by an independent steering committee to detect unexpectedly high levels of abuse. The surveillance program needed to estimate the monthly rate of abuse, defined as the number of abuse cases per 100,000 patients prescribed the drug during the month. The number of abuse cases was obtained from reports received through the FDA MedWatch system. To estimate the monthly rate of abuse, the program needed to estimate the number of patients prescribed tramadol on a monthly basis.

Cicero et al. (1999) estimated the number of individuals exposed to tramadol every month during a 3-year period (April 5, 1995 to June 30, 1998) after tramadol's introduction in the United States. Cicero et al. gave an example of how the calculation was carried out for June 1998 (last month of the program). The calculation requires several assumptions and information from several data sources. It can be described in the following steps:

1. According to the manufacturer, the number of tablets sold for June 1998 was 48,938,000.
2. Data from the National Prescription Audit (IMS American, Ltd.) suggested that the average number of tablets per prescription for June 1998 was 51.52. Dividing 48,938,000 by 51.52 yields 949,884 as the estimated number of prescriptions filled for the month.
3. The National Disease and Therapeutic Index data (IMS American, Ltd.) suggested that 53% of the prescriptions were for new patients. Multiplying 53% and 47% to 949,884 yields 503,438 prescriptions for new patients and 446,445 prescriptions for continuing patients, respectively.
4. Free samples are regularly given to prescribers by manufacturers. The National Disease and Therapeutic Index database (IMS American, Ltd.) estimated that for June 1998, sold prescriptions made up approximately 85% of total prescription-equivalents among new patients. In other words, free samples contribute to 15% of tramadol use among new patients. For continuing patients, prescription-equivalents from free samples is 75% less compared to new patients, that is, free samples made up 3.75%

(= 0.25 × 0.15) of the total tramadol use. This means that the total number of prescriptions for new patients and continuing patients, when taking free samples into account, is estimated to be 503,438/0.85 = 592,280 and 446,445/0.963 = 463,839, respectively.

5. Assuming that the average number of tablets per day is 4.6, the average 51.52 tables per prescription in Step 2 corresponds to 11.2 days of coverage. If a patient took the average number of tramadol tablets for an entire month, he or she would need 2.714 prescriptions (= 30.4/11.2) during an average month. However, this number must be adjusted because of the following reasons.
   a. Assume that new patients start their tramadol uniformly over the month. This means that the average number of prescription for new patients per month is 50% of (30.4/11.2). In addition, the authors assume that, on average, new patients take only 85% of their medications. This means that they would need, on average, 0.5 × (30.4/11.2) × 0.85 = 1.154 prescriptions a month only.
   b. For continuing patients, the authors assume that they take 70% of their medication. Therefore, they would need (30.4/11.2) × 0.70 = 1.900 prescriptions a month.
6. Dividing 1.154 into 592,280 produces the number of new patients for June (513,432). Similarly, dividing 1.900 into 463,839 produces the number of continuing patients for the same period (244,126). Adding these two numbers together gives 757,558, the estimated number of patients exposed to tramadol in June 1998.

The above steps were admittedly complex. They were proposed before access to large administrative (claims and electronic medical record) databases became a common practice. Moving forward, it will be possible to query, for example, claims databases to estimate the exposure to a medication in a population with a demographic composition similar to that in the United States. To do this, we can first estimate the extent of exposure within each major demographic (e.g., age, sex) stratum. Once we obtain the exposure rates within the various strata, we can combine the rates using weights that reflect the composition of the population in the United States. As pointed out earlier, it is important to remember that distribution (dispensing) is not equal to consumption when using claims databases to estimate drug exposure/usage.

7.4 Observational Studies as Data Source for Risk–Benefit Analysis

As noted above, RCTs are generally considered to provide the most valid assessments of causal relationships between drugs and either benefits or adverse events, by ensuring that, on average, confounding factors (such as demographic status and comorbidities) are distributed equally across all treatment groups. However, as we discussed earlier, use of RCTs to fully understand drug safety is limited by several factors. RCTs for product approval usually exclude important segments of the population who may be at higher risk of adverse events, such as the elderly, pregnant women, people with impaired liver or kidney function or other significant comorbidities, and those who are taking concomitant medications. Because trials often have short follow-up duration and limited sample size, most RCTs, and even the entire development programs, are frequently underpowered to detect any increased risk of rare drug adverse events (Qiu et al. 2015), especially for subgroups.

Observational studies using large-scale health care databases, such as administrative claims and electronic health records (EHRs), have the potential to support B–R assessment. Observational studies can range from population-based cohort studies with prospective data collection to targeted patient registries to retrospective case–control studies, and to studies conducted in administrative data sources, such as health insurance claims. Many potential biases and sources of variability threaten the validity of such studies and a substantial literature documents these concerns (Ioannidis 2005).

7.4.1 Study Designs

Case–control studies and cohort studies are two primary types of observational studies that aid in evaluating associations between diseases and exposures.

7.4.1.1 Case–Control

Case–control studies compare the probability of exposure prior to outcomes among cases with the probability of exposure in patients without outcomes (Madigan et al. 2013a). This design permits estimation of odds and odds ratios, but not of risks and risk differences. Allowance may be made for potential confounding factors by measuring them and making appropriate adjustments in the analysis. This statistical adjustment may be rendered more efficient by matching cases and controls with respect to confounders, either on an individual basis (e.g., by pairing each case with one or more controls of the same age and sex, or other matching factors) or in groups (e.g., stratifying by age and sex and filling strata with controls based on the age and sex distribution of the cases). Case–control studies are particularly suited to studying uncommon outcomes, because the study groups are defined by outcome, and statistical power is determined to a large extent by the number of cases in a study.

7.4.1.2 Cohort Method

Typically, in pharmacoepidemiology studies, the cohort method is used in a new-user cohort design. New users of the target drug are identified using a predefined minimum period of nonuse and are compared to new users of a comparator drug or group of drugs. Relative risk can be estimated with adjustment for baseline covariates through various strategies, including propensity score matching (Ryan et al. 2013a). Because exposure is identified before the outcome, cohort studies have a temporal framework that is sometimes assumed to be more valid than case–control studies with respect to assessing causality and thus have the potential to provide the strongest scientific evidence (Green and Byar 1984) next to the RCTs. Cohort studies are particularly advantageous for examining rare events because subjects are selected by their exposure status. Additionally, the investigator can examine multiple outcomes simultaneously. Disadvantages include the need for a large sample size and the potentially long follow-up duration of the study design, resulting in a costly endeavor.

The nested case–control study is something of a compromise between the cohort and case–control studies. In this setting, the cohort is established and defines the population from which both cases and controls are sampled (although often, a 100% sample of cases is taken). Because the cohort is defined, data collection took place before the cases became cases; hence, the temporality is the same as it would be under the cohort design. The efficiency is gained from having to get detailed information only for a sample of the noncases. Sampling of controls often uses a technique called incidence-density sampling, under which controls are sampled at the same point in follow-up as the corresponding matched case. For example, a case with the defining event after 2 years in the cohort would be matched with a control who has been in the cohort for at least 2 years and has not had the event. Information is collected from both the case and control over the same period, looking backward at exposures before that shared time point.

7.4.1.2.1 Self-Controlled Cohort

The self-controlled cohort (SCC) design is an extension of a traditional cohort design in which the rate of adverse drug events can be compared across groups of patients exposed to different medications, allowing comparisons within a cohort population, between treatments, and relative to the overall population at large. SCC estimates the strength of association by comparing the post-exposure incidence rate with the pre-exposure incidence rate in the same patients exposed to the target drug of interest (Ryan et al. 2013b; Suchard et al. 2013).

7.4.1.2.2 Self-Controlled Case Series

The self-controlled case series (SCCS) design focuses on time exposed/unexposed to the target drug and occurrences of the target condition. The method estimates the association between a transient exposure and adverse event using only cases; no separate controls are required because each case acts as its own control. By considering a patient's entire profile through the study follow-up period, SCCS is based on the principle of a cohort study, although it relies solely on patients who have experienced the event of interest (i.e., cases only). Each case's observation time is divided into a "control" period and an "at risk" period. As such, each participating patient acts as his or her own control, and confounding factors that do not vary with time, such as sex, some chronic comorbidities, or genetics, are implicitly adjusted for (Whitaker et al. 2006).

Although estimated on the basis of cases only, the design provides consistent estimates of the relative incidence. It also allows an effective control of all fixed confounders, including both observable and unobservable confounders. Moreover, under certain circumstances, the model is highly efficient compared with the retrospective cohort method from which it is derived (Whitaker et al. 2006). Besides the need for the occurrence of events of interest to be independent, one of the fundamental assumptions underpinning SCCS is that censoring of patients during follow-up is independent of the risk of future occurrence of the event (i.e., the probability of exposure is not affected by the occurrence of an outcome event). This assumption could be a problem for certain types of exposures, for which terminating exposure is explicitly tied to occurrence of an event. In the case of hormonal contraceptives to be discussed in Section 7.7, the occurrence of a venous thromboembolism (VTE) becomes a specific contraindication for subsequent exposure. Although SCCS is based on the principle of cohort design, the patient's follow-up time does not need to end at the time of an event. Moreover, the subsequent follow-up time after the occurrence of the event should be independent of the occurrence of that event. Case-based methods for dealing with confounders have the potential for effectively controlling both measured and unmeasured confounders and therefore should be strongly considered in situations where unmeasured and probably nonmeasurable confounders are strongly suspected, at least as part of a sensitivity analysis (Ryan et al. 2013b).

7.4.2 Data Sources

One type of data source that has provided fertile ground for epidemiologic investigation has been observational health care databases.

7.4.2.1 Administrative Claims

Administrative claims databases have been the most actively used observational health care data source. They typically capture data elements used within the reimbursement process. Providers of health care services (i.e., physicians, pharmacies, hospitals, and laboratories) submit encounter information so that they will be paid for services delivered (Hennessy 2006). This commonly includes pharmacy claims for prescription drug fills (providing what drug was dispensed, the dispensing date, and the amount of supply) and medical (inpatient and outpatient) claims that detail the date and type of service rendered. Medical claims typically contain diagnosis codes used to justify reimbursement for the procedures (also coded). Age and gender can also commonly be obtained from the available data.

In these databases, data are recorded only when a patient has a reimbursable encounter with the health care system that has been properly filed, coded, and adjudicated by the payer (Schneeweiss and Avorn 2005). As a result, many key data elements may not be available. Information on over-the-counter drug use and in-hospital medication is usually unavailable and the patient's actual consumption pattern of the prescription medication is generally unknown (Suissa and Garbe 2007). Retail pharmacy claims data can be used to study drug utilization pattern, but the completeness of these data can vary by patient age (Polinski et al. 2009) or other unobservable characteristics. Also of note, many potential benefits are not typically captured in claims. For example, if a schizophrenic patient takes an antipsychotic and experiences symptomatic benefit, that isn't captured directly. Only reimbursable events are captured, such as rehospitalization.

One potential issue with claims data is the possibility of upcoding of a diagnostic code to justify a higher reimbursement amount (see, e.g., Bonewit-West et al. 2013). This has the potential of downgrading a patient's health state before an intervention and thus making the intervention appear to be more effective than it actually is.

7.4.2.2 Electronic Health Records

EHRs generally contain data captured at the point of care, with the intention of supporting the clinical care process. A patient chart may include demographics (birth date, gender, and race), height and weight, and family and medical history. Many EHR systems support provider entry of diagnoses, signs, and symptoms and also capture laboratory values and imaging reports (Schneeweiss and Avorn 2005). EHR systems usually have the capability to record other important health status indications, such as alcohol use and smoking status (Lewis and Brensinger 2004), but these data may be missing in many patient charts (Hennessy 2006).

EHR systems are generally maintained independently by physician practices or individual hospitals. Drug exposure may be inferred from various sources. For example, providers may use the EHR system to capture patient-reported medication history and to write prescriptions. It should be noted that there might be no confirmation that a prescription was actually filled at a pharmacy. Since multiple health care providers may deliver care to a patient without a central tracking system, a patient may have multiple EHRs scattered across these providers. Rarely are these multiple records integrated. As a result, each EHR may reflect a different and incomplete perspective of a patient's health care experience.

To estimate potential drug exposures, for example, researchers can make inferences from administrative claims sources based on pharmacy dispensing records, whereas inferences for EHR systems rely on patient self-report and physician prescribing orders (Hennessy 2006). Neither approach reflects the timing, dose, or duration of drug ingested; hence, assumptions are required in interpretation of all study results. There are a number of linked databases becoming available recently, in which claims data are linked for each patient to EHR data, providing a more complete and richer source of data, potentially, than either source alone.

For both administrative claims and EHRs, B–R analyses are considered a secondary use of the data. Therefore, the onus is on the researcher to fully understand and assess the relative strengths and limitations of each potential source before conducting an evaluation (US FDA 2013a). Data recorded in either system reflect data used for its primary intent and therefore may not necessarily represent the optimal information for study.

7.4.3 Distributed Network Approach

Mini-Sentinel is a pilot project, initiated by the FDA in 2010, to test the FDA's plan to create the Sentinel System. Mini-Sentinel uses preexisting electronic health care data from multiple sources. In general, collaborating institutions offer scientific and organizational expertise. Some of the databases are administrative databases. Mini-Sentinel uses a distributed data model. Upon receiving a query from the FDA, data partners will transform their own data to the Mini-Sentinel common data model. The coordinating center distributes analytic codes (e.g., SAS codes) to data partners via the distributed querying portal. Data partners use the codes to analyze their own data and return summary data to the coordinating center via the secured distributed query portal. The coordinating center reviews and analyzes the summary data. It then provides a detailed report to the FDA. The coordinating center does not have access to patient-level data, which remain with individual data partners. In 2015, the FDA began the process to transition Mini-Sentinel to a fully operational Sentinel System.

7.4.4 Bias and Confounding

Identifying and controlling systematic error (bias) in observational studies is a critical concern in ensuring the validity of the study results. Bias can arise from a number of sources and can be classified into three types: inappropriately selected study subjects (selection bias), errors during data collection/definition (information bias), and confounding. Most prominent in pharmacoepidemiology is confounding that arises when the indication for treatment is an independent risk factor for the outcome of interest (known as "confounding by indication"). For example, a treatment for diabetes may be under investigation for CV events, but diabetes itself confers an increased risk of the same events. Proton pump inhibitors are given to patients with gastrointestinal (GI) symptoms that may represent early signs of GI bleeding; thus, the medication may appear to be associated with increased risk of bleeding, despite having demonstrated efficacy at preventing GI bleeding in randomized trials (Hernán et al. 2004). A full discussion of the various sources of bias in epidemiologic studies is beyond the scope of this chapter. For a more thorough understanding of these issues, a number of standard textbooks would provide a useful starting point (Hartzema et al. 2008; Varadhan et al. 2013).

7.5 Registries as a Data Source to Enable B–R Assessment

A patient registry is an organized system that uses observational study methods to uniformly collect data (clinical and other) to evaluate specified outcomes for a population defined by a particular disease, condition, or exposure, and that serves a predetermined scientific, clinical, or policy purpose (Polygenis 2013). The registry database is the file(s) derived from the registry.

Registries are particularly important for understanding real-world treatment use of a drug. They provide an opportunity to assess patient responses to treatment, in terms of safety and effectiveness. Registries allow for a wide variety of observational study design options including prospective cohort studies with nested case–control analysis, new-user cohort design, retrospective cohorts for events with short induction times, natural history studies, cohort studies with internal comparators, linkage or supplementary data collection, and case–control studies. Disease registries can also be used as a source of subjects for RCTs. When a medicine is already on the market and there is adequate follow-up information in many patients taking the medicine in the registries, then registries could be used to supply a nonrandomized comparator group of patients using the medicine for another study.

Registries allow for a large number of subjects to be followed, which is an asset for rare safety events and for studying treatment heterogeneity. They are especially beneficial when information is not available in other settings and for events that would not come to the attention of traditional care providers or health care systems. Furthermore, registries are valuable when data on patient-reported information are needed and for rare conditions. For these reasons, registries are often thought of as having great depth of data, but they can also be limited in the breadth of data they collect. In some settings, then, it might be desirable to be able to link registry data to claims data or to EHRs.

Because patients in registries typically are not randomized to the treatments they received, observational studies using registry data face the same challenges as described in Section 7.4. Depending on how diligent a registry owner is in collecting data on registry patients, data quality could vary substantially across registries. (Hence, a well-done registry may not be much less expensive than a randomized trial.) Data quality could clearly influence B–R assessment. In some registries, one may not be able to robustly define comparison groups and information provided about the external validity of a registry sample may be limited. These factors must be considered when attempting to draw inferences based on analyses of registry data (Sedrakyan et al. 2010). In addition, it is important to consider whether most or all important covariates were collected, how complete and accurate the data were, and how missing information was handled in the registry.

7.6 Principles of Using Information from Different Data Sources for B–R Assessment

We have shown that data from different sources could be used to provide information needed for B–R assessment. A natural question is how data from different sources should be used to supplement each other. In this section, we list a set of principles in addressing this question.

7.6.1 Hierarchy of Evidence from Different Data Sources

We can group safety data into three categories, those from clinical trials, those from spontaneous reports, and those from observational studies including registries. The primary objective of looking at data from these different data sources is to check for consistency in information across data sources and to look for information that is unique to certain sources.

Green and Byar (1984) discussed the hierarchy of strength of evidence concerning efficacy of a treatment. They list confirmed randomized controlled clinical trials as providing the highest level of strength, followed by a single randomized controlled clinical trial, series based on historical control groups, case–control observational studies, analyses using computer databases, series with literature controls, and case series without controls. At the bottom of this pyramid are anecdotal case reports. There are notable sublevels in the above hierarchy. For examples, double-blinded RCTs are generally considered to offer higher-quality evidence than open-label randomized RCTs, and cohort studies are considered to have a higher validity than case–control studies.

The above hierarchy is not directly applicable to safety because different data sources often offer different types of information that, when viewed together, helps us understand the risk of a product. While RCTs provide the best characterization of product-induced common adverse reactions, one may not observe drug-related rare events in these trials because of limited exposure and highly selected trial populations. On the other hand, a couple of spontaneous reports of an event that is uncommon but known to be strongly associated with drug exposure (e.g., angioedema, hepatic injury, Stevens-Johnson syndrome, and agranulocytosis) by patients using a product strongly suggest the drug–event relationship (Wittes et al. 2015).

7.6.2 Strategies in Using Data from Different Sources

In general, we do not recommend combining data from uncontrolled trials (e.g., extension trials) with those from controlled trials. Data from the uncontrolled trials could offer additional information and can check if rates from the uncontrolled trials are generally similar to those obtained in randomized trials or those observed in claims or medical records data. However, the lack of a randomized control could lead to issues such as the Simpson's paradox (confounding) (Chuang-Stein and Beltangady 2011) if we pool data from trials with and without a control group.

For rare and serious events that appear only in uncontrolled extension trials, we can compare the rates of these events (adjusted for exposure) with the background rates obtained from epidemiologic studies. Nevertheless, this comparison must be made with caution since background rates from epidemiologic studies are appropriate as a reference only if we can identify the right population, that is, a population that is similar to the clinical trial sample, with respect to disease severity and risk factors so that a comparison is more likely to be valid. We discussed this point briefly in Section 7.2.

Spontaneous reports are particularly useful to identify rare events or adverse reactions in high-risk populations. Spontaneous report systems remain the source in which a rare adverse reaction is often first identified. For spontaneous reports, we can evaluate reporting rates over time since product launch (see Section 7.3.1). Spontaneous report systems offer information concerning risk but do not offer information on benefit.

Observational studies using administrative databases or EHRs have gained popularity. They constitute an increasing percentage of postauthorization safety studies required by regulators. There are several major findings from the Observational Medical Outcomes Partnership (OMOP), which was a public–private partnership established to inform the appropriate use of observational health care databases for studying the effects of medical products (see http://omop.org/). One lesson is the substantial heterogeneity across different observational databases. OMOP researchers found that for the same design and analytical method, different databases may yield very different treatment effect estimates (Madigan et al. 2013b). Next, for the same database, different analytic design choices may yield quite different estimates (Madigan et al. 2013c). Furthermore, on the basis of empirical evaluation, most observational methods were found not to have the nominal statistical operating characteristics these methods are set out to achieve (Ryan et al. 2013c). Issues identified by OMOP researchers are likely to be relevant to findings from the Mini-Sentinel or Sentinel System as well.

Because of the above, we do not recommend combining results from published observational studies as a general principle. However, meta-analyses or systematic reviews of observational studies may be warranted for the following situations:

- To assess the need to conduct a randomized trial because of weaknesses of available observational studies or the inability of observational studies to answer an important question
- To provide evidence of the comparative effect of treatments that cannot be randomized or of outcomes that are unlikely to be studied in randomized trials (e.g., birth defects in newborns)
- To gain information on treatment effect in subgroups typically not studied in clinical trials

We can display results from different data sources using some of the B–R graphs discussed by Wen et al. (2016). For example, results from different sources could be noted by different colors in the same forest plot and compared visually for consistency. We could use data from different sources to create a range of values for a clinical endpoint in a tornado diagram. As stated earlier, we do not recommend combining data across different types of data sources. In other words, we do not recommend combining RCTs with spontaneous reports, combining RCTs with observational studies, and combining spontaneous reports with observational data.

There may be unique situations when combining results from different data sources may be justified in order to improve the precision in estimating a treatment effect. For example, if a manufacturer observed two cases of PML in clinical trials and there were seven spontaneous reports of PML over a period after product launch, is there a reasonable way to combine the information quantitatively to better estimate the rate of PML if (1) there is a mechanism to closely track the postlaunch patient population and (2) the postlaunch patient population is reasonably similar to the clinical trial population? While this sounds reasonable and may even be desirable, combining data in this fashion will require a great deal of care because of the heterogeneity existing between the patient populations and other factors. Methods for this type of formal combination of data, to our knowledge, have not yet been broadly researched and developed.

7.7 Examples

7.7.1 Example 1. The Case of Terfenadine

Terfenadine (trade name: Seldane in the United States; Triludan in the United Kingdom; and Teldane in Australia) was the first nonsedating antihistamine approved in the United

States for the treatment of allergic rhinitis in 1985. Because of its nonsedating feature, it quickly became a market leader for allergic rhinitis. According to terfenadine's manufacturer, more than 100 million people worldwide used the drug by mid-1990. For the year 1991 alone, 17 million new and refill prescriptions were written for terfenadine (Thompson et al. 1996).

Thompson et al. (1996) stated that reports of serious ventricular arrhythmias associated with terfenadine use began to surface after the product launch. In June 1990, the Pulmonary–Allergy Drugs Advisory Committee of the FDA issued a report identifying risk factors for these events. The risk factors included concomitant use of macrolide antibiotics and the antifungal ketoconazole. In August 1990, under the FDA's directive, the manufacturer sent a "Dear Doctor" letter to all practicing physicians in the United States notifying them of the problem. In July 1992, a black-box warning and new contraindication were added to terfenadine's label to inform the public of the potential for terfenadine users to experience drug–drug interactions. In the years before 1997, the FDA documented 40 cases of serious cardiac dysrhythmias and 17 deaths associated with the use of terfenadine (Hughes et al. 2007).

Temple (2007) stated that it did not take long for regulators and researchers to realize that the reported torsade de pointes ventricular arrhythmias occurred almost solely in people taking inhibitors of cytochrome P450 3A4. These P450 3A4 inhibitors blocked the metabolism of terfenadine to fexofenadine. Because of the near-complete metabolism of terfenadine to fexofenadine by the liver immediately after leaving the gut, terfenadine normally is not measurable in the plasma. However, in the presence of a P450 3A4 inhibitor, terfenadine level in the plasma rises. Unfortunately, terfenadine itself is cardiotoxic at higher doses. It was also found that the active metabolite fexofenadine was responsible for virtually all the antihistamine activity of terfenadine without the arrhythmic risk (see, e.g., Roy et al. 1996).

With the above discovery, the FDA took steps to decrease concomitant use of 3A4 inhibitors with terfenadine, as described above. The measure succeeded to some extent, but not completely. Reports of fatalities continued to come in. The FDA kept terfenadine on the market even after the approval of another nonsedating antihistamine, loratadine, in 1993. Loratadine does not have proarrhythmic potential. The FDA's decision to keep terfenadine on the market after loratadine's approval was attributed to its reluctance to leave patients with only one relatively new nonsedating antihistamine choice. It is well recognized that patients' responses to drugs differ and there was limited experience with loratadine then. It is understandable that the FDA was cautious about loratadine after the experience with terfenadine. Eventually, terfenadine's manufacturer was able to synthesize fexofenadine and develop it into a drug. Fexofenadine was approved by the FDA in 1998. Upon fexofenadine's approval, terfenadine was removed from the market.

Considering that terfenadine was used by hundreds of millions of people, the number of registered cases of torsade de pointes was low. A significant challenge in conducting B–R assessment in the case of terfenadine is how to weigh a rare, serious adverse event against a non-lifesaving benefit of symptomatic improvement that is present in a large percentage of terfenadine users. Symptomatic improvement can be very important to many users afflicted by the debilitating allergy. In making regulatory decisions about terfenadine, Temple (2007) emphasized that in making decisions about terfenadine, the FDA (1) recognized the importance of nonsedating antihistamine to patients; (2) concluded that giving patients only a single nonsedating choice, loratadine, would not meet patients' needs; (3) realized that the regulatory actions to remove concomitant use of terfenadine with 3A4 inhibitors did not achieve the zero occurrence goal concerning torsade de pointes; and (4) recognized that the availability of fexofenadine made terfenadine superfluous.

The steps of aggregating individual case reports, identifying risk factors, and managing the identified risk have become part of the standard procedure to understanding spontaneous reports. Statistical methods such as the disproportionality analysis have been regularly used to help identify potential safety signals. Once a safety signal is identified and refined, determining whether benefit still outweighs risk becomes the next critical step.

7.7.2 Example 2. The Case of Hormonal Contraceptives

Combination hormonal contraceptives contain the synthetic hormones estrogen and progestin. When administered exogenously, these hormones inhibit the natural production of ovarian hormones. Pregnancy is prevented by a combination of preventing ovulation, increasing cervical mucus viscosity to make it less penetrable to sperm, and making the uterine endometrial lining inhospitable for implantation of an embryo. Hormonal contraceptives offer multiple benefits, but they also come with some risk. For example, all of the currently available hormonal contraceptives, including oral contraceptives (OCs), transdermal patches, and vaginal rings, carry a labeling warning of the risk of blood clots, specifically VTE. VTE risk increases with age, cigarette smoking, and other underlying risk factors. There are several different types of OCs, and numerous epidemiologic studies have been performed to characterize the risk of VTE associated with them. Both estrogen dose and the type of progestin contained in combination hormonal contraceptives appear to be associated with VTE risk.

Despite the known risks of these drugs, otherwise safe and effective contraceptive options are necessary to prevent unintended pregnancies. Despite family planning efforts, almost half of the approximately 6.4 million pregnancies in the United States are unintended. Many women who conceive do so while using contraceptives, and pregnancy is often associated with lack of adherence to the contraceptive regimen. In one study, the proportion of OC users who missed at least three birth control pills during a treatment cycle ranged from 30% to 51% over three cycles (Potter et al. 1996). We will return to the question of using real-world data for examining effectiveness of hormonal contraceptives below.

Information on risks of various CV events, including myocardial infarction, VTE, and cerebrovascular events, is incorporated into product labeling for all hormonal contraceptives. For example, the "Warnings" section of the Lessina (levonorgestrel and ethinyl) label (http://www.drugs.com/pro/lessina.html) starts with

> Cigarette smoking increases the risk of serious cardiovascular side effects from oral contraceptive use. This risk increases with age and with heavy smoking (15 or more cigarettes per day) and is quite marked in women over 35 years of age. Women who use oral contraceptives should be strongly advised not to smoke.

The above is followed by

> The use of oral contraceptives is associated with increased risks of several serious conditions including myocardial infarction, thromboembolism, stroke, hepatic neoplasia, gallbladder disease, and hypertension, although the risk of serious morbidity or mortality is very small in healthy women without underlying risk factors. The risk of morbidity and mortality increases significantly in the presence of other underlying risk factors such as hypertension, hyperlipidemias, obesity and diabetes.

In the same section, the label states that "Throughout this labeling, epidemiologic studies reported are of two types: retrospective or case control studies and prospective or cohort studies." It goes on to explain what these types of studies can offer and refer readers to a text on epidemiologic studies. In other words, the information included in the product labels is exclusively based on epidemiologic studies, mostly using large administrative databases (either health insurance claims or electronic medical records databases).

Epidemiologic studies are needed to study VTE because it is a relatively infrequent event in a generally healthy population. Phase III trials are typically not large enough to study the incidence of VTE. Consider ORTHO EVRA (norelgestromin and ethinyl), a contraceptive patch, which is no longer available as a branded product in the US market (for reasons unrelated to risk of VTE) but is still available outside the United States as EVRA. Of the 3330 subjects who received ORTHO EVRA in the Phase III studies, only two events of pulmonary embolus occurred that the investigators judged to be possibly, probably, or very likely related to study drug treatment (see http://www.fda.gov/downloads/advisorycommittees/committeesmeetingmaterials/drugs/reproductivehealthdrugsadvisorycommittee/ucm282636.pdf).

Epidemiologic studies were also used to compare the so-called third-generation OCs with second-generation OCs for their VTE risk. Second-generation OCs are OCs that contain progestins such as levonorgestrel and norgestimate. Third-generation OCs contain progestins such as desogestrel, gestodene (not available in the United States), or etonogestrel, which were introduced to the contraceptive market years after the second-generation OCs. A published meta-analysis (Hennessy et al. 2001) found a summary relative risk of 1.7 (third generation over second generation) with a 95% confidence interval of (1.3, 2.1). This is noted in the product labeling for third-generation OCs as an "approximate 2-fold increased risk" (http://www.fda.gov/downloads/advisorycommittees/committeesmeetingmaterials/drugs/reproductivehealthdrugsadvisorycommittee/ucm282636.pdf). Despite this labeled increased risk of VTE among women who use third-generation OCs, these drugs are kept on the market by health authorities and used by many women because of other product attributes. Women and their health care providers weigh the benefits and risks of various hormonal contraceptive options and compare them with other options available to them.

Because epidemiologic studies are exclusively used to assess the risk of rare events associated with OCs, it will be informative to look more closely at the scientific issues when using these studies to compare third-generation versus second-generation OCs. Beyond the general concerns about biases as discussed in Section 7.4, there is an additional concern that an observed association is spurious because of a phenomenon known as "depletion of susceptibles." This occurs when the risk of an outcome appears to decline as duration of exposure increases, because those at highest risk for the event experience it early in the course of treatment, leaving fewer high-risk individuals remaining in the population at later periods. Because desogestrel and gestodene were introduced into the market more recently than levonorgestrel, any given group of desogestrel and gestodene users is likely to contain a higher proportion of new starters of OCs than any given group of levonorgestrel users. If that were true, the implication would be that the desogestrel and gestodene users would contain a higher proportion of individuals with an elevated risk for VTE, because the "susceptibles" have not yet been depleted. Thus, the observed associations might have been an artifact of making a comparison between new users of desogestrel and gestodene with longer-term users of levonorgestrel.

To address the issue of depletion of susceptibles, Hennessy et al. (2001) conducted a meta-analysis comparing the risk for VTE for OCs containing desogestrel or gestodene versus levonorgestrel among first-time users with <1 year use. Three of the 12 studies contained the needed data. A meta-analysis of these three studies suggested an increased relative risk in the first year of use, with an estimated relative risk of 2.7 (95% confidence interval, 1.4–5.4) for desogestrel or gestodene versus levonorgestrel. This finding did not support the depletion-of-susceptibles theory in explaining the estimated relative risk of 1.7 obtained earlier.

7.7.3 Example 3. The Case of Natalizumab

Natalizumab (TYSABRI) is the first monoclonal antibody treatment for patients with relapsing forms of multiple sclerosis (MS) to reduce the frequency of clinical exacerbations. It received accelerated approval on November 23, 2004, based on results after approximately 1 year of treatment in two ongoing controlled trials designed with a treatment duration of 2 years. The first trial investigated natalizumab as a monotherapy versus placebo while the second trial investigated natalizumab as an add-on to another MS product, interferon beta-1a (AVONEX). The monotherapy trial showed that natalizumab reduced the risk for MS exacerbations by 66% when compared to placebo. The add-on trial showed that natalizumab, when added to AVONEX, reduced the risk of exacerbations by 54% compared to AVONEX alone. These results represented an important and meaningful benefit for patients with MS. At the time of the approval, approximately 1100 patients with MS had received Tysabri for 1 year or longer. As a condition for the approval, the manufacturer was required to continue the above two trials to show that the natalizumab continues to provide benefit.

On February 18, 2005, the FDA was notified of one fatal case of PML and another possible case of PML (which was later confirmed) that occurred in patients in the continuation phase of the above trials. On February 28, 2005, the manufacturer suspended marketing of natalizumab and stopped all dosing in clinical trials. At the time of marketing suspension, there were 5000 new patients receiving natalizumab postmarketing. These patients had received only a few doses and no PML was reported by them.

The manufacturer began a phase of extensive investigations to identify the link between Tysabri and PML. With some initial understanding of the risk factors, the manufacturer submitted an application to have the product reintroduced. After a thorough review of the manufacturer's Risk Management Plan and proposed changes to its original marketing application, the FDA determined that natalizumab should be made available, but under a restricted distribution program called TOUCH. The program contains the following features:

- Natalizumab will only be prescribed, distributed, and infused by prescribers, infusion centers, and pharmacies registered with the program.
- Natalizumab will only be administered to patients who are enrolled in the program.
- Before initiating the therapy, health care professionals are to obtain the patient's magnetic resonance imaging scan to help differentiate potential future MS symptoms from PML.
- Patients on natalizumab are to be evaluated at 3 and 6 months after the first infusion and every 6 months after that, and their status will be reported regularly to the manufacturer.

Ultimately, the manufacturer identified duration of therapy, prior use of immunosuppressants, and presence of anti-JC virus antibodies as the major risk factors for PML in patients receiving natalizumab. These risk factors were included in a boxed Warning and the "Warnings and Precautions" section of the label.

Through the restricted distribution implemented by the TOUCH Program, natalizumab patients are registered and regularly followed for PML. As a result, cases of observed PML in patients enrolled in the TOUCH Program can be used to estimate the incidence proportion of PML in natalizumab patients. The incidence proportions based on postmarketing data are included in Table 1 of the natalizumab label (TYSABRI 2013).

The natalizumab example shows the steps taken to keep a valued medicine on the market for patients in need. In this process, data from different sources were used together to develop a strategy to manage the risk of a product. By carefully managing the risk, the company was able to make the B–R profile for natalizumab more favorable. Natalizumab is not alone in this regard. Nevertheless, it is a clear example of the role of different data sources in optimizing the use of a pharmaceutical product.

7.7.4 Example 4. The Case of Hydroxyethyl Starches

Hydroxyethyl starch (HES) is a class of synthetic colloids that have been widely used for volume expansion and fluid resuscitation in critically ill patients with extensive blood loss, as well as for intraoperative fluid management during surgery. A number of HES products of varying molecular weights have been licensed around the world and in the United States. Preapproval trials for HES products were generally small RCTs in surgical patients. For example, the primary Phase III trial for US approval of Voluven (HES 130/0.4) was a randomized controlled equivalence study comparing HES 130/0.4 to HES 450/0.7 in 100 adult patients undergoing major elective orthopedic surgery (US FDA 2007).

For many years, there was considerable debate in the literature regarding the relative B–R profiles of colloid solutions including HES versus crystalloid solutions, such as saline, for volume expansion (Phillips et al. 2013). A small clinical trial published in 2001 suggested a possible association between use of HES and acute renal failure in patients with severe sepsis or septic shock (Schortgen et al. 2001). Over the next decade, a series of observational studies and small clinical trials investigating this association as well as associations between HES use and increased overall mortality in acutely ill patients were published. This in turn led to the publication of a number of meta-analyses of the safety and effectiveness of HES in critically ill patients. One systematic analysis of HES reviews identified 12 meta-analyses published between 2000 and 2010, 10 of which made unfavorable recommendations about HES (Hartog et al. 2012).

A larger clinical trial, Efficacy of Volume Substitution and Insulin Therapy in Severe Sepsis (VISEP) published in 2008, investigated intensive versus conventional insulin therapy and HES 200/0.5 versus modified Ringer's lactate in a 2 × 2 factorial design in patients with severe sepsis (Brunkhorst et al. 2008). That study was stopped early for safety, finding that HES was associated with increased incidence of renal failure. After publication of the VISEP trial, two large clinical trials were initiated in 2009, attempting to definitely resolve the question of the safety of HES use in critically ill patients. Results from both trials were published in 2012. The Scandinavian Starch for Severe Sepsis/Septic Shock (6S) trial, which included 804 patients, found a 17% increased risk of 90-day mortality and a 35% increased risk of need for renal replacement therapy for HES 130/0.42 versus Ringer's acetate in patients with severe sepsis (Perner et al. 2012). Both results were statistically significant. The Crystalloid versus Hydroxyethyl Starch Trial (Myburgh et al. 2012), which included just under 7000 patients, found a statistically nonsignificant 6% increased risk of 90-day mortality and a statistically significant 21% increased risk of need for renal replacement therapy for HES 130/0.4 in 0.9% saline versus 0.9% saline alone in a more heterogeneous population of patients admitted to an intensive care unit.

Regulatory agencies initiated public actions on HES risks starting in 2012. The FDA convened a public workshop on the risks and benefits of HES solutions (US FDA 2012). While a great deal of discussion at that workshop focused on the renal and mortality risks associated with HES, several participants also stressed the general lack of strong evidence of increased benefit of HES versus crystalloid solutions. The FDA released a Safety Communication on June 24, 2013 (subsequently revised on November 25, 2013), discussing a boxed warning for the entire class of HES products regarding the risk of increased mortality and need for renal replacement therapy in critically ill adult patients treated with HES and an additional warning of excessive bleeding associated with HES use in patients undergoing open heart surgery in association with cardiopulmonary bypass (US FDA 2013b). The EMA's Pharmacovigilance Risk Assessment Committee initiated a review of HES products on November 29, 2012, and issued a recommendation on June 13, 2013, that use of HES products be suspended in all patient populations (EMA 2013a,b). This recommendation was subsequently revised to allow for use of HES products in patients with hypovolemia caused by acute blood loss, "provided that appropriate measures are taken to reduce potential risks and that additional studies are carried out." The EMA explained its decision to continue to allow use of HES in certain settings by citing a series of studies showing volume-sparing effects and other hemodynamic advantages of HES products in surgical and trauma patients. Before issuing a final assessment report, the EMA solicited opinions from an ad-hoc expert group, who agreed that HES may have short-term benefit in managing perioperative bleeding.

This example highlights the effect of a slow accumulation of sometimes-ambiguous safety information postlicensure for a widely used class of products that were generally considered to be safe at the time of approval, despite limited premarket trial data. A series of observational studies, clinical trials, and meta-analyses ultimately led to the undertaking of multiple consensus clinical trials, which in turn supported imposition of boxed warnings in HES labels in the United States and indication restrictions in Europe.

While the postmarket safety concerns accumulated, decisive evidence of counterbalancing benefits for HES products relative to other available volume expanders generally failed to emerge, despite the opinions that HES may have benefits in certain settings.

7.8 Summary

In this chapter, we discuss the unique roles different data sources could play in B–R assessment. Different sources are important as they provide critical information at different stages during the life cycle of a pharmaceutical product. We use four examples to illustrate how clinical trials, spontaneous reports, and observational studies have been used to arrive at B–R decisions in real life. The examples help drive our messages, which can be summarized briefly as follows:

1. It is important to think how well an outcome of interest is captured in a particular data source.
2. Phase III clinical trials generally aim at assessing benefit. Safety assessment, while routinely conducted for these trials, is limited by treatment duration and the potential lack of heterogeneity among patients in these trials.

3. The incidence of a common drug-related AE can generally be characterized with reasonable precision based on data from Phase III clinical trials. This is not true with uncommon events.
4. Spontaneous report systems offer the first opportunity for risk assessment in the real-world setting after product launch.
5. Observational studies are subject to a range of potential biases, which need to be taken into account when evaluating risks and benefits.
6. So far, researchers have more experience using observational studies to assess safety. Experience using observational studies to investigate treatment effectiveness is nevertheless increasing.
7. We need to use all the data sources for B–R assessment at any particular point in time, staying fully aware of the limitations and specific biases associated with the data sources. While general principles are fine, each situation has its own unique aspects.

References

Alvarez-Requejo A, Carvajal A, Bégaud B, Moride Y, Vega T, Arias LH (1998) Under-reporting of adverse drug reactions. Estimate based on a spontaneous reporting scheme and a sentinel system. *Eur J Clin Pharmacol* 54(6):483–448.

Bonewit-West K, Hunt SA, Applegate E (2013) *Today's Medical Assistant: Clinical and Administrative Procedures*, 2nd edition. Elsevier.

Brunkhorst FM, Engel C, Bloos F, Meier-Hellmann A, Ragaller M, Weiler N, Moerer O, Gruendling M, Oppert M, Grond S, Olthoff D, Jaschinski U, John S, Rossaint R, Welte T, Schaefer M, Kern P, Kuhnt E, Kiehntopf M, Hartog C, Natanson C, Loeffler M, Reinhart K, German Competence Network Sepsis (SepNet) (2008) Intensive insulin therapy and pentastarch resuscitation in severe sepsis. *NEJM* 358(2):125–139.

Chuang-Stein C, Beltangady M (2011) Reporting cumulative proportion of subjects with an adverse event based on data from multiple studies. *Pharmaceutical Statistics* 10(1):3–7.

Cicero TJ, Adams EH, Geller A et al. (1999) A postmarketing surveillance program to monitor Ultram (tramadol hydrochloride) abuse in the United States. *Drug and Alcohol Dependence* 57:7–22.

CIOMS Working Groups III and V (1999) *Guidelines for Preparing Core Clinical-Safety Information on Drugs*. Council for International Organizations of Medical Sciences.

Daggumalli JSV, Martin IG (2012) Are pharmaceutical market withdrawals preventable? A preliminary analysis. *Drug Information Journal* 46(6):694–700.

European Medicines Agency (2013a) Press Release: PRAC confirms that hydroxyethyl-starch solutions (HES) should no longer be used in patients with sepsis or burn injuries or in critically ill patients, October 11, 2013. http://www.ema.europa.eu/ema/index.jsp?curl=pages/news_and_events/news/2013/10/news_detail_001917.jsp&mid=WC0b01ac058004d5c1 (accessed May 8, 2015).

European Medicines Agency (2013b) Assessment report for solutions for infusion containing hydroxyethyl starch, November 11, 2013. http://www.ema.europa.eu/docs/en_GB/document_library/Referrals_document/Hydroxyethyl_starch-containing_medicines_107/Recommendation_provided_by_Pharmacovigilance_Risk_Assessment_Committee/WC500154254.pdf (accessed May 11, 2015).

Gould AL, Lystig TC, Lu Y, Fu H, Ma H (2015) Methods and Issues to Consider for Detection of Safety Signals From Spontaneous Reporting Databases. A Report of the DIA Bayesian Safety Signal Detection Working Group. *Therapeutic Innovation & Regulatory Science* 49(1):65–75.

Green SB, Byar DP (1984) Using observational data from registries to compare treatments: The fallacy of omnimetrics. *Statistics in Medicine* 3:361–370.

Hammad TA, Neyarapally GA, Iyasu S, Staffa JA, Dal Pan G (2013) The future of population-based postmarket drug risk assessment: A regulator's perspective. *Clinical Pharmacology & Therapeutics* 94:349–358.

Hartog CS, Skupin H, Natanson C, Sun J, Reinhart K (2012) Systematic analysis of hydroxyethyl starch (HES) reviews: Proliferation of low-quality reviews overwhelms the results of well-performed meta-analyses. *Intensive Care Med* 38(8):1258–1271.

Hartzema AG, Tilson HH, Chan KA (editors) (2008) *Pharmacoepidemiology and Therapeutic Risk Management*. Cincinnati OH, Harvey Whitney Books Co.

Hazell L, Shakir SA (2006) Under-reporting of adverse drug reactions: A systematic review. *Drug Saf* 29(5):385–396.

Hennessy S (2006) Use of health care databases in pharmacoepidemiology. *Basic Clin Pharmacol Toxicol* 98:311–313.

Hennessy S, Berlin JA, Kinman JL, Margolis DJ, Marcus SM, Strom BL (2001) Risk of venous thromboembolism from oral contraceptives containing gestodene and desogestrel versus levonorgestrel: A meta-analysis and formal sensitivity analysis. *Contraception* 64:125–133.

Hernán MA, Hernández-Díaz S, Robins JM (2004) A structural approach to selection bias. *Epidemiology* 15(5):615–625.

Hughes D, Bayoumi AM, Pirmohamed M (2007) Current assessment of risk–benefit by regulators: Is it time to introduce decision analyses? *Clinical Pharmacology & Therapeutics* 82(2):123–127.

ICH E2C(R2). Periodic Benefit–Risk Evaluation Report (PBRER) (2012) Available at http://www.ich.org/fileadmin/Public_Web_Site/ICH_Products/Guidelines/Efficacy/E2C/E2C_R2_Step4.pdf (accessed April 12, 2015).

Ioannidis JP (2005) Why most published research findings are false. *PLoS Med* 2:e124.

Ishiguro C, Hinomura Y, Uemura K, Matsuda T (2014) Analysis of the factors influencing the spontaneous reporting frequency of drug safety issues addressed in the FDA's drug safety communications, using FAERS data. *Pharmaceutical Medicine* 28:7–19.

Kim JH, Scialli AR (2011) Thalidomide: The tragedy of birth defects and the effective treatment of disease. *Toxicological Sciences* 122(1):1–6.

Lewis JD, Brensinger C (2004) Agreement between GPRD smoking data: A survey of general practitioners and a population-based survey. *Pharmacoepidemiol Drug Saf* 13:437–441.

Lu G, Ades A (2004) Combination of direct and indirect evidence in mixed treatment comparisons. *Statistics in Medicine* 23(20):3105–3124.

Lumley T (2002) Network meta-analysis for indirect treatment comparisons. *Statistics in Medicine* 21(16):2313–2324.

Madigan D, Schuemie MJ, Ryan PB (2013a) Empirical performance of the case–control design: Lessons for developing a risk identification and analysis system. *Drug Saf* 36(1):73–82.

Madigan D, Ryan PB, Scheumie MJ (2013b) Does design matter? Systematic evaluation of the impact of analytical choices on effect estimates in observational studies. *Therapeutic Advances in Drug Safety* 4(2):53–62.

Madigan D, Ryan PB, Schuemie MJ et al. (2013c) Evaluating the Impact of Database Heterogeneity on Observational Study Results. *American Journal of Epidemiology* 178(4):645–651.

Marchenko O, Qi J, Chakravarty A, Ke C, Ma H, Maca J, Russek-Cohen E, Sanchez-Kam M, Zink RC, Chuang-Stein C (2015) Evaluation and review of strategies to assess cardiovascular risk in clinical trials in patients with type 2 diabetes mellitus. To appear in *Statistics in Biopharmaceutical Research* 7(4):253–266.

Matter G (2013) Problems in Research: Regulations—The Diethylstilbestrol Tragedy https://www.themedicalbag.com/article/problems-in-research-regulations-the-diethylstilbestrol-tragedy (accessed May 14, 2015).

Myburgh JA, Finfer S, Bellomo R, Billot L, Cass A, Gattas D, Glass P, Lipman J, Liu B, McArthur C, McGuinness S, Rajbhandari D, Taylor CB, Webb SA, CHEST Investigators, Australian and

New Zealand Intensive Care Society Clinical Trials Group (2012) Hydroxyethyl starch or saline for fluid resuscitation in intensive care. *NEJM* 367(20):1901–1911.

Ohlssen D, Kerman J, Fu H, Quartey G, Heilmann C, Ma H, Carlin B (2013) Guidance on the implementation and reporting of a drug safety Bayesian network meta-analysis. *Pharmaceutical Statistics* 2013. doi: 10.1002/pst.1592.

Perner A, Haase N, Guttormsen AB, Tenhunen J, Klemenzson G, Åneman A, Madsen KR, Møller MH, Elkjær JM, Poulsen LM, Bendtsen A, Winding R, Steensen M, Berezowicz P, Søe-Jensen P, Bestle M, Strand K, Wiis J, White JO, Thornberg KJ, Quist L, Nielsen J, Andersen LH, Holst LB, Thormar K, Kjældgaard AL, Fabritius ML, Mondrup F, Pott FC, Møller TP, Winkel P, Wetterslev J, 6S Trial Group, Scandinavian Critical Care Trials Group (2012) Hydroxyethyl starch 130/0.42 versus Ringer's acetate in severe sepsis. *NEJM* 367(2):124–134.

Phillips DP, Kaynar AM, Kellum JA, Gomez H (2013) Crystalloids vs. colloids: KO at the twelfth round? *Crit Care* 17(3):319.

Polinski, Jennifer M., Schneeweiss, Sebastian, Levin, Raisa, Shrank, William H (2009) Completeness of retail pharmacy claims data: Implications for pharmacoepidemiologic studies and pharmacy practice in elderly patients. *Clinical Therapeutics* 31(9):2048–2059.

Polygenis D (editor) (2013) *ISPOR Taxonomy of Patient Registries: Classification, Characteristics and Terms*. Lawrenceville, NJ.

Potter L, Oakley D, de Leon-Wong E, Cañamar R (1996) Measuring compliance among oral contraceptive users. *Family Planning Perspectives* 28:154–158.

Qiu H, Berlin JA, Stang PE (2015) Observational safety study design, analysis and reporting. In Jiang Q, Xia HA (eds.). *Quantitative Evaluation of Safety in Drug Development: Design, Analysis and Reporting*. CRC Press, Boca Raton FL, pages 125–140.

Quartey G, Ke C, Chuang-Stein C et al. (2016) Overview of benefit–risk evaluation methods: A spectrum from qualitative to quantitative. In *Benefit-Risk Assessment Methods in Medicinal Product Development: Bridging Qualitative and Quantitative Assessments*, in press.

Roy ML, Dumaine R, Brown AM (1996) HERG, a primary human ventricular target of the nonsedating antihistamine terfenadine. *Circulation* 94:817–823.

Ryan PB, Schuemie MJ, Gruber S, Zorych I, Madigan D (2013a) Empirical performance of a new user cohort method: Lessons for developing a risk identification and analysis system. *Drug Saf* 36(1):59–72.

Ryan PB, Schuemie MJ, Madigan D (2013b) Empirical performance of the self-controlled cohort design: Lessons for developing a risk identification and analysis system. *Drug Saf* 36(1):83–93.

Ryan PB, Stang PE, Overhage JM et al. (2013c) A Comparison of the Empirical Performance of Methods for a Risk Identification System. *Drug Saf* 36(1):143–158.

Schneeweiss S, Avorn J (2005) A review of uses of health care utilization databases for epidemiologic research on therapeutics. *J Clin Epidemiol* 58:323–337.

Sedrakyan A, Marinac-Dabic D, Normand SL et al. (2010) A framework for evidence evaluation and methodology studies. *Med Care* 48 (6 suppl):S121–S128.

Schortgen F, Lacherade JC, Bruneel F, Cattaneo I, Hemery F, Lemaire F, Brochard L (2001) Effects of hydroxyethylstarch and gelatin on renal function in severe sepsis: A multicentre randomised study. *Lancet* 357(9260):911–916.

Suchard MA, Zorych I, Simpson SE, Schuemie MJ, Ryan PB, Madigan D (2013) Empirical performance of the self-controlled case series design: Lessons for developing a risk identification and analysis system. *Drug Saf* 36(1):83–93.

Suissa S, Garbe E (2007) Primer: Administrative health databases in observational studies of drug effects—Advantages and disadvantages. *Nat Clin Pract Rheumatol* 3:725–732.

Telfair T, Mohan AK, Shahani S, Klincewicz S, Atsma WJ, Thomas A, Fife D (2006) Estimating post-marketing exposure to pharmaceutical products using ex-factory distribution data. *Pharmacoepidemiology and Drug Safety* 15:749–753.

Temple R (2007) Quantitative decision analysis: A work in progress. *Clinical Pharmacology & Therapeutics* 82(2):127–130.

Thompson D, Oster G (1996) Use of terfenadine and contraindicated drugs. *Journal of the American Medical Association* 275(17):1339–1341.

TYSABRI® label December 2013. Available at http://www.accessdata.fda.gov/drugsatfda_docs/label/2013/125104s840s847s889lbl.pdf (accessed April 1, 2015).

U.S. Food and Drug Administration Statistical Review and Evaluation for 6% hydroxyethyl starch 130/0.4 in 0.9% sodium chloride (Voluven®), November 16, 2007. http://www.fda.gov/BiologicsBloodVaccines/BloodBloodProducts/ApprovedProducts/NewDrugApplicationsNDAs/ucm163911.htm (accessed May 8, 2015).

U.S. Food and Drug Administration Guidance to Industry. Diabetes Mellitus—Evaluating Cardiovascular Risk in New Antidiabetic Therapies to Treat Type 2 Diabetes, December 2008. Available at: http://www.fda.gov/downloads/Drugs/GuidanceComplianceRegulatoryInformation/Guidances/ucm071627.pdf (accessed May 14, 2015).

U.S. Food and Drug Administration, Public Workshop on the Risks and Benefits of Hydroxyethyl Starch Solutions, Bethesda, MD, September 6–7, 2012. http://www.fda.gov/BiologicsBloodVaccines/NewsEvents/WorkshopsMeetingsConferences/ucm313370.htm (accessed May 8, 2015).

U.S. Food and Drug Administration (2013a), Guidance for Industry and FDA Staff—Best Practices for Conducting and Reporting Pharmacoepidemiologic Safety Studies Using Electronic Healthcare Data, May 2013. http://www.fda.gov/downloads/Drugs/GuidanceComplianceRegulatoryInformation/Guidances/UCM243537.pdf (accessed May 15, 2015).

U.S. Food and Drug Administration (2013b), Safety Communication: Boxed Warning on increased mortality and severe renal injury, and additional warning on risk of bleeding, for use of hydroxyethyl starch solutions in some settings, November 25, 2013. http://www.fda.gov/BiologicsBloodVaccines/SafetyAvailability/ucm358271.htm (accessed May 8, 2015).

Varadhan R, Segal JB, Boyd CM et al. (2013) A framework for the analysis of heterogeneity of treatment effect in patient-centered outcomes research. *Journal of Clinical Epidemiology* 66(8):818–825.

Wen S, He W, Evans S et al. (2016). Graphical presentations of benefit–risk profile. In *Benefit-Risk Assessment Methods in Medicinal Product Development: Bridging Qualitative and Quantitative Assessments*, in press.

Whitaker HJ, Farrington CP, Spiessens B, Musonda P (2006) Tutorial in biostatistics: The self-controlled case series method. *Statistics in Medicine* 25:1768–1797.

Wittes J, Crowe B, Chuang-Stein C et al. (2015) The FDA's final rule on expedited safety reporting: Statistical considerations. To appear in *Statistics in Biopharmaceutical Research* 7(3):174–190.

Section IV

Benefit–Risk Assessment Methods and Visual Tools

8

Overview of Benefit–Risk Evaluation Methods: A Spectrum from Qualitative to Quantitative

George Quartey, Chunlei Ke, Christy Chuang-Stein, Weili He, Qi Jiang, Kao-Tai Tsai, Guochen Song, and John Scott

CONTENTS

ABSTRACT It has long been understood that the benefits of a medical product should be assessed in the context of the risks or harms associated with that product, and vice versa. Until recently, however, drug development and regulatory decisions were usually based on informal, qualitative weighing of benefits and risks, often leading to opaque decisions. Now, pharmaceutical companies and other clinical organizations are increasingly using structured benefit–risk assessments (BRAs), sometimes including sophisticated quantitative methods, as part of their decision-making processes. There are also vast efforts from health authorities and academia to standardize, streamline, and improve the BRA process. In the wake of these initiatives, the field of structured BRA has blossomed, with major advances in methodology and implementation. As a result, a large number of methods have been proposed to facilitate the BRA, which also further complicates the BRA picture. In this chapter, we will discuss these different BRA methodologies and recommend a set of systematic methods for general use in the pharmaceutical industry. We will also describe some criteria to select the methods as well as challenges in applying them.

8.1 Introduction

It has long been understood that the benefits of a medical product should be assessed in the context of the risks or harms associated with that product, and vice versa. Until recently, however, drug development and regulatory decisions were usually based on informal, qualitative weighing of benefits and risks, often leading to opaque decisions. For example, although two experts may agree on a set of facts regarding the benefits and risks of a drug, the experts may not agree on accepting the risks given the demonstrated benefits of the drug.

Now, pharmaceutical companies are increasingly using structured benefit–risk assessment (BRA), sometimes including sophisticated quantitative methods, as part of their internal decision-making processes. Efforts are underway within the drug development community to enhance the evaluation and communication of the benefits and risks associated with pharmaceutical products, aimed at increasing the consistency, predictability, transparency, and efficiency of pharmaceutical regulatory decision making.

There are also vast efforts from health authorities and academia to standardize, streamline, and improve the BRA process. For example, the Prescription Drug User Fee Act (PDUFA) V commits the Food and Drug Administration (FDA) to a series of meetings and workshops during 2013–2018 to develop a BRA framework. The FDA released a 2013 draft benefit–risk (B–R) implementation plan entitled "Structured Approach to Benefit–Risk Assessment in Drug Regulatory Decision-Making" (FDA 2013). The European Medicines Agency (EMA) Benefit–Risk Methodology Project was aimed at the development and testing of tools and processes for balancing multiple benefits and risks, which could be used as an aid to informed, science-based regulatory decisions about medicinal products (EMA Methodology Project 2013; EMA Reflection Paper 2008). The Institute of Medicine recommended that the FDA create a publicly available BRA management plan with periodic updates. In addition, several other proposed structured BRA initiatives developed by the PhRMA BRAT (Pharmaceutical Research and Manufacturers of America Benefit–Risk Action Team) (Coplan et al. 2011), the Universal Methodology for Benefit–Risk Assessment (UMBRA) framework by the Centre for Innovation in Regulatory Science organization (Walker et al. 2015), the PrOACT-URL framework recommended by the EMA (Phillips et al. 2013), FDA Center for Devices and Radiological Health (CDRH) Decision Analysis Initiative and CDRH/Center for Biologics Evaluation and Research Benefit–Risk Guidance, and the Periodic Benefit–Risk Evaluation Report based on the International Conference on Harmonization of Technical Requirements for Registration of Pharmaceuticals for Human Use (ICH) Guidance (ICH E2C(R2) 2012) have placed a descriptive approach as a critical part of BRA.

In the wake of these initiatives, the field of structured BRA has blossomed with major advances in methodology and implementation. As a result, a large number of methods have been proposed to facilitate the BRA process, which also further complicates the BRA picture (Guo et al. 2010; Mt-Isa et al. 2014; Phillips et al. 2013). For example, the EMA Benefit–Risk Methodology Project Work Package 2 examined the applicability of 18 quantitative approaches for assessing the B–R balance and three qualitative frameworks (Phillips et al. 2013); the Innovative Medicines Initiative Pharmacoepidemiological Research on Outcomes of Therapeutics by a European Consortium WP5 recommended 13 methodologies for further examination in BRA of medicines (Mt-Isa et al. 2014); and the International Society for Pharmacoeconomics and Outcomes Research Risk-Benefit Management Working Group recommended 12 methods for use in BRA (Guo et al. 2010).

Although numerous approaches and frameworks have been proposed in recent years, there is no single approach or framework that can be applied and utilized in every setting. This is because BRA is often multifaceted and complex, and the goals of BRA in different settings (e.g., disease areas, clinical development stages) may be different. The suitability of the recommended methods still needs to be further explored in structured systematic BRAs to determine the circumstances they best fit and whether they could be used in clinical development settings. At the same time, the limitations of each proposed approach have not been well studied, and therefore, those carrying out the assessment often have difficulty in selecting an appropriate methodology. Also, the complexity of BRA increases with multiple data sources (i.e., electronic health records/claims databases from observational studies, spontaneous reporting data, and randomized clinical trial data), and synthesis of these different data sources into one assessment is very challenging because of differences in data quality, high heterogeneity, and the presence of diverse biases (Ioannidis 2005). Hence, better guidance on selecting and combining data sources is needed within these frameworks. Chapter 7 provides an excellent discussion on sources of data to enable BRA and will not be further discussed here.

There is therefore the need to define criteria to select a BRA method, make recommendations on appropriate methods for pharmaceutical industry, and address key challenges in applying these methods. Moreover, there is a desire to be more transparent and clearer in communicating the reasoning behind BRA decisions, including which benefits and risks are considered, how the evidence is interpreted, and what the implications of the evidence are for the BRA.

The Quantitative Sciences in the Pharmaceutical Industry B–R Working Group (QSPI BRWG) was formed in early 2013 with a vision to help ensure that BRA methods are well understood and broadly used by statisticians and quantitative scientists through training/education and to increase the role of statistical leadership in BRA through cross-functional collaboration as well as work with regulatory agencies to promote structured BRA. The group is composed of individuals from academia, industry, and regulatory agencies with a mission to facilitate the appropriate use and contribute to the progress of BRA methodology. In this chapter, the Methods subteam proposes some criteria to select BRA methods and recommends a set of systematic methods for general use in the pharmaceutical industry. Illustrative case studies are included to assist the readers with the use of relevant methods.

Following this introduction, the criteria for selecting BRA methods throughout the life cycle of a product are provided. Section 8.3 presents the recommended approach from the QSPI BRWG along with illustrative case studies/examples. Section 8.4 describes some challenges in applying the recommended methods. The chapter ends with discussions and conclusions in Section 8.5.

8.2 Criteria to Select BRA Methods

A large number of methods have been proposed or adapted to perform BRA in the literature (Guo et al. 2010; Mt-Isa et al. 2014; Phillips et al. 2013). There is no defined and agreed methodology to combine benefits and risks to allow direct comparisons. Various criteria have been used to evaluate the existing BRA methods. For example, in the EMA's evaluation of quantitative approaches, the appraisal was based on the following criteria: *Logical soundness*, *Comprehensiveness*, *Acceptability of results*, *Practicality*, and *Generativeness* (Phillips et al. 2013). The IMI PROTECT initiative also undertook a systematic review and classification of methodologies for BRA, where appraisal of existing methods was based on four predefined criteria: *Principle* (if the reasoning is theoretically correct), *Features* (number of criteria, number of options, capacity to deal with uncertainty), *Accessibility* (if it is easy to use or not), and *Visualization* (the proposed visual representation of the results and if there is software to implement them). None of the BRA approaches satisfied all the criteria used by both the EMA WP2 project and the IMI PROTECT. Indeed, many of the criteria are not even relevant to some of the approaches. Thus, we will propose the following simplified criteria in selecting and recommending BRA methods for use in a pharmaceutical setting.

8.2.1 Intuitive

The BRA method should be easy to understand and able to integrate benefits and risks in a direct and natural way. Graphical presentation should be used whenever applicable. The BRA method should allow communication of the B–R conclusion to the general public. The B–R conclusion should be interpretable. The B–R method can be standardized, can be readily implemented, and is easy to extend to more complex situations. It should be practical, with ease of use and available computer software.

8.2.2 Comprehensive

The B–R approach should allow for the incorporation of many important aspects of BRA, that is, include discussion of factors that affect B–R decision and steps to perform B–R assessment; should accommodate multiple benefit and risk endpoints; and handle all relevant data types (i.e., qualitative or quantitative, objective or subjective discrete data). The approach should allow for more systematic accounting of various sources of uncertainty.

8.2.3 Scientifically Sound

The steps and components of the B–R evaluation should be theoretically and clinically meaningful and relevant. Integration of benefits and risks can be made in a sensible and logically sound way. The method should be internally consistent and coherent. The B–R conclusion should be interpretable and viable.

8.2.4 Broadly Applicable

The BRA method should be applicable throughout the life cycle of a drug and in different therapeutic areas by capturing the full range of decisions and critical issues from premarket to postmarket setting.

8.3 The QSPI BRA Approach

Based on the set of criteria described in Section 8.2, we present six key BRA approaches that satisfy these requirements and provide guidance and cautions on the use of them. For the purposes of this chapter, a "qualitative BRA" is defined as a descriptive approach that focuses on the individual benefits and risks, including their frequency and duration, and fully describes how that information weighs into decision making. The term *quantitative BRA* encompasses approaches that seek to quantify benefits and risks, as well as the weight that is placed on each of the components. A quantitative BRA uses the weights to combine benefits and risks into a B–R measure (or utility index). The B–R measure together with its variability and how the measure varies as a function of the weights forms the basis for B–R decisions.

Figure 8.1 provides an illustration of the QSPI-recommended approach: The descriptive qualitative benefit–risk framework (DBRF) forms the centerpiece, starting point, or foundation of any BRA. It can be used to select, organize, summarize, and communicate data relevant to a B–R decision. A DBRF may be complemented with quantitative BRA methods when appropriate. For example, when there are major benefit or risk issues on which decision makers have divergent views, quantification could capture the issues of contention that a qualitative B–R framework alone is unable to. Also, as interventions are given to individuals, it is important to look at benefit and risk at the patient level to help us identify subgroups of patients who may experience greater benefits without associated increase in risks.

Therefore, a DBRF may be complemented with the other five BRA methods when appropriate. These include (i) methods for evaluating benefits and risks at each patient level to provide important insight on the interaction of benefits and risks across subsets and over time, (ii) methods for quantifying patient preference and satisfaction, (iii) methods that handle a single benefit and a single risk endpoint, (iv) methods for synthesizing multiple

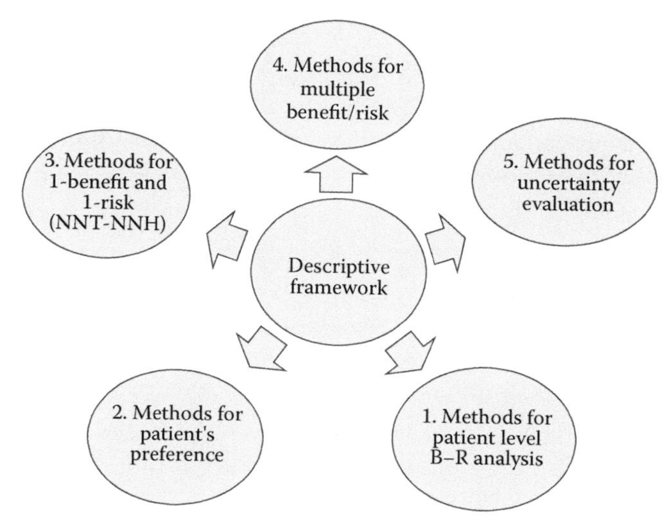

FIGURE 8.1
QSPI BRA approach.

benefit and risk criteria, and finally (v) methods for characterizing uncertainty in B–R evaluation.

We provide brief descriptions of the recommended methods together with examples/case studies.

8.3.1 Descriptive Benefit–Risk Framework

A DBRF is a set of tools to select, organize, and summarize the relevant facts, uncertainties, and key areas of judgment, and communicate data relevant to any B–R decision. The DBRF provides an explicit process (systematic, transparent, consistent, predictable) that can be used to implement other BRA methods and to articulate the reasoning behind BRA decisions. The DBRF can incorporate both evaluative judgments from different perspectives (e.g., sponsor, physician, patient) as well as quantitative data (e.g., statistical analysis outputs) to inform trade-offs between multiple benefit and multiple risk elements in a logically consistent and transparent manner. This approach can handle all relevant data types (i.e., qualitative or quantitative, objective or subjective discrete data) and can be adapted to any stage of product development (pre- and postmarket) and updated as new information emerges. For DBRF, explicit trade-off is not required, and tabular and visual summary of key benefits and risks (Coplan et al. 2011; Walker et al. 2015) can support discussion around overall B–R balance.

Several DBRFs are proposed (Coplan et al. 2011; FDA 2013; Phillips et al. 2013; Walker et al. 2015). For example, the FDA has adopted a five-step structured qualitative approach that is designed to support the identification and communication of the key considerations in FDA's BRA (FDA 2013). The EMA eight-step PrOACT-URL (problem, objectives, alternatives, consequences, trade-offs, uncertainty, risk, and linked decisions) provides a framework for addressing the necessary elements in decision problems and has also been repeatedly used as the basis for other methodologies (Phillips et al. 2013). BRAT was developed to standardize and communicate BRA between the pharmaceutical companies and the regulators and presents B–R results of individual criteria as forest plots (Coplan et al. 2011). The UMBRA follows the same principles and contains all the key features of the other frameworks (Walker et al. 2015).

These approaches are quite similar in their most basic forms (Figure 8.2): defining the context in which the decision is being made, identifying the important relevant information and data regarding benefits and risks, assessing that information with respect to its bearing on the decision, drawing conclusions from the information based on expert judgment, and communicating the decision and its rationale.

We illustrate the use of a DBRF in BRA with data from the FDA Arthritis Advisory Committee meeting in 2012 (FDA Advisory Committee 2012). In this example, we followed a structured systematic approach for tofacitinib 3-month placebo-controlled trial data in order to produce a graphical representation of the B–R profile in patients with moderate to severe rheumatoid arthritis (RA) who had an inadequate response or intolerance to nonbiologic and/or biologic DMARDs (disease-modifying antirheumatic drugs). Five Phase 3 and

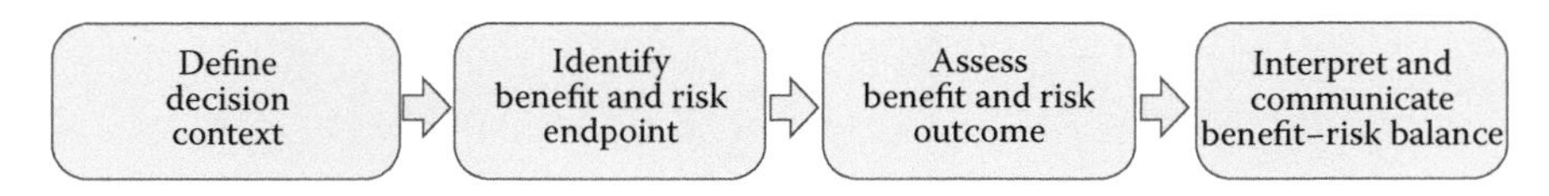

FIGURE 8.2
Basic structure of DBRF.

four Phase 2 randomized, placebo-controlled studies (one study with adalimumab as active control) and data from two open-label long-term extension studies with continued exposure to up to 3 years as well as published data of other antirheumatic drugs on the market such as adalimumab, certolizumab, etanercept, golimumab, infliximab, tocilizumab, abatacept, and anakinra were used (see http://www.fda.gov/downloads/AdvisoryCommittees/CommitteesMeetingMaterials/Drugs/ArthritisAdvisoryCommittee/UCM302960.pdf). We described the basic four-step DBRF for tofacitinib as follows:

Step 1. Define the decision context

The first step in using a DBRF is to provide the context for the analysis (including the disease or condition, the patient population, the time frame, and the stakeholder perspective). For this example, the decision context was whether tofacitinib should be given marketing approval at the time of registration.

Population and indication: Patients with moderate to severe RA who had an inadequate response or intolerance to nonbiologic or biologic DMARDs.

Unmet medical need: Multiple therapeutic options to treat RA; there is limited treatment success rate and the need for additional therapeutic options. Tofacitinib is an oral agent with novel mechanisms of action.

Decision questions: Is the drug effective regarding clinically relevant parameters? What are the safety risks for 5- and 10-mg doses? Are the risks compelling compared to the approved biologics? Are the risks manageable?

Step 2. Identify benefit and risk endpoints

Key considerations of benefits and risks of tofacitinib, as measured by efficacy responses and safety events of special interest, were identified and displayed in a value tree graph (Figure 8.3): The value tree contains identified/potential outcomes and serves as a basis for a transparent discussion of underlying assumptions about B–R of a drug and underlying data. The benefits of tofacitinib treatment in the DMARD population were defined as endpoints for signs and symptoms, progression of joint damage and disability. For signs and symptoms, improvement from baseline as measured by the American College of Rheumatology (ACR) criteria was selected. Disease Activity Score in 28 joints (DAS28) and health-related quality of life or disability as measured by Health Assessment Questionnaire-Disability Index (HAQ-DI) and Functional Assessment of Chronic Illness Therapy-Fatigue scales (FACIT) were also included. The risks for this exercise included all-cause mortality, serious infections, lymphoma, lung cancer, gastrointestinal perforation, myocardial infarction, serious adverse events (AEs), herpes zoster, and malignancies.

Value trees should ideally be developed before known clinical trial results. The development should incorporate clinical judgment on the importance of the various potential benefits and risks. Nevertheless, the initial value tree may be modified to reflect data availability and emerging risks.

Step 3. Assessing benefit and risk

A graphical display of key benefit and risk elements was generated based on meta-analysis results. Results of the elements identified in the value tree are visually presented in Figure 8.4. The data displays illustrate how a DBRF can be used to compare key efficacy and safety endpoints. The goal is to present efficacy and safety data side by side to facilitate BRA.

Tofacitinib
Benefits
ACR20
ACR50
ACR70
DAS28 <= 3.2
DAS28 < 2.6
HAQ-DI improvement >= 0.3
FACIT >= 4
Risks
All-cause mortality
Serious infections
Malignancy (excl. NMSC)
Lymphoma
Lung cancer
Myocardial infarction
GI perforation
Herpes zoster

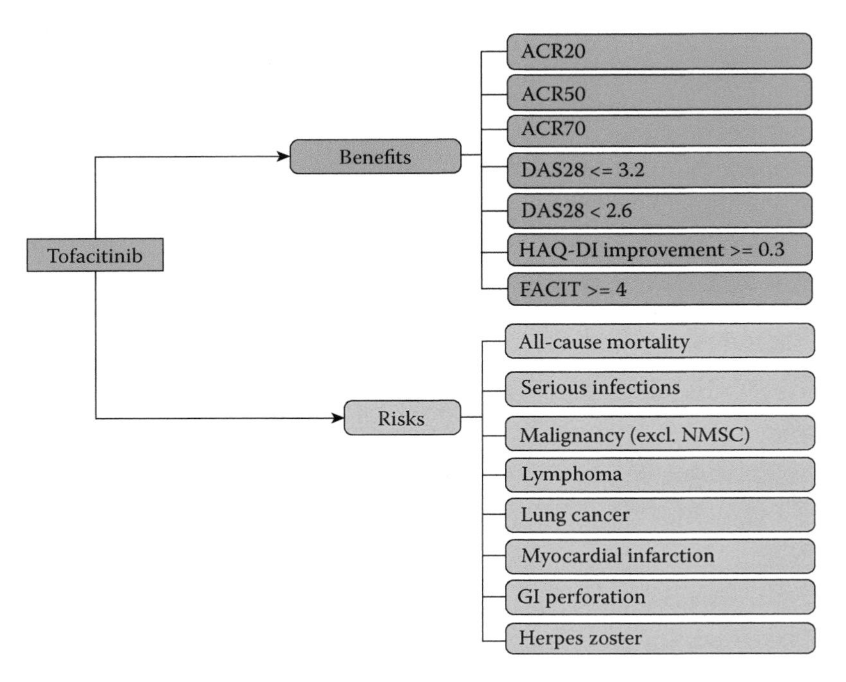

FIGURE 8.3
Value tree showing key benefits and risk endpoints.

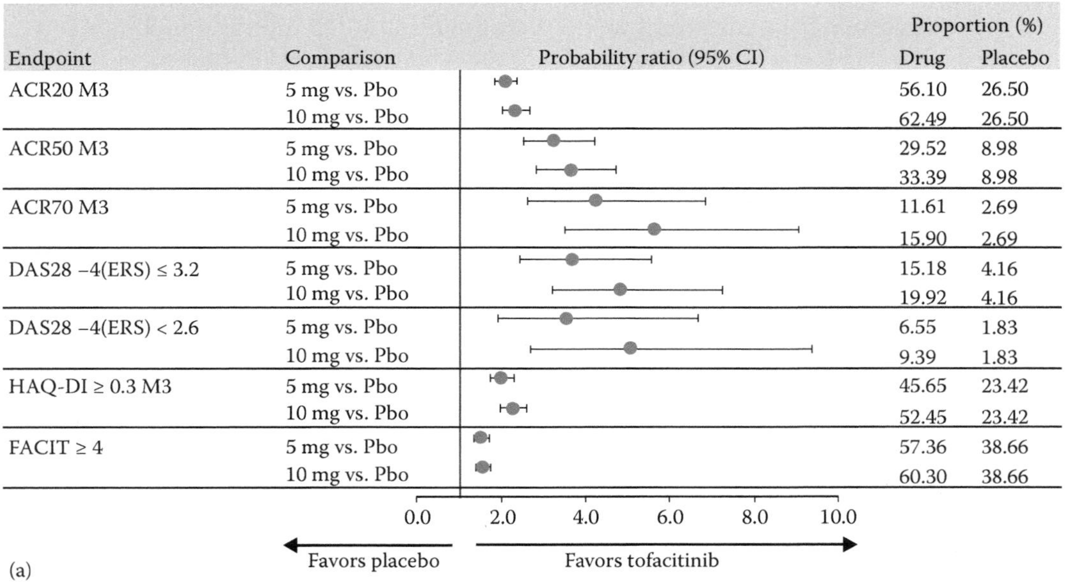

Endpoint
Comparison
Probability ratio (95% CI)
Proportion (%)
Drug
Placebo
ACR20 M3
5 mg vs. Pbo 56.10 26.50
10 mg vs. Pbo 62.49 26.50
ACR50 M3
5 mg vs. Pbo 29.52 8.98
10 mg vs. Pbo 33.39 8.98
ACR70 M3
5 mg vs. Pbo 11.61 2.69
10 mg vs. Pbo 15.90 2.69
DAS28 −4(ERS) ≤ 3.2
5 mg vs. Pbo 15.18 4.16
10 mg vs. Pbo 19.92 4.16
DAS28 −4(ERS) < 2.6
5 mg vs. Pbo 6.55 1.83
10 mg vs. Pbo 9.39 1.83
HAQ-DI ≥ 0.3 M3
5 mg vs. Pbo 45.65 23.42
10 mg vs. Pbo 52.45 23.42
FACIT ≥ 4
5 mg vs. Pbo 57.36 38.66
10 mg vs. Pbo 60.30 38.66
0.0
2.0
4.0
6.0
8.0
10.0
Favors placebo
Favors tofacitinib
(a)

FIGURE 8.4
Concise benefit and risk summary. (a) Clinical efficacy of tofacitinib 5 mg BID versus placebo and tofacitinib 10 mg BID versus placebo in Phase 3 studies (see http://www.fda.gov/downloads/AdvisoryCommittees/CommitteesMeetingMaterials/Drugs/ArthritisAdvisoryCommittee/UCM302960.pdf). *(Continued)*

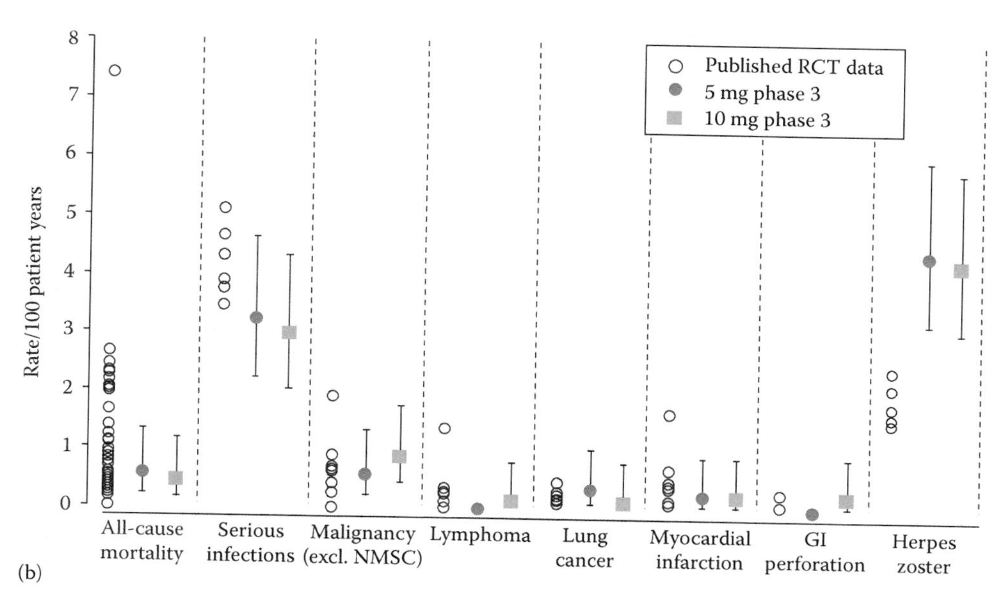

FIGURE 8.4 (CONTINUED)
Concise benefit and risk summary. (b) Safety profile of tofacitinib (5 mg and 10 mg dose) in Phase 3 studies versus clinical trial data of TNF inhibitors and other biologic DMARDs (see http://www.fda.gov/downloads/AdvisoryCommittees/CommitteesMeetingMaterials/Drugs/ArthritisAdvisoryCommittee/UCM302960.pdf).

Comparative risk–benefit plots were produced showing the probability difference (95% confidence interval [CIs]) between the tofacitinib and placebo groups in the percentage of patients with an ACR20/50/70 response at 3 months and the difference between tofacitinib and placebo in the rate per 100 patient-year (PY) (95% CI) of adverse events of special interest for the tofacitinib 5 mg/10 mg group (Figure 8.4a and b) (see http://www.fda.gov/downloads/AdvisoryCommittees/CommitteesMeetingMaterials/Drugs/ArthritisAdvisoryCommittee/UCM302960.pdf). For both doses of tofacitinib, clear improvements in efficacy endpoints are shown compared with placebo while differences in the rates of adverse events of special interest per 100 PY appear to be small except for herpes zoster.

Another key consideration is to identify and evaluate sources of uncertainty, including the sources of evidence, the strength of each piece of evidence, and how the uncertainty weighs on the decision. Uncertainty is shown with CIs. Although weighting is possible within a DBRF, weight was not described explicitly for this analysis. Variables can be rank ordered by levels of severity, or for different audiences in a DBRF. Value judgments can be displayed through rank ordering of variables, or through inclusion and exclusion of variables.

Step 4. Interpretation and communication

The results of this semiquantitative BRA of the tofacitinib clinical trial data show that the efficacy benefits of tofacitinib compared to placebo are robust, while the observed differences in safety event rates between tofacitinib and placebo-treated patients appear to be small except for herpes zoster. These observations support the overall positive BRA of tofacitinib treatment in patients with moderate to severe RA.

Overall, the DBRF has accomplished its purpose in framing the B–R problem and in clearly displaying the probability differences for the outcomes of interest. The framework is intended to guide users through framing and communicating their analyses.

8.3.2 Methods for Patient-Level Data Analysis

8.3.2.1 Discounting Benefit by Risk within an Individual

Since interventions are given to individuals, it is natural to look at benefit and risk experience at an individual level to decide if the total experience for the individual is more positive than negative. If the benefit outweighs adverse experience, the treating physician will likely advise the individual to stay on the intervention if other considerations are also positive (e.g., convenience of dosing, cost, and the nature of the adverse reaction). Looking at benefit and risk at the patient level can help us identify subgroups of patients who may experience greater benefits without associated increase in risks. If such subgroups could be characterized by biologically plausible factors and identified before the initiation of a treatment, this will make the treatment particularly appealing to these subgroups. The biologic factors to identify the subgroups could be prognostic, predictive, or both.

What are some measures to assess the net benefit within an individual? An early measure is quality-adjusted life-years (QALYs) used in cancer trials (Gelber et al. 1989). Discounting survival gain by the loss in quality of life is a natural way to incorporate treatment-induced toxicity into the overall assessment. Interestingly, QALYs have become the metric that some health technology agencies (e.g., the National Institute for Health and Care Excellence 2013) use to assess the cost-effectiveness of a new health technology even though we have not seen this measure used in any regulatory decision.

A measure similar to QALYs is time without symptoms of disease and toxic effects due to treatment (TWiST) (Gelber et al. 1989), again in evaluating cancer treatments. Instead of discounting survival by a factor (utility) that reflects the quality of life at different periods of the total survival, TWiST dismisses days when a patient experienced disease symptoms or toxic effects from the total survival days. One can combine the concept of quality of life with that of TWiST to arrive at quality-adjusted TWiST (Q-TWiST) (Glasziou et al. 1990). For Q-TWiST, QALYs lost because of disease symptoms and treatment toxicities are subtracted from the total QALYs.

Because quality of life is generally subjective, sensitivity analysis is often conducted when using QALYs and Q-TWiST as the net benefit measures. For example, Glasziou et al. (1990) suggested a threshold utility analysis that compares treatments across all combinations of the utility used to describe the quality of life at predefined time intervals in constructing Q-TWiST.

QALYs, TWiST, and Q-TWiST use time as the basic scale to measure benefit and risk. Benefit measured in survival is discounted to account for compromised quality of life or toxicities associated with treatment. The idea of discounting benefit by treatment-associated risk was used by Chuang-Stein (1994) to construct a benefit-less-risk (BLR) score for each individual when benefit and risk are measured on different scales. To construct the BLR, Chuang-Stein used an approach proposed by Chuang-Stein et al. (1992) to consolidate important safety experience on an intervention into a risk score for each individual. The decision on what safety experience to include in constructing the risk score depends on the disease being treated. For a disorder such as cancer, serious adverse reactions may be the only risks that need to be considered. On the other hand, adverse reactions such as slight liver function elevation can be of substantial concern when treating patients with mildly elevated cholesterol but otherwise healthy.

The risk score for an individual is based on the individual's adverse reaction experience using prespecified rules. The severities of the reactions as well as the relative importance of the adverse reactions jointly determine an individual's risk score. Once a risk score is determined for an individual, Chuang-Stein (1994) proposed to bring the risk score to the scale as the benefit through a conversion factor f. Denote the risk score by R and the benefit by B. In the example considered by Chuang-Stein (1994), B is the increase in the treadmill exercise tolerance test time (in seconds) from baseline at the end of 4 weeks of treatment. As for the risk score, Chuang-Stein considered 10 system organ classes and used a prespecified rules to assign scores (0–3) to the overall safety experience within each system organ class. In addition, Chuang-Stein assigned weights to the 10 classes to reflect their relative importance to the overall well-being of patients. The risk score for each patient was derived as a linear combination of the weights and the scores within each class. Chuang-Stein proposed to construct a BLR score for each individual and offered a rationale for determining the conversion factor f in the treadmill example.

$$BLR = B - f \times R$$

Once a BLR score is constructed for each individual, treatments can be compared using the BLR scores. Sensitivity analysis should be conducted to see how results change as a function of the conversion factor f.

8.3.2.2 Classifying Benefit and Risk Jointly into Categorical Responses

Another approach to summarize benefit and risk at an individual level is to classify them jointly into B–R categories. Chuang-Stein et al. (1991) consider five categories: efficacy and no serious side effects, efficacy and serious side effects, no efficacy and no serious side effects, no efficacy and serious side effects, and side effects leading to withdrawal as displayed in Table 8.1. In Table 8.1, "serious side effects" could be replaced by "side effects of special interest" or a group of side effects determined to be important to the patient population. Under the classification, the observed proportions of the five categories for each treatment follow a multinomial distribution.

If one accepts that the five categories in Table 8.1 can be ordered (e.g., Category 1 > Category 2 ≥ Category 3 > Category 4 > Category 5), one can test if the distribution of the B–R response for one treatment is stochastically smaller than that of the other treatment. In other words, one can test the hypothesis that patients receiving one treatment have a higher probability to have their responses in a lower (the more desirable) category than patients receiving another treatment.

TABLE 8.1

Five B–R Categories to Describe Benefit and Risk Jointly at an Individual Level

		Efficacy	
		Yes	**No**
Serious side effects	No	Category 1	Category 3
	Yes	Category 2	Category 4
Side effects leading to withdrawal		Category 5	

Norton (2010, 2011) displays the distribution of the five categories over time graphically. Labeling the five outcomes as "Benefit Only" (Category 1), "Benefit + AE" (Category 2). "Neither" (Category 3), "AE only" (Category 4), and "Withdraw" (Category 5), Norton plotted each individual's outcome category at each of the six postrandomization assessment points for the two treatment groups in a 12-week trial. For ease of visualization, individuals in Figure 8.5 are arranged in such a way that dropouts are grouped together. Except for individuals who dropped out of the study, individuals could stay in or move to another B–R category from one assessment period to the next. For individuals who missed an intermediate B–R classification, one needs to decide in advance how to display the intermediate results for these individuals. One option is to take the worst of the two adjacent classifications surrounding the missing assessment period.

The display in Figure 8.5 clearly shows patients' B–R experience in a trial. Some descriptive statistics could be constructed for Figure 8.5. For example, one can compute the percentages of area occupied by the various colors and examine if one group has a higher percentage for the area in green.

One can include more than five B–R categories. For example, Entsuah and Gorman (2002) considered six categories: response with no AEs (Category 1); response with mild AEs (Category 2); response with moderate to severe AEs (Category 3); no response and no AEs, or discontinuation for lack of efficacy or a reason unrelated to treatment (Category 4); no response with mild AEs (Category 5); and no response and moderate to severe AEs, or discontinuation for AEs regardless of response (Category 6). Pritchett and Tamura (2008)

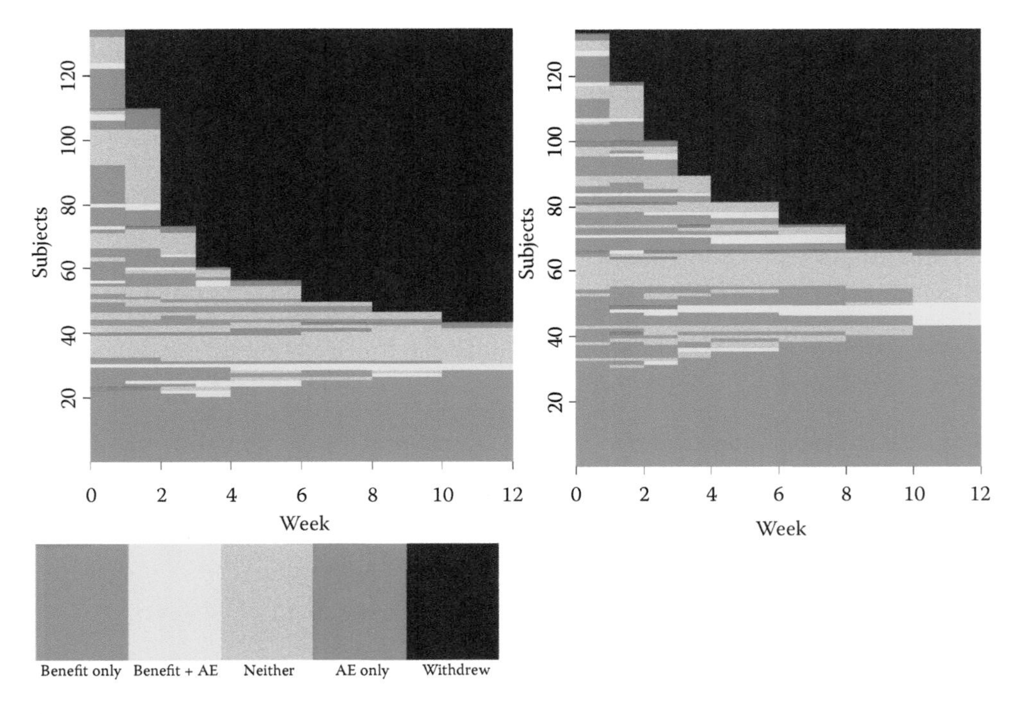

FIGURE 8.5
Display of five joint B–R classifications over time. The left panel pertains to the control group while the right panel pertains to the investigational treatment group (Courtesy of Norton, J. A longitudinal model for medical benefit–risk analysis, with case study. Presented at the 19th Annual International Chinese Statistical Association Applied Statistics Symposium, Indianapolis IN, June 20–23, 2010.)

used remission status to categorize benefit and four possible adverse event outcomes to describe risk (no adverse events, mild or moderate adverse events, severe adverse events, or discontinued because of adverse events).

In addition to describing the distribution of patients' response in the chosen B–R categories, Chuang-Stein et al. (1991) propose to assign weights to B–R categories and construct linear or ratio B–R score. The same idea was later used by Entsuah and Gorman (2002) and Pritchett and Tamura (2008) with expanded B–R categories. We will use the five B–R categories to illustrate. Assume $\{p_i, i = 1, \ldots, 5\}$ are the observed proportions of the five B–R categories for one treatment group and $\{w_i, i = 1, \ldots, 5\}$ are the weights chosen to reflect the relative desirability of the five categories. One example for $\{w_i, i = 1, \ldots, 5\}$ is to set $w_1 = 2$, $w_2 = 1$, $w_3 = 0$, $w_4 = 1$, $w_5 = 2$. Chuang-Stein et al. (1991) proposed the two sets of statistics in Equation 8.1. One is a linear score and the other is a ratio score. The exponent "e" in the numerator in the ratio score allows further calibration of efficacy relative to risk.

$$\text{Linear score} = w_1p_1 + w_2p_2 - w_3p_3 - w_4p_4 - w_5p_5$$

$$\text{Ratio score} = \frac{(w_1p_1 + w_2p_2)^e}{w_3p_3 + w_4p_4 + w_5p_5} \tag{8.1}$$

One can calculate the sampling variability associated with the linear and ratio score. In addition, one can compare two groups with respect to the mean linear or mean ratio score. Because weights are used, sensitivity analysis is recommended.

Other extensions of the concept of B–R categories are possible. For example, if there are two separate serious AEs of equal importance and having both of them is twice as bad as having one of them, we could construct a net B–R measure of "benefit response (0 or 1) – (no. of the two serious AEs)." This measure can take on values of 1, 0, –1, –2, and withdrawal. For example, if an individual experienced the benefit but also one of the two serious AEs, then the individual will have a net measure of 0. The same value can be achieved by someone experiencing no benefit and none of the two serious AEs. If there are two equally important and distinct categorical responses to assess benefit and two distinct serious AEs, we could construct a net measure of "no. of benefit responses – no. of the AEs." In this case, the net B–R measure can take on values of 2, 1, 0, –1, –2, and withdrawal. One can display the net B–R values graphically.

It is important to be aware of the assumptions behind the net B–R measures described in the preceding paragraph. The measure assumes that each beneficial response is equivalent to one serious AE experience. Of course, one can enhance the B–R measure by weighing beneficial responses and the AEs of interest differently. However, introducing additional complexity may reduce the attractiveness of these measures because of their simplicity and ease to communicate.

8.3.3 Methods for Eliciting Patient Preference

When the trade-off between benefit and risk has to be made, it seems obvious that the end user, that is, the patient, should play a key role in the decision-making process. Although there is substantial research in the health economic field about soliciting patient preferences, or what is more formally known as stated preference or stated choice, its application is more focused on marketing (e.g., cost vs. benefit) than a B–R perspective. However, in recent years, researchers as well as regulatory agencies have become more and more aware that patients' preferences should be taken into consideration in B–R decisions. For example, the FDA Guidance on Factors to Consider When Making Benefit–Risk Determinations in Medical Device Premarket Approval and De Novo Classifications (FDA CDRH 2012) states: "When assessing such data in a PMA application or de novo petition, FDA realizes that some patients are willing to take on a very high risk to achieve a small benefit, whereas others are more risk averse. Therefore, FDA would consider evidence relating to patients' perspective of what constitutes a meaningful benefit when determining if the device is effective, as some set of patients may value a benefit more than others. It should also be noted that if, for a certain device, the probable risks outweigh the probable benefits for all reasonable patients, FDA would consider use of such a device to be inherently unreasonable."

Because preference is not directly observable, separate studies and different study designs are needed. Conjoint analysis (CA), which was invented by economists and mathematical psychologists, can be applied for such studies. CA is a tool that collects information and analyzes and draws conclusions on people's preference of a set of attributes by forcing people to make trade-offs among different combinations of the attributes under study. Its original form, the full-profile CA, requires study subjects to rank and rate all possible combinations of different levels of attributes under study, which is often impractical unless the number of attributes and levels are very small. In practice, a subset of such combinations is selected and study subjects are asked to rate and rank the select combinations only. The categories and levels of attributes used for B–R study are determined through existing publications and expert opinions, with a pilot study carried out to assist the final study design.

Table 8.2 illustrates the structure of the selected attributes and their associated levels in a B–R study for patients' preference in non–small-cell lung cancer treatment (NSCLC) conducted by Mühlbacher and Bethg (2014).

In this example, there are seven attributes in total: one benefit attribute, five risk attributes, and one attribute about convenience of administration. Each of the attributes has three levels except for the administration attribute, which has two levels. The total number of possible combinations of attribute levels is $3^6 \times 2 = 1458$ and the number of possible choice sets is $\binom{1458}{2}$. The study selected 24 choice sets as two blocks, and each patient is asked to make 12 choices. To rate and rank the different combinations of the attributes, the discrete choice experiments (DCE) method was used. This method asks the patient to

TABLE 8.2

Structure of Selected Attributes and Levels in Patients with NSCLC

Attributes	Level 1	Level 2	Level 3
Time without tumor progression	High	Medium	Low
Side effect of skin	None	Mild	Moderate
Nausea and vomiting	Mild	Moderate	Severe
Diarrhea	Mild	Moderate	Severe
Tiredness/fatigue	Mild	Moderate	Severe
Tumor-related symptoms	Mild	Moderate	Severe
Mode of administration	Tablet	Infusion	

Source: Adapted from Mühlbacher, A. and Bethg, S. (2014). Patients' preferences: a discrete-choice experiment for treatment of non-small-cell lung cancer. *The European Journal of Health Economics.*

TABLE 8.3

Example Choice Question for Comparing Hypothetical Medicines

Attributes	Treatment A	Treatment B
Time without tumor progression	Medium	Medium
Side effect of skin	Moderate	None
Nausea and vomiting	Mild	Severe
Diarrhea	Moderate	Moderate
Tiredness/fatigue	Mild	Severe
Tumor-related symptoms	Severe	Mild
Mode of administration	Infusion	Tablet

Source: Adapted from Mühlbacher, A. and Bethg, S. (2014). Patients' preferences: a discrete-choice experiment for treatment of non-small-cell lung cancer. *The European Journal of Health Economics.*

choose (instead of ranking) between two (or more) treatments that have different combinations of attributes with different benefit and risk profiles. With a preferable benefit coupled with unpreferable risk, this method reveals the level of risk a patient is willing to take to gain a certain benefit. Table 8.3 illustrates a choice set that the patients were asked in the NSCLC study example.

Using the collected patient choice (for each choice set, each patient) as the response variable, and the associated attribute levels as covariate variables, regression models such as generalized linear latent and mixed model (GLLMM) can be applied to estimate coefficients for each attribute (for attributes that have more than two levels, for each attribute level). Statistical inferences such as magnitude or significance of each coefficient can shed light on the decision process of B–R. In the example above, Mühlbacher and Bethg (2014) found that all the seven attributes were statistically significant in the main effect model, where a GLLMM with multinomial logit link for response variable was applied. In contrast with the common belief that progression free survival is the most important attribute in efficacy, they found that the tumor-associated symptom was as important. This study suggested that in future design of NSCLC studies, tumor-associated symptom might be considered as one of the key efficacy variables.

It is very difficult to include numerous patient preference type endpoints in B–R assessment. The DCE method can integrate multiple benefits and harms by allowing the patient to specify their risk tolerances and preferences for various treatment profiles. The results from these studies can help with understanding the analysis condition and decision contexts and may eventually translate to the decision contexts and important clinical thresholds that we could use to make final B–R decisions. For example, it might help determine the weight for methods such as the weighted number needed to be treated (see Section 8.3.4) and multicriteria decision analysis (MCDA, see Section 8.3.5).

8.3.4 Methods for One Benefit and One Risk

In this subsection, we assume that selection of key efficacy and safety endpoints for BRA resulted in one efficacy and one safety endpoint. For one efficacy and one safety endpoint, BRA generally comes to a pairwise comparison between benefit and risk. The advantages are that the approach is easy to understand, clearly shows the main benefit and risk tradeoff, and can use a simple measure for BRA, such as the ratio of number needed to treat for benefit (NNT) and number needed to treat for harm (NNH). The disadvantages are that the approach does not distinguish between many events within an efficacy or safety endpoint. For example, if a composite event is used for either efficacy or safety, the approach assumes similar clinical impact of the components making up the composite endpoint. For another example, time to first event analysis of a composite efficacy event of cardiovascular (CV) death, nonfatal myocardial infarction (MI), or stroke does not distinguish between the clinical importance of CV death, nonfatal MI, and stroke since only the component that occurred first is counted in the analysis.

Below, we describe a few metrics and associated methods that can be used for one benefit and one risk endpoint and provide guidance and cautions on their use.

8.3.4.1 NNT and NNH

NNT measures benefits in terms of number of patients needed to treat so that one additional patient derived the benefit (e.g., preventing one additional patient from experiencing a clinical event of interest), and NNH is similarly defined as number of patients needed to treat to cause one additional adverse event. IMI PROTECT WP5 BRWG (Mt-Isa et al. 2014) provided a comprehensive discussion of NNT and NNH, along with several extensions of the measures, such as Utility and Time Adjusted NNT (UT-NNT) that incorporates utility and time, Adverse Event Adjusted NNT (AE-NNT) that integrates one benefit with multiple risks, and Relative-Value Adjusted NNT (RV-NNT) that may include utilities and multiple risks. However, these extensions are not recommended by PROTECT because of potential for implausible interpretations or difficulty in obtaining individual patient-level data to derive the measures. On the basis of the criteria to select BRA methods as mentioned in Section 8.2, the QSPI BRWG also feels that these extensions of NNT and NNH are not broadly applicable in BRA settings.

NNT is derived as the reciprocal of an absolute risk reduction or a difference in response rates between two treatment groups. NNH is similarly derived for the safety endpoint. In a B–R assessment, NNT and NNH are calculated independently and directly compared against favorite and unfavorite effects of similar clinical impact. If the single efficacy endpoint is as important as the single safety endpoint, then a treatment with NNT < NNH will have its benefit outweigh its harm. Derivation of NNT or NNH is simple but requires explicitly stating and justifying the source of data used for rates or probabilities. The interpretation of NNT or NNH aligns well with clinical perspective. Limitations of NNT and NNH include difficulty in estimating uncertainty associated with the NNT and NNH estimates and an unstable ratio estimate for NNT/NNH when the risk difference between two treatment groups is close to zero. In addition, it should be cautioned that comparing NNT directly to NNH (i.e., claiming favorable B–R when NNT/NNH < 1) may not be logically sound in many situations as this comparison implicitly assumes equal importance between the efficacy and safety endpoints. A different threshold from 1 could be used but requires subjective judgment on the relative importance.

Figure 8.6 presents an example with the use of NNT and NNH shown at the FDA Cardiovascular and Renal Drugs Advisory Committee for Vorapaxar on January 15, 2014 (FDA Advisory Committee 2014). Using CV death (efficacy) and fatal bleeding (safety) as an example, the NNT and NNH, calculated as the reciprocal of an exposure adjusted risk difference in 10,000 PY, showed that treatment with vorapaxar plus standard of care in 918 patients would prevent one CV death, whereas treatment with vorapaxar plus standard of care in 2971 patients would cause one fatal bleeding. In this example, it may be reasonable for a clinician to compare NNT for CV death with NNH for fatal bleeding, as both would result in death and therefore should have equal clinical significance. On the

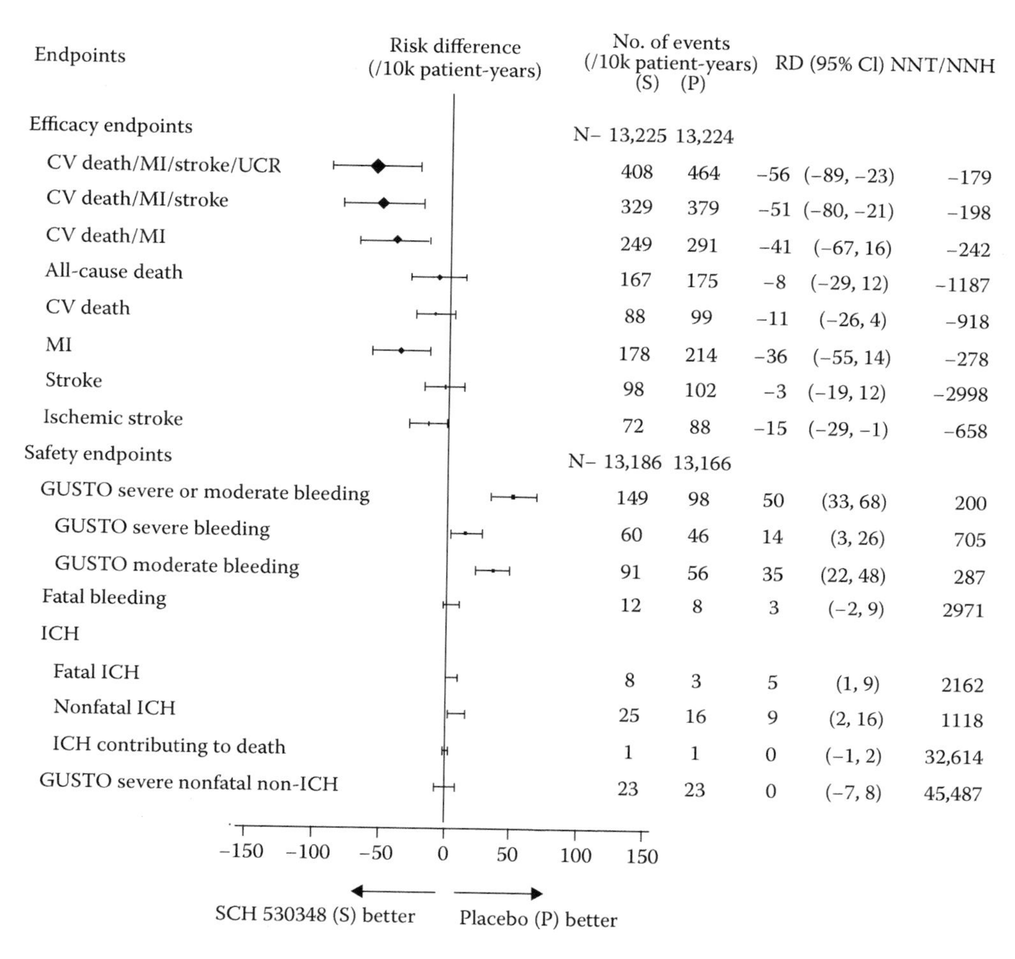

FIGURE 8.6
Benefit and risk endpoints, risk differences, and NNT/NNH (see http://www.fda.gov/downloads/AdvisoryCommittees/CommitteesMeetingMaterials/Drugs/CardiovascularandRenalDrugsAdvisoryCommittee/UCM386272.pdf).

basis of the results, a clinician may reasonably conclude that vorapaxar plus standard of care demonstrated better B–R profile as compared to the standard of care alone.

8.3.4.2 Joint Evaluation of B–R

He et al. (2012) proposed a joint evaluation framework using one efficacy and one safety endpoint, via Bayesian method. The framework assesses B–R by comparing efficacy and safety data with clinically meaningful thresholds that are chosen with the consideration of medical condition and current treatment options. This joint evaluation approach should be useful as a quantitative method for BRA in the setting of one efficacy and one safety endpoint. Chapter 9 provides a detailed review of the proposed approach. A real case application of one efficacy and one safety endpoint can be found in Section 9.5.1 of Chapter 9.

Although the joint evaluation framework is quantitative, it fits well with a structured B–R evaluation framework as detailed in the FDA Draft PDUFA V Implementation Plan.

Further, the approach provides a common unit by quantifying judgments about clinical relevance and trade-offs between the effects by aggregating all effects and presenting an overall B–R assessment via a probability. Lastly, the approach accommodates uncertainties by quantifying uncertainty about all effects via posterior distributions of the estimated treatment effects. Once a clinical team selects key favorable or unfavorable effects for evaluation and narrows them to a few items, this joint evaluation approach would be very useful to support key B–R decisions.

8.3.5 Methods for Multiple Benefits/Risks

Clinical trials usually collect large quantity of data regarding both efficacy and safety, namely, benefit and risk, of an experimental drug. The pharmaceutical companies and the regulatory agencies can then evaluate the merits of the experimental drug on the basis of the data collected. The evaluation processes are both extensive and complicated as they take into consideration all relevant data for an aggregated evaluation of the potential merits of the experimental drug to the general public and to make a decision of whether to grant the marketing approval. One quantitative B–R approach that allows the integration of multiple benefits and risks is the MCDA framework.

The construct of MCDA very much coincides with the principles of the descriptive/qualitative methods for BRA, such as the PrOACT-URL and BRAT. In addition, with proper derivations and simplifications, the MCDA framework can also include many other univariate or multivariate methods as special cases (Belton and Stewart 2002; Mussen et al. 2009; Nixon and Oliveira 2011; Nutt et al. 2010; Tsai and Bruce 2015). In this section, we describe the theoretical derivation of MCDA, the advantages of the method, and the cautionary disadvantages followed by an example.

8.3.5.1 Applications of MCDA

For the general applications of MCDA, one needs to identify a list of relevant benefit and risk endpoints or criteria that are used to determine the B–R profile and the potential utilization. The steps of MCDA can be outlined as follows.

For each criterion, define the benchmark reference points that represent practically (instead of theoretically) the best and worst possible scenarios of benefit and risk for both the experimental drug and comparator to be evaluated. One can then evaluate and score each criterion result against the reference points. The scoring can be based on certain functions reflecting the relative preference. The functions can be linear or nonlinear, and they do not need to be the same for all the criteria under evaluation.

A set of weights (or utilities) need to be specified, based on clinical considerations, for each criterion to reflect its relative importance among the factors considered in the decision. Compute the weighted sum of the scores by multiplying the score with weight for each criterion and add them together for all the factors considered. This is the primary MCDA statistic or index to be used for evaluations or comparisons.

Because of the subjective nature of the choices of value functions (i.e., function that converts the input data [parameters] in all criteria into a preference value or utility for the options under evaluation) and weight, sensitivity analyses should be conducted by varying the feasible value functions and weights to obtain an extensive distribution of the MCDA statistic for inferences, either for the evaluation of a single product or for the comparison of multiple products, and to derive a decision.

Mathematically, let the response of the ith endpoint be x_i, the best possible response for this endpoint be b_i, the worst possible response for this endpoint be c_i, and the weight (or utility) associated with this endpoint be μ_i. Suppose that we are considering a total of k endpoints with a mixture of both benefit (efficacy) and risk (safety), and a linear score function. The MCDA index or score can be calculated as

$$\text{MCDA index} = \sum_{i=1}^{k} \mu_i (x_i - c_i)/(b_i - c_i).$$

This index can be estimated for each treatment and the quantities can be compared. It can be viewed as composed of weighted preference scores corresponding to the benefit endpoints and weighted preference scores corresponding to the risk endpoints. For sensitivity analysis, one can perturb the values of μ_i, c_i, and b_i within a certain range and gauge the variation of the MCDA index.

8.3.5.2 Advantages of MCDA

There are many advantages of the MCDA method. The following highlights a few of them.

The method is able to numerically integrate qualitative judgments and quantitative data by assigning weights to the scores, which provide greater transparency about how the criteria are scored and weighted.

MCDA is able to incorporate a comprehensive and structured list of possible benefit and risk criteria considered to be of potential relevance clinically and scientifically. It also offers the flexibility to include any additional benefit and risk criteria and thus could be extended to comparable clinical situations in any ad hoc basis.

It allows performing the subsequent sensitivity analyses, exploring the dependency of the conclusions on the chosen weights and scoring functions, and gaining an extensive understanding of the distribution of MCDA statistics under various scenarios. The successful applications of MCDA require multidisciplinary discussions about the subjective weights, scores, and qualitative measures and allow the assessors to consider a comprehensive B–R profile of new medicines or any health technology products.

8.3.5.3 Disadvantages of MCDA

Below are some potential disadvantages of MCDA. The decision makers should not unduly rely on the numerical outcome of the analysis from the method because of the fact that no model can sufficiently represent the whole scope of complexities of the BRA of a new product.

A common criticism of the MCDA method is the subjectivity of the scoring function and weights. The sensitivity analysis via the variety of scoring functions and weights is able to provide some simulated scenarios to aid decision making to a certain degree. The medical community and regulatory agencies may establish certain consensus guidance on this aspect for different products in different therapeutic areas. Another criticism is that the MCDA method does not provide the measure of uncertainties and treats the benefits and risks criteria as independent factors. This concern can be alleviated if the MCDA is conducted on the subject-level data. At the subject level, one can jointly estimate the covariance matrix of the criteria and produce an inferential statistic following the chi-square distribution for comparisons between products (Tervonen et al. 2011; Tsai and Bruce 2015).

Finally, there could be significant divergences between stakeholders for the choice of weights. The discussion on BRA may be distracted and shifted to discussions on values and weighting factors instead. This has the potential to derail important conversations and reduce complex issues to oversimplified abstract quantities instead.

8.3.5.4 Example

The following is an example with a clinical trial data set to illustrate the computation of the preference scores for benefit and risk, as well as the overall MCDA score.

As shown in Table 8.4, four benefit (efficacy) variables and five risk (safety) variables are selected for the overall consideration of the joint benefit and risk evaluation for three treatments, namely, Placebo, Treatment A, and Treatment B in patients with rheumatic arthritis (see Section 8.3.1). Table 8.4 also includes the best feasible and worst feasible scores for the scenarios under consideration. Note that, theoretically, the best possible score for benefit is 100%; however, that may not be feasible. A similar rationale applies to the worst possible score. Additionally, Table 8.3 also includes the weights for all the variables. The weights subjectively reflect the relative importance of the variables considered and need to be normalized so that the total weights sum up to 100%.

Following the equation shown above for the calculation of the MCDA score and the data in Table 8.4, Table 8.5 shows the benefit preference score, risk preference score, and the total MCDA score for the three treatment groups. Treatment B shows the highest preference score for benefit; however, it also exhibits the least preference for the risk variables. Taking into account the benefit and risk variables together, the MCDA score clearly shows an increasing preference order of Placebo, Treatment A, and Treatment B. It can also be shown graphically in Figure 8.7.

As discussed above, a common criticism of the MCDA method is the subjectivity of the scoring function and the weights. An extensive sensitivity analysis with varieties of scoring functions and weights is conducted using the data in Table 8.3 and the results are shown graphically in Figures 8.8 and 8.9.

Figure 8.8 shows the distribution of MCDA scores generated from the sensitivity analysis for Placebo, Treatment A, and Treatment B, respectively. The red vertical lines indicate the median MCDA score of the distributions. Figure 8.9 shows the MCDA score difference between the treatments. The red vertical lines indicate the median of the differences and the cyan lines indicate the 95% empirical CI of the MCDA score differences. The CIs can assist the readers in assessing the clinical relevance and significance on the basis of the MCDA score differences and its distributions. One should be careful not to equate the CI of MCDA score differences with the common statistical CIs, which are usually derived based on an underlying distribution.

Another variant of MCDA, the stochastic multicriteria acceptability analysis (SMAA) proposes a way to overcome these limitations through simulations (Tervonen and Figueira 2008; Tervonen et al. 2011). SMAA can be seen as an extension of MCDA with an added advantage of being able to include parameter uncertainties owing to sampling variations and the ability to characterize typical B–R trade-offs without using a set of specific weights. The choices of weights across criteria can be in a range or follow some probability distributions. Therefore, the B–R balance for an alternative is also a distribution. SMAA calculates the probabilities that a treatment enjoys various ranks (from top to bottom) among a group of treatments, on the basis of the overall B–R balance. A treatment with a very high probability to be top ranked will be considered favorably. The calculation of the probabilities is done through simulation.

TABLE 8.4

Data for Example

Score/Weight/Group	ACR20	ACR50	ACR70	HAQ-DI	Severe AE	Dropout	Serious AE	Life-Threatening	Death
Best feasible response	0.6	0.45	0.3	0.55	0	0	0	0	0
Worst feasible response	0.05	0	0	0	0.5	0.4	0.3	0.2	0.1
Weight	16.7	16.7	16.7	16.7	3.33	4.44	5.55	8.88	11
Placebo	0.1875	0.0645	0.0141	0.068	0.0343	0.0358	0.0328	0	0
Treatment A	0.3200	0.1420	0.0480	0.162	0.0298	0.0453	0.0237	0.00103	0.00103
Treatment B	0.3944	0.1811	0.1449	0.211	0.0360	0.0647	0.1644	0.00206	0.00206

TABLE 8.5

Benefit Preference, Risk Preference, and MCDA Scores

Groups	Benefit Preference Score	Risk Preference Score	MCDA Score
Placebo	9.42	31.97	41.39
Treatment A	21.06	31.90	52.96
Treatment B	31.65	28.88	60.53

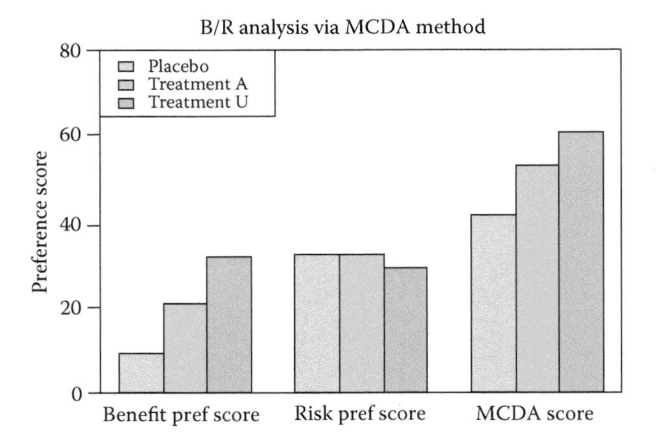

FIGURE 8.7
Value-added graphs: preference scores for benefit, risk, and MCDA.

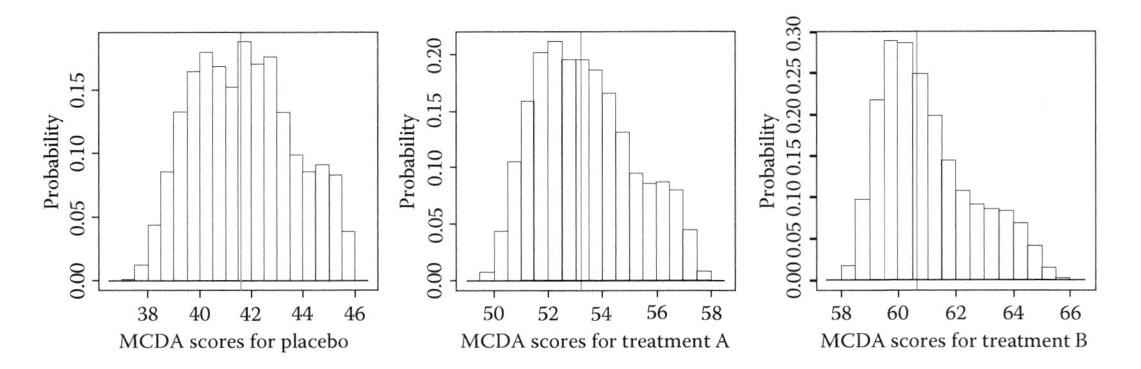

FIGURE 8.8
Value-added graphs: preference scores for placebo, treatment A, and treatment B.

Many of the current B–R analysis methods can be considered as special cases of MCDA, namely, the BLR method discussed in Section 8.3.2.1; the Clinical Utility Index (CUI), which is defined as the weighted sum of benefits and risks with a similar definition as MCDA; the Desirability Index (DI), which is a geometric equivalence of CUI; and many other methods (Ouellet 2010; Ouellet et al. 2009; Poland et al. 2009; Renard et al. 2009).

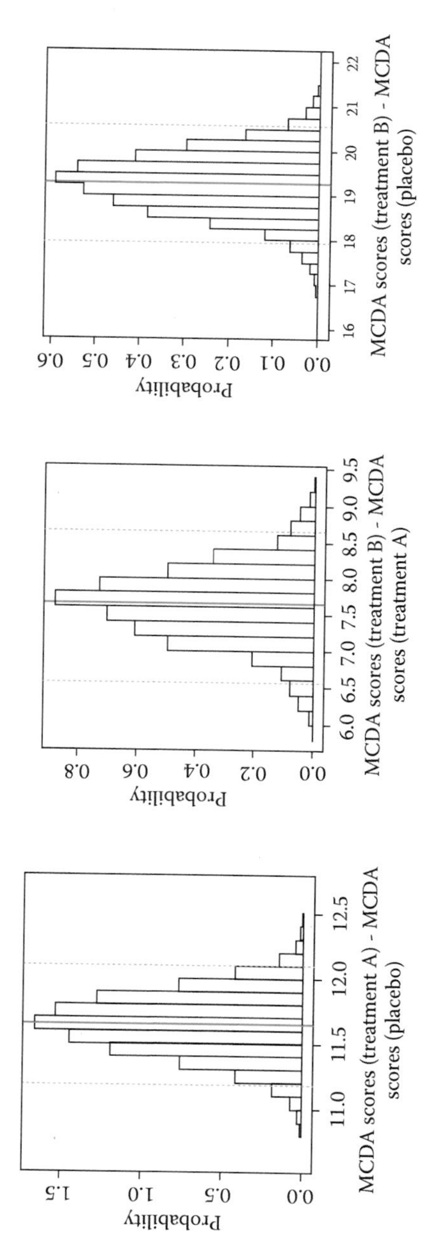

FIGURE 8.9
Value-added graphs: preference scores for treatment A-placebo, treatment B-treatment A, and treatment B-placebo.

MCDA was used in few occasions in the pharmaceutical industry in various settings, for example, Tsai and Bruce (2015), Mussen et al. (2009), and the illustrative examples in various publications (EMA WP2 Report; IMI PROTECT WP5 Report). However, quantitative BRA is not expected to replace qualitative evaluation because not all information can be summarized into numeric terms, and a single mathematical construct generally cannot adequately substitute for the intellectual process of assessing the empirical evidence, accommodating risks, and balancing risks and benefits. The expert judgment is expected to remain the cornerstone of B–R evaluation for the authorization of medicinal products. The quantitative evaluation should not convey a false sense of precision and shift the focus on overall numerical summaries at the expense of information on the qualitative differences.

8.3.6 Methods for Uncertainty Evaluation

Uncertainty is an important aspect to consider in the BRA regardless of qualitative or quantitative methods. The FDA framework has five decision factors: analysis of condition, current treatment option, benefit, risk, and risk management. For each of these five factors, evidence and uncertainties need to be considered. Similarly, the Committee for Medicinal Products for Human Use (CHMP) BRA includes background, benefits and associated uncertainties, and risks and associated uncertainties. CHMP recommendations are largely similar to those from FDA and it is important to describe sources of uncertainty and variability and their impact on the B–R (EMA Reflection Paper 2008; FDA 2013).

Uncertainty exists in BRAs since available information is limited. There are many potential sources of uncertainties. Some of these uncertainties are "known knowns." For example, we know that efficacy estimates from clinical trials are often robust. Some of the uncertainties are "known unknowns" such as adverse events with low frequency, which may not be well characterized in clinical trials. The others are "unknown unknowns." For example, very rare drug-induced adverse reactions may only be observed in postmarketing after broad usage and wide patient exposure.

There are many ways to categorize these uncertainties. One way is to consider them during the pre- and postmarketing. During the premarketing phase, some uncertainties could come from the level of evidence for benefit and for risk in clinical development and from the relative importance of benefits versus risks. In addition, uncertainties could arise from BRA in the postmarket setting.

First, for the level of evidence for benefit and for risk in clinical development, as we know, clinical trial populations are finite. Because of the limited sample sizes, there is uncertainty associated with estimated drug effects. In particular, safety endpoints often have low power and therefore greater uncertainty associated with them. In addition, there has been much increased discussion on missing data. Random missingness may not be a big issue since it just reduces the effective sample size, but nonrandom missingness could be problematic since it can introduce unknown bias. Inconsistencies are also a source of uncertainty. For example, does B–R vary across patient characteristics, across geographic region, and across studies? There can also be inconsistencies when evaluating B–R using different metrics, such as absolute risk versus relative risk. Which metrics to use for B–R endpoints introduces uncertainty that is reflected through associated statistical variability? Second, a source of uncertainty comes from translating from the premarket to the postmarket setting since the population in the real world could be somewhat different from the patient population in the premarket. Third, drawing conclusions in the face of uncertainty can be complex and challenging. Lastly, in order to deal with uncertainties, we need to understand them. One way to help understand them is to illustrate them with graphics.

Uncertainty associated with study design and conduct such as missing data could be addressed by proactive planning and prevention of issues. Sometimes, analytical remedies are possible. Estimates of benefit and risk could be provided with measures of uncertainty. In addition, well-designed and well-conducted meta-analyses for safety endpoints can be used to synthesize information from different sources. Graphical tools are also helpful to illustrate uncertainty. Furthermore, subgroup analysis can be used to examine consistency of effects and to identify subpopulations with a favorable B–R profile. Analyses can be characterized with CIs or probability distributions. Predictive models help inform patients and physicians about the future course of an illness or the risk of developing an illness and, thereby, help guide individual BRA. Chapter 4 provides a detailed review of the methods for understanding and evaluating uncertainties in the assessment of B–R in pharmaceutical drug development.

8.4 Challenges in Applying BRA Methods

There are many challenges to performing BRAs, some common to all approaches and some specific to one or more of the approaches described above. Before enumerating these challenges, it may be helpful to ask: what would an easy BRA look like? First, we would have a clear decision context, perhaps one requiring a binary decision. We would have high-quality data relevant to benefits and to risks. All stakeholders would have a shared set of values that could be directly applied to interpret the data on benefits and risks. We would be able to quantify all major sources of uncertainty and clearly communicate the decision, the decision-making process, and the uncertainties to the general public.

8.4.1 Decision Context Challenges

Having described the ideal circumstances for a BRA, it is now relatively straightforward to imagine potential difficulties under the less-than-ideal circumstances in which we usually find ourselves. Starting with the decision context, there can be a surprising amount of ambiguity in the task at hand. A single medical product may go through several BRAs in different decision contexts: manufacturers will use BRA to plan development programs, regulatory agencies will use BRA to guide approval and labeling decisions, health technology assessment organizations may use BRA—with the added dimension of cost—in developing formularies and determining reimbursement, and medical societies will use BRA to develop practice guidelines. Sadly, none of these are typically binary decisions. Consider, as an example, a BRA used to support a regulatory decision for a new medical product, rather than a seemingly binary decision of approval versus nonapproval, a complete description of the decisions to be made for an "approvable" product would encompass indication, dose, warnings and other risk communications, mandates for postmarketing studies and surveillance, and many other factors. Even for a product that will not be approved, BRA is required to determine what, if any, additional data should be requested before reconsidering an application.

Another decision context challenge in regulatory uses of BRA is determining how to incorporate information on other treatments. For instance, should licensure of a new product be an occasion for revisiting BRAs of existing treatments? Simply identifying all the dimensions of a decision context is a major challenge, even before attempting to understand how the BRA fits into the decision. One final issue is that choice of BRA approach(es) is itself part of a decision context, and there may not be sufficient experience with many of the approaches described earlier in this chapter to give decision makers confidence. Encouraging wider adoption of structured BRA approaches is a critical challenge for statisticians and physicians working in this field.

8.4.2 Data Challenges

Many of the challenges associated with collecting and interpreting data on risks and benefits were discussed in Section 8.3.6 and are further elaborated in another chapter in this book. Briefly, we highlight again differential ascertainment of safety and efficacy information. In premarket BRA, safety information is less likely than efficacy information to come from specifically targeted endpoints, and follow-up may not be long enough to understand delayed risks or risks associated with long-term use. This situation is, to some degree, reversed in the postmarket setting where systematic data collection for efficacy largely ceases while safety information continues to accumulate. This asymmetry of information, together with regression to the mean, may tend to lead to increasingly equivocal BRAs as products age through their life cycle.

Another, more technical, challenge arises from having multiple data sources, such as more than one Phase 3 clinical trial. Determining how to approach evidence synthesis is a critical and, perhaps, often overlooked step in the BRA process. For instance, should meta-analyses for efficacy and safety be performed before forming an overall BRA? Or should BRA be performed at the trial level and then synthesized to form the overall picture?

8.4.3 Challenges in Incorporating Values

Measuring and quantifying values is often cited as the greatest challenge for the various BRA approaches that explicitly incorporate value judgments. Although there have been many worthwhile efforts—several of which have been described above—to provide procedures for quantifying values through endpoint weighting or other means, they all fundamentally rely on a certain amount of medical judgment and subjectivity. Furthermore, no statistical procedure can answer fundamental questions such as "Whose values?" Manufacturers, regulators, payers, and individual physicians, patients, and caregivers may all have different values and priorities, suggesting that there often may be no one correct weighting and no one right answer to a development or approval decision.

It is also important to note that, while qualitative methods that do not explicitly incorporate values may seem to sidestep these thorny issues, this is a superficial advantage only. All decisions based on BRA involve value judgments, either explicit or implicit. What we might gain in simplicity by not quantifying value judgments, we lose in transparency. However, one additional challenge for quantitative methods that incorporate value judgments is general acceptability: it may be difficult to communicate such approaches and there may be reluctance among patients and providers to adopt their results.

8.4.4 Challenges in Uncertainty and Communication

Section 8.3.6 provided considerable detail on sources of and challenges associated with uncertainty. There are many good practices for quantifying and communicating uncertainty, including use of CIs and sensitivity analyses. These tools are not without their own difficulties, however. CIs are widely misunderstood and may be particularly misleading in graphical displays of many endpoints, many subgroups, or both. This considerably limits their usefulness as a communication tool, and, while sensitivity analyses are indispensable for evaluating the effect of various assumptions on a BRA, they can complicate the decision-making process. It is not always clear how to proceed when sensitivity analyses show that there is indeed sensitivity to assumptions in a given context.

8.5 Discussions and Conclusions

Although numerous approaches and frameworks have been proposed in recent years, there is no single approach or framework that can be applied and utilized in every setting and a combination of methods may be needed for each BRA. This is because BRA is often multifaceted and complex, and the goals of BRA in different settings may be different. A large number of methods, mostly descriptive and informal, have been proposed or adapted to perform BRA in the literature (Guo et al. 2010; Mt-Isa et al. 2014; Phillips et al. 2013). In this chapter, we laid out some criteria for selecting a BRA method, made recommendations on appropriate methods for pharmaceutical industry, and addressed some key challenges in applying the methods.

On the basis of the proposed criteria, a set of quantitative and qualitative approaches were recommended under different scenarios. We consider that a structured descriptive qualitative framework is key to the assessment and that some semiquantitative or quantitative approaches are able to provide valuable support for the B–R decision maker. Important issues of uncertainties and challenges were also highlighted.

Because of the nature of the BRA, the B–R decision is informed by evidence from various sources but inevitably requires expert judgment. Some therefore argue against the use of quantitative methods. It should be noted that quantitative methods such as MCDA are powerful to synthesize a large amount of data that are not easy to grasp qualitatively. Quantitative methods can either account for uncertainties or be used to demonstrate the impact of uncertainties on the overall B–R results through sensitivity analysis. In addition, methods such as CA and patient survey can directly quantify the uncertainties and integrate multiple benefits and harms by allowing patients to specify their risk tolerances and preferences for various treatment profiles. Therefore, in the structured BRA, appropriate quantitative evaluation is necessary and should be used to support and facilitate the judgment of the B–R profile. However, it is not possible to substitute judgment for quantitative analyses only.

As in study endpoints and study design where there exist many standards across the industry, stakeholders will also benefit from standardization of some aspects of BRA for a specific class of drugs or specific therapeutic area, such as methods to be employed and weights to be given to each benefit or risk. Prespecifying these aspects in either the study protocol or Statistical Analysis Plan may provide more formal and consistent assessment. Furthermore, to a broader extent, it will be beneficial to consider the BRA as an end outcome in designing a clinical study or a clinical development program so that more relevant and complete evidence is accumulated for the BRA. For example, novel endpoints combining benefits and risks can be developed for clinical studies. Preference or weight data can be collected from the patients and physicians together with efficacy and safety data to inform the balancing of benefits and risks.

The methods for patient-level BRA provide a means to evaluate the B–R profile for specific subpopulations. Although the drug evaluation is primarily at the population level, the disease and patient responses to the drug are usually heterogeneous. More personalized medicines are being developed for complex diseases such as cancer, and it is important to identify the right populations for such treatments. Therefore, patient-level BRA should be considered not only for the regulatory approval but also for the treatment of patients. In this chapter, methods based on several scores or indices were proposed. More applications to the real data are needed to demonstrate their use.

The recommended methods are for the general purpose and need to be tailored for specific cases. For example, in oncology, the endpoints are typically based on time-to-event endpoints, and corresponding methods need to be adapted. We encourage readers to experiment with methods recommended in this chapter.

There usually are large amount of data available for the BRA, at different development phases, including postmarketing or real-world setting. Although not covered in this chapter, approaches such as meta-analyses and mixed treatment comparisons are useful to combine and synthesize data from various sources.

Finally, BRA should be performed throughout the life cycle of a drug. The BRA methods may differ at various stages. To put in place, a BRA strategic plan is helpful in guiding periodic evaluation.

References

Belton V, Stewart T. Multiple criteria decision analysis: An integrated approach. Norwell, MA: Kluwer Academic Publishers, 2002.

Chuang-Stein C, Mohberg N, Sinkula M. Three measures for simultaneously evaluating benefits and risks using categorical data from clinical trials. *Stat Med* 1991; 10:1349–1359.

Chuang-Stein C, Mohberg N, Musselman D. Organization and analysis of safety data using a multivariate approach. *Stat Med* 1992; 11:1075–1089.

Chuang-Stein C. A new proposal for benefit-less-risk analysis in clinical trials. *Control Clin Trials* 1994; 15:30–43.

Coplan PM, Noel RA, Levitan BS, Ferguson J, Mussen F. Development of a framework for enhancing the transparency, reproducibility and communication of the benefit–risk balance of medicines. *Clin Pharmacol Ther* 2011; 89(2):312–315.

Entsuah R, Gorman J. Global benefit–risk assessment of antidepressants: Venlafaxine XR and fluoxetine. *J Psychiatric Res* 2002; 36:111–118.

European Medicines Agency. Reflection paper on benefit–risk assessment methods in the context of the evaluation of marketing authorization applications of medicinal products for human use. http://www.ema.europa.eu/docs/en_GB/document_library/Regulatory_and_procedural_guideline/2010/01/WC500069634.pdf. Published 2008. Accessed November 20, 2013.

European Medicines Agency. Benefit–risk methodology project: Development and testing of tools and processes for balancing multiple benefits and risks as an aid to informed regulatory decisions about medicinal products. http://www.ema.europa.eu/docs/en_GB/document_library/Report/2011/07/WC500109477.pdf. Published 2009. Accessed November 20, 2013.

FDA, 2013, Structured approach to benefit–risk assessment in drug regulatory decision-making draft PDUFA V implementation plan—February 2013, fiscal years 2013–2017. Silver Spring, MD: FDA; February 2013. Available at: http://www.fda.gov/downloads/ForIndustry/UserFees/PrescriptionDrugUserFee/UCM329758.pdf.

FDA Advisory Committee Meeting. Pfizer Briefing Information, for the Arthritis Advisory Committee Meeting May 9, 2012. http://www.fda.gov/downloads/AdvisoryCommittees/CommitteesMeetingMaterials/Drugs/ArthritisAdvisoryCommittee/UCM302960.pdf.

FDA Advisory Committee Meeting. Merck Presentations for the January 15, 2014 Meeting of the Cardiovascular and Renal Drugs Advisory Committee. http://www.fda.gov/downloads/AdvisoryCommittees/CommitteesMeetingMaterials/Drugs/CardiovascularandRenalDrugsAdvisoryCommittee/UCM386272.pdf.

FDA CDRH, 2012 Guidance for industry and Food and Drug Administration staff—Factors to consider when making benefit–risk determinations in medical device premarket approvals and de novo classifications. Silver Spring, MD: FDA CDRH; March 28, 2012.

Gelber R, Gelman R, Goldhirsch A. A quality of-life oriented endpoint for comparing treatments. *Biometrics* 1989; 45:781–795.

Glasziou P, Simes R, Gelber R. Quality adjusted survival analysis. *Stat Med* 1990; 9:1259–1276.

Guo JJ, Pandey S, Doyle J, Bian B, Lis Y, Raisch DW. A review of quantitative risk–benefit methodologies for assessing drug safety and efficacy-report of the ISPOR risk–benefit management working group. *Value Health* 2010; 13(5):657–666.

He W, Cao X, Xu L. A framework for joint modeling and joint assessment of efficacy and safety endpoints for probability of success evaluation and optimal dose selection. *Statistics in Medicine* 2011; 31:401–419.

IMI Pharmacoepidemiological Research on Outcomes of Therapeutics by European ConsorTium (PROTECT). WP5: Benefit–risk integration and representation. http://www.imiprotect.eu/wp5.html.

International Conference on Harmonization Guideline: Periodic Benefit–Risk Evaluation Report (PBRER) E2C(R2), 2012.

Ioannidis JP. Why most published research findings are false. *PLoS Med* 2005; 2:e124.

Mt-Isa S, Hallgreen C, Wang N, Callréus T, Genov G, Hirsch I, Hobbiger H, Hockley K, Lucian D, Phillips L, Quartey G, Sarac S, Stoeckert I, Tzoulaki I, Micaleff A, Ashby D. Review of methodologies for benefit and risk assessment of medication Pharmaco-epidemiological Research on Outcomes of Therapeutics by a European Consortium *Pharmaco-epidemiology and Drug Safety* 2014; doi: 10.1002/pds.3636.

Mühlbacher A, Bethg S. (2014). Patients' preferences: A discrete-choice experiment for treatment of non-small-cell lung cancer. *The European Journal of Health Economics*. Published online: 19AUG2014. http://rd.springer.com/article/10.1007%2Fs10198-014-0622-4.

Mussen F, Salek S, Walker S. Development and Application of a Benefit–Risk Assessment Model Based on Multi-Criteria Decision Analysis. Benefit–Risk Appraisal of Medicines. John Wiley & Sons, Ltd.; 2009.

National Institute for Health and Care Excellence, 2013, "Guide to the methods of technology appraisal," UK, NHS. Available at: http://www.nice.org.uk/article/PMG9/chapter/Foreword, published April 2013 (accessed December 22, 2014).

Nixon R, Oliveira P. Benefit–Risk of Multiple Sclerosis Treatments: Lessons Learnt in Multi-Criteria Decision Analysis BBS Spring Conference Comparative Quantitative Assessments: Benefit–Risk & Effectiveness, May 10, 2011.

Norton J. A longitudinal model for medical benefit–risk analysis, with case study. Presented at the 19th Annual International Chinese Statistical Association Applied Statistics Symposium, Indianapolis IN, June 20–23, 2010.

Norton J. A longitudinal model and graphic for benefit–risk analysis, with case study. *Drug Information Journal* 2011; 45:741–747.

Nutt DJ, King LA, Phillips LD, *Drug harms in the UK: A multicriteria decision analysis*, on behalf of the Independent Scientific Committee on Drugs, *Lancet* 2010; 376:1558–65.

Ouellet D, Werth J, Parekh N, Feltner D, McCarthy B, Lalonde RL. The use of a clinical utility index to compare insomnia compounds: A quantitative basis for benefit–risk assessment. *Clin Pharmacol Ther* 2009; 85(3):277–282.

Ouellet D. Benefit–risk assessment: The use of clinical utility index. *Expert Opin Drug Saf* 2010; 9(2):289–300.

Phillips LD, Fasolo B, Zafiropoulos N, Beyer A. Benefit–risk Methodology Project Work Package 2 Report: Applicability of Current Tools and Processes for Regulatory Benefit–risk Assessment. European Medicines Agency: London, 2010. Report No.: EMA/549682/2010. http://www.ema.europa.eu (accessed July 8, 2013).

Poland B, Hodge FL, Khan A, Clemen RT, Wagner JA, Dykstra1 K, Krishna R. The clinical utility index as a practical multi-attribute approach to drug development decisions. *Clinical Pharmacology & Therapeutics* 2009; 86:105–108.

Pritchett Y, Tamura R. The application of global benefit–risk assessment in clinical trial design and some statistical considerations. *Pharm Stat* 2008; 7(3):170–178.

Renard D, Wu K, Wada R, Flesch G. Using desirability indices for decision making in drug development. Population Approach Group Europe (PAGE); 2009 June 23; St. Petersburg, Russia: Novartis Pharma AG, Basel, Switzerland; 2009.

Tervonen T, van Valkenhoef G, Buskens E, Hillege HL, Postmus D. A stochastic multi-criteria model for evidence-based decision making in drug benefit–risk analysis. *Stat Med* 2011; 30(12):1419–1428.

Tervonen T, Figueira JR. A survey on stochastic multi-criteria acceptability analysis methods. *Journal of Multi-Criteria Decision Analysis* 2008; 15(1–2):1–14.

Tsai K, Bruce D. *Multi-Criteria Decision Analysis for Benefit–Risk Analysis and Pharmaceutical Pricing*. ASA Proceeding of the Biopharmaceutical Section; 2015.

Walker S, McAuslane N, Liberti L, Leong J, Salek S. "A Universal Framework for the Benefit-Risk Assessment of Medicines: Is This the Way Forward?" *Therapeutic Innovation & Regulatory Science* 2015; 49(1):17–25.

9

Benefit–Risk Evaluation Using a Framework of Joint Modeling and Joint Evaluations of Multiple Efficacy and Safety Endpoints

Weili He and Bo Fu

CONTENTS

ABSTRACT Structured benefit–risk (B–R) assessment has gained increased focus and interest in recent years. Pharmaceutical companies and regulatory agencies are increasingly using structured B–R assessments as part of their internal decision-making processes or for review of regulatory filings. However, amid numerous proposed frameworks, metrics, estimation techniques, and utility survey techniques in B–R assessment, quantitative approaches that separate fact from judgment, aggregate all effects with a common unit, and quantify uncertainties about all effects via a model approach are still lacking. In this chapter, we propose a B–R framework that incorporates efficacy and safety data simultaneously for joint modeling and joint evaluation of clinical proof of concept (POC), optimal dose selection, phase 3 probability of success, and an overall B–R evaluation. Simulation studies were conducted to evaluate the properties of our proposed methods. The proposed approach was applied to a real clinical study. On the basis of the true outcome of the clinical study, the assessment based on our proposed approach suggested a reasonable path forward for the clinical programs.

9.1 Introduction

Structured benefit–risk (B–R) assessment has gained increased focus and interests in recent years with the efforts by the European Medicines Agency (PrOACT-RUL framework), the Food and Drug Administration (FDA) (Center for Devices and Radiological Health B–R Guidance, Center for Drug Evaluation and Research B–R Structured Framework), and several other working groups including the Benefit–Risk Action Team, the Unified Methodology for Benefit–Risk Assessment Framework by the Centre for Innovation in Regulatory Science, and the Periodic Benefit–Risk Evaluation Report based on ICH Guidance. Although most B–R frameworks or methods to date are qualitative in nature and final B–R decisions may be made subjectively, the decision is often supported by quantitative evidence. The Pharmacoepidemiological Research on Outcomes of Therapeutics by a European ConsorTium (PROTECT) methodology review[1] reports a classification system of four headings: frameworks (with subcategories of descriptive frameworks and quantitative frameworks), metrics (threshold indices, health indices, and trade-off indices), estimation techniques, and utility survey techniques.[1] Of particular interest to the authors of this chapter, the authors of the PROTECT report recommended two quantitative frameworks (multicriteria decision analysis [MCDA] and stochastic multicriteria acceptability analysis [SMAA]). In discussing the PROTECT review report, Phillips[2] provides four pragmatic criteria for the characteristics that quantitative B–R methods should possess:

1. Comprehensive: Provides for any number of favorable and unfavorable effects to be considered and accepts any performance measures (measurable quantities, scoring systems, relative frequencies, health outcomes, etc.)
2. Separates fact from judgment: Distinguishes measured data about favorable and unfavorable effects from the clinical relevance of the effects
3. Provides a common unit: Quantifies clinical judgments about clinical relevance and about trade-offs between the effects, thereby establishing a common unit that enables comparison of combinations of effects, and can aggregate all effects
4. Accommodates uncertainty: Quantifies uncertainty about all effects

Phillips[2] concludes that a fully comprehensive, explicit, and quantitative model would satisfy all four criteria, but indicates that the recommended quantitative frameworks, MCDA and SMAA, by PROTECT fell short. We feel that while it may be optimal to identify a quantitative method that fits all the criteria described above, additional quantitative methods, even those that do not fit all the checkboxes for the above pragmatic criteria, may still be useful and play a critical role in supporting certain aspects of B–R evaluation.

In clinical development, we are often faced with two questions after phase 2 study data become available. First, can we assess the probability of success (POS) of a phase 3 program incorporating both phase 2 efficacy and safety information? Second, how should we select a phase 3 dose or doses among a few based on phase 2b dose range finding study data? In addition, when phase 3 studies are completed, we also face the question of whether or not the B–R profile of the proposed product meets regulatory standards for approval. In important regulatory decisions, such as for new drug approvals and post-market assessments, the concept of B–R is the fundamental yardstick for deliberations. Among other requirements, a drug cannot be brought to market unless the FDA finds that there is "substantial evidence" establishing the drug as both safe and effective.[3] In the past, the decision to move to phase 3, to select a phase 3 dose or doses, or to demonstrate that benefits outweigh risks in premarketing applications were often made based on subjective and qualitative assessment of efficacy and safety profiles. This has led to quite a few failed phase 3 programs at very late stages or premarketing applications that failed to gain regulatory approvals, raising the critical needs to utilize more quantitative approaches as additional measures to provide and supplement overall B–R evidence. As a result, appropriate utilization and application of available B–R framework and methods, along with any newly proposed B–R methods, should be considered to provide substantial evidence for new drug approval.

This research investigates a joint modeling and joint evaluation framework to assess the POS of a phase 3 program, to assist phase 3 dose selections, and to provide quantitative evidence to support regulatory approval. He et al.[4] proposed a joint modeling and joint evaluation framework for one efficacy endpoint and one safety endpoint. We extend the proposed framework by He et al.[4] to multiple efficacy and safety endpoints. This chapter is arranged as follows. In Section 9.2, we briefly describe the joint model and joint evaluation framework using one efficacy and one safety endpoint as proposed by He et al.[4] We then extend the joint model approach to multiple efficacy and safety endpoints. We propose a joint evaluation framework in Section 9.3 along with its extension to multiple efficacy and safety endpoints via Bayesian methods. Section 9.4 presents a simulation study setting and results for the proposed framework. We illustrate the framework with a real case study in Section 9.5. Section 9.6 includes some discussions.

9.2 Joint Modeling Approach

9.2.1 Joint Model Approach Using One Efficacy and One Safety Endpoint

He et al.[4] proposed a joint modeling and joint evaluation framework for B–R assessment with one efficacy and one safety endpoint. We summarize the main point of their proposed framework in this section.

The primary application of joint modeling approaches has been in the area of modeling a primary endpoint and a longitudinal process.[5] The chief interest is to characterize the association between the primary endpoint and a longitudinal process and to also understand the inherent features of the longitudinal process. In the early clinical development stage, the primary question of interest is whether or not a phase 3 development program will be successful and how early phase clinical study information can be utilized to evaluate the POS of a phase 3 program. In the late clinical development stage, on the other hand, the primary interest lies in whether or not the results of pivotal trials have provided sufficient and substantial evidence to establish the safety and effectiveness of a drug for regulatory approval. In the past, the approaches for evaluating the success of a phase 3 program, for dose selection, or for B–R evaluation for regulatory approval were quite subjective, and safety and efficacy data were often evaluated separately without consideration of their intricate relationships. This has resulted in failures of quite a few phase 3 programs in the past that either failed close to the end of clinical development programs or was unsuccessful in obtaining regulatory approval for the indication, owing to unfavorable B–R profiles. One noticeable example was rimonabant,[6] which failed to gain FDA approval for obesity indication because of safety concerns of suicidality and other adverse side effects that outweighed the benefit of weight loss. The joint model He et al.[4] proposed is described below.

For each of the $i = 1,\ldots, N$ subjects, let Y_{ij} be the observed efficacy response at time t_{ij}, $j = 1,\ldots,n_i$, where n_i is the total number of visits of patient i; $s_i(t)$, $i = 1,\ldots, N$, be the time-to-safety-event-of-interest or a binary random variable with a value of 0 or 1, 0 being no safety event and 1 otherwise. If we consider modeling safety endpoint as a binary variable, then $s_i(t) = s_i$. Suppose X_i is a vector of the fixed effects, which include possibly times of measurements and fixed covariates, such as treatment group assignments. Under the latent process models framework,[4] the joint model of $\tilde{y}_i = (y_{i1},\ldots,y_{in_i})$ and $S_i(t)$ can be expressed as follows:

$$
\begin{aligned}
f(\tilde{y}_i, s_i(t) \mid X_i) &= \int f(\tilde{y}_i, s_i(t), \eta_i(t)|X_i)\, d\eta_i(t) \\
&= \int f(s_i(t)|\eta_i(t), X_i) f(\tilde{y}_i|\eta_i(t), X_i) f(\eta_i(t)|X_i)\, d\eta_i(t),
\end{aligned}
$$

where $\eta_i(t)$ is a latent process that represents the health or disease status of patient i that is imperfectly measured by $\tilde{y}_i$. $f(s_i(t)|\eta_i(t), X_i)$ is a model for the safety response, and $f(\tilde{y}_i|\eta_i(t), X_i)$ is a model for the efficacy response. Under the latent process models assumption, $s_i(t)|\eta_i(t), X_i$ and $\tilde{y}_i|\eta_i(t), X_i$ are conditionally independent given $\eta_i(t)$. The relationship between $\tilde{y}_i$ and $\eta_i(t)$ is established by specifying that given $\eta_i(t)$, $\tilde{y}_i$'s are independent observations from a generalized linear model (GLM)[4] with linear predictor $\eta_i(t)$:

$$
g[E\{\tilde{y}_i|\eta_i(t)\}] = \eta_i(t),
$$

where g can be an arbitrary but known link function. Next, He et al. assume that $\eta_i(t)$ follows a Gaussian stochastic process:

$$
\eta_i(t) = X_i^T\beta + D_iU_i + W_i(t), \quad i = 1,\ldots,N,
$$

where X_i is a vector of the known fixed covariates, β is a vector of the regression coefficients of the fixed covariates, D_i is the design matrix, and the elements of U_i are the associated Gaussian random effects. If $D_i = (1, t)$, then $U_i = (U_{i1}, U_{i2})$ represents the random intercept and random slope for each subject. $W_i(t)$ is a zero mean stationary Gaussian process to introduce serial autocorrelation that dies away to 0 as two observations for an individual subject become further separated in time.

For the safety model, $f(s_i(t)|\eta_i(t), V_i)$, where V_i can be the same set of fixed effects or a subset of X_i. If the safety endpoint is a time-to-safety-event endpoint, then He et al. assume that the conditional hazard of a safety event given V_i and $\eta_i(t)$ is

$$h\{t|\eta_i(t), V_i\} = h_0(t, \alpha_0)\exp\left[\eta_i(t)\alpha_1 + V_i^T\alpha_2\right],$$

where $h_0(t, \alpha_0)$ is the baseline hazard, and α_1 and α_2 are the effects of $\eta_i(t)$ and V_i on the hazard of $s_i(t)$, respectively. If the safety endpoint is binary, indicating the presence or absence of a safety event of interest, the safety event indicator s_i is either 1 or 0. The authors then assume that the conditional model of S_i follows a logit model:

$$E(s_i) = p_i, \quad \log\frac{p_i}{1-p_i} = V_i^T\alpha + U_i^T\gamma,$$

where p_i is the probability of having a safety event of interest for patient i, α is the regression coefficient of the fixed effects, and γ is the regression coefficient of the random effects U_i. In the case of a binary endpoint not dependent on time, s_i cannot be written directly as a function of $\eta_i(t)$. It is, though, still correlated with efficacy data $\tilde{Y}_i$ through both fixed and the random effects.

He et al. employed the Markov chain Monte Carlo (MCMC) approach using BRugs, an R package calling OpenBUGS from R to obtain estimates of model parameters.

9.2.2 Extension of Joint Modeling Framework to Multiple Efficacy and Safety Endpoints

In clinical development programs, B–R evaluation is often multifaceted, supported by multiple efficacy and safety endpoints. We extend the joint modeling approach by He et al. to multiple efficacy and safety endpoints.

For each of the $i = 1,\ldots, N$ subjects, let $\tilde{y}_{1i}$ and $\tilde{y}_{2i}$ be the vectors of observed efficacy response over time for efficacy endpoints 1 and 2, respectively; $s_{1i}(t)$ and $s_{2i}(t)$, $i = 1,\ldots, N$, be the time-to-safety-event-of-interest or binary random variables with a value of 0 or 1, 0 being no safety event and 1 otherwise for observed safety endpoints 1 and 2, respectively. If we consider modeling safety endpoint as a binary variable, then $s_{1i}(t) = s_{1i}$, and $s_{2i}(t) = s_{2i}$. Suppose X_i is a vector of the fixed effects, which include possibly times of measurements and fixed covariates, such as treatment group assignments. Under the latent process models framework,[4] the joint model of $\tilde{y}_{1i}$, $\tilde{y}_{2i}$, $s_{1i}(t)$, and $s_{2i}(t)$ can be expressed as follows:

$$\begin{aligned}
&f\left(\tilde{y}_{1i}, \tilde{y}_{2i}, s_{1i}(t), s_{2i}(t)\middle|\eta_i(t)\right)\\
&= \int f\left(\tilde{y}_{1i}, \tilde{y}_{2i}, s_{1i}(t), s_{2i}(t), \eta_i(t)\middle| X_i, X_{ki}, V_{ki}, \eta_i(t)\right)d\eta_i(t)\\
&= \int\prod_{k=1}^{2}\left\{f\left(\tilde{y}_{ki}\middle|\eta_i(t), X_i, X_{ki}\right)f\left(s_{ki}(t)\middle|\eta_i(t), X_i, V_{ki}\right)\right\}f\left(\eta_i(t)\middle|X_i\right)d\eta_i(t)
\end{aligned}$$

where $k = 1, 2$ for kth endpoint, and similar to notations in Section 9.2, $\eta_i(t)$ is a latent process that represents the health or disease status of patient i that is imperfectly measured by $\tilde{y}_{ki}$. $f(s_{ki}(t)|\eta_i(t), X_i, V_{ki})$ is a model of the safety response, and $f(\tilde{y}_{ki}|\eta_i(t), X_i, X_{ki})$ is a model of the efficacy response. Similarly, X_{ki} and V_{ki} can be the same set of fixed effects or a subset of X_i. Under latent process assumption, $s_{ki}(t)|\eta_i(t), X_i, V_{ki}$ and $\tilde{y}_{ki}|\eta_i(t), X_i, X_{ki}$ are conditionally independent given $\eta_i(t)$. Similar to the descriptions in Section 9.2.1, $\tilde{y}_{ki}$'s are independent observations from a GLM with linear predictor $\eta_i(t)$:

$$g\left[E\left\{\tilde{y}_{ki}|\eta_i(t)\right\}\right] = \eta_i(t) + X_{ki}^T\beta_k,$$

where $\eta_i(t) = X_i^T\beta + D_iU_i + W_i(t)$, $i = 1,\ldots,N$. The parameters in $\eta_i(t)$ are similarly defined as in Section 9.2.1.

For a time-to-event type safety endpoint with model $f(s_{ki}(t)|\eta_i(t), V_{ki})$, a Cox model can be assumed as

$$h\left\{t|\eta_i(t), V_{ki}\right\} = h_0(t, \alpha_0)\exp\left\{\eta_i(t)\alpha_1 + V_{ki}^T\alpha_2\right\},$$

where $h_0(t, \alpha_0)$ is the baseline hazard and α_1 and α_2 are the effects of $\eta_i(t)$ and V_{ki} on the hazard of $s_{ki}(t)$, respectively. If the safety endpoints are binary, indicating the presence or absence of a safety event of interest, the safety event indicator s_{ki} is either 1 or 0. We then assume that the conditional model of s_{ki} follows a logit model:

$$E(S_{ki}) = p_{ki}, \ \log\frac{p_{ki}}{1-p_{ki}} = V_{ik}^T\alpha + \gamma_k U_i,$$

where p_{ki} is the probability of having a safety event of interest for patient i and endpoint k, α is the regression coefficient of the fixed effects, and γ_k is the regression coefficient of the random effects U_i for the kth safety model. In the case of a binary endpoint not dependent on time, s_{ki} cannot be written directly as a function of $\eta_i(t)$. It is, though, still correlated with efficacy data $\tilde{y}_{ki}$ through both fixed and the random effects.

We employ similar computation methods as in He et al. to obtain estimates of model parameters.

9.3 Joint Evaluation and Importance of Clinical Meaningful Thresholds

9.3.1 Importance of Clinical Meaningful Thresholds

Aspiration levels play an important role in everyday decision making. New York cab drivers are motivated to earn a daily target return. On rainy, busy days, their earnings per hour are high and they go home early. Likewise, in the pharmaceutical industry, when management has to decide which projects or portfolios to invest in, they are keen on achieving a target rate of return as well.[7] Once an aspiration level is decided, the probabilities of success and failure are naturally identified: these are the overall probabilities that the aspiration will be reached or will fall short of.

In drug development, the test drug is often compared to either placebo or an active comparator, which is in the market for the same indication the test drug is being developed for. In early clinical development phase, a pharmaceutical company that is developing the test drug often has the following goals under different development paradigms: (a) if the test drug is being compared to placebo, then the test drug should achieve a clinically meaningful threshold versus placebo, or (b) if the test drug is being compared to an active comparator for superiority, then the test drug should be better than the active comparator in efficacy by a certain threshold if safety profile is similar or the test drug should be better than the active comparator in safety by a certain threshold if efficacy profile is similar.[7] For drug products that are ready for premarketing applications, the FDA Draft PDUFA V Implementation Plan[8] provides excellent guidance on the key elements that are needed for a structured B–R evaluation. Specifically to our research interest are the key factors with regard to analysis of condition and current treatment options. These two key factors require a summary and assessment of the severity of the condition that the product is intended to treat and other therapies that are available to treat the condition. This represents the context of the decision that can provide useful information for weighing the benefits and risks of the drug under review. Clinical meaningful thresholds in the context of our proposed joint evaluation framework are consistent in concept with the analysis of condition and current treatment options as recommended by the FDA Implementation Plan and are used quite similarly to the weighting of endpoints in the aforementioned B–R literature in Section 9.1. Moreover, we believe that the clinical meaningful thresholds have added advantage, since they come from a real clinical setting and are selected with current treatment options in mind, reducing the subjectivity in the selection of weights.

9.3.2 Joint Evaluation Framework Using One Efficacy and One Safety Endpoint

He et al.[4] proposed a joint evaluation framework using one efficacy and one safety endpoint, via Bayesian methods, that assesses B–R by comparing efficacy and safety data with clinical meaningful thresholds that are chosen with the consideration of analysis of condition and current treatment options. We briefly summarize the main point of the proposed joint evaluation framework in this section but also extend their framework to incorporating multiple efficacy and safety endpoints in the next section.

For one efficacy endpoint only, let θ denote the treatment effect (i.e., test drug vs. placebo or test drug vs. an active comparator) and δ denote a clinical meaningful threshold of which substantial evidence of efficacy has been achieved if $\theta > \delta$. Using Bayesian methods, the probability of technical success (POTS) is defined as the posterior probability that the treatment effect, θ, is larger than δ; that is,

$$\text{POTS} = \Pr(\theta > \delta \mid y),$$

where y represents data from a clinical trial or trials. POTS depends only on completed clinical trial data and can be used as a metric for the assessment of substantial evidence of efficacy. Using a similar definition as Chuang-Stein[9] and Liu,[10] we define POS as the expected probability of rejecting the null hypothesis over the posterior distribution of θ; that is,

$$\text{POS} = E\{\Pr(\text{reject } H_0) | y\},$$

where H_0 tests whether $\theta - \delta \leq 0$ in a phase 3 trial. In other words, POS is a weighted average of conditional power, which depends on both the early clinical trial data and also the planned phase 3 sample size. POS is bounded by POTS (POTS is an upper bound of POS) in cases where POTS is sufficiently large. In simulation studies, we found that only in situations where the estimate of POTS is extremely small (e.g., less than 0.0001) can the estimate of POS exceed the estimate of POTS. Theoretically, the values of POTS and POS rely on the posterior distribution of θ. In one extreme case where the posterior distribution is only supported on the null hypothesis space $\Theta_0 = \{\theta : \theta - \delta \leq 0\}$, the definition of POTS and POS suggests that POTS = 0 < POS. Hence, when POTS is extremely small, we cannot guarantee that POTS > POS. However, if the posterior distribution favors the alternative space $\Theta_1 = \{\theta : \theta - \delta > 0\}$, POTS can serve as an upper bound of POS. This is a reasonable conclusion because in a real clinical development paradigm, new chemical entities being tested in phase 2 clinical trials are strongly supported by animal models, biologic plausible evidence, and early phase clinical trials for the potential efficacy in the treatment of a disease of interest. Therefore, in this paradigm, we conclude that POS is bounded by POTS. Finally, it can be shown that POS approaches POTS when n, the phase 3 sample size, approaches infinity.

When a phase 2 trial or trials are completed, it is important to first establish whether or not proof of concept (POC) of the test drug for the intended indication is achieved. POTS is a useful tool in that regard. If the POTS is high, for example, in the range of >80%, it gives a clear indication that the probability that the treatment effect of a test drug versus placebo or a comparator surpasses a clinically meaningful threshold is high, providing assurance that the test drug works for the intended indication. Once POC is achieved, planning for the phase 3 program can begin. Related to this, evaluation of POS is critical in the assessment of the success rate of the planned phase 3 program.

For one efficacy and one safety endpoints, let θ_e denote the treatment effect for an efficacy endpoint (i.e., test drug vs. placebo or test drug vs. an active comparator), θ_s denote the treatment effect for a particular safety endpoint of interest, δ_e denote a clinically meaningful threshold for efficacy of which the success of a phase 3 trial can be achieved from efficacy prospective if $\theta_e > \delta_e$, and δ_s denote a safety threshold of which the safety of the test drug is considered acceptable if $\theta_s < \delta_s$. Similar to the one endpoint case and without loss of generality, POTS for one efficacy endpoint and one safety endpoint can be defined as follows:

$$\text{POTS} = \Pr(\theta_e > \delta_e \quad \text{and} \quad \theta_s < \delta_s | y, s),$$

where y and s represent the efficacy and safety endpoints from a previous trial, respectively. POS for one efficacy endpoint and one safety endpoint case can be defined as

$$\text{POS} = E\{\Pr(\text{reject } H_0) | y, s\},$$

where H_0 tests whether $\theta_e - \delta_e \leq 0$ OR $\theta_s - \delta_s \geq 0$ in a phase 3 trial.

The above framework also provides a useful tool for the selection of an optimal dose or doses for the phase 3 trial(s). Presumably, once POC is achieved based on high POTS in one or more test drug doses, the optimal dose or doses that correspond to the highest POTS could be chosen.

9.3.3 Joint Evaluation Framework Using Multiple Efficacy and Safety Endpoints

In clinical development, assessment of B–R is often multifaceted, necessitating the incorporation of multiple key efficacy or safety factors into B–R assessment. We extend the joint evaluation framework by He et al. to multiple efficacy and safety endpoints.

Let θ_{e1} and θ_{e2} denote the treatment effect for efficacy endpoints 1 and 2, respectively; θ_{s1} and θ_{s2} denote the treatment effect for safety endpoints 1 and 2, respectively; δ_{e1} and δ_{e2} denote clinically meaningful thresholds, respectively, for efficacy endpoints 1 and 2 of which clinical meaningful efficacy can be achieved if $\theta_{ek} > \delta_{ek}$, $k = 1, 2$; and δ_{s1} and δ_{s2} denote safety thresholds of which the safety of the test drug is considered acceptable if $\theta_{sk} < \delta_{sk}$, $k = 1, 2$. POTS for multiple efficacy and safety endpoints can be defined as follows:

$$\text{POTS} = \Pr(\theta_{e1} > \delta_{e1}, \theta_{e2} > \delta_{e2}, \theta_{s1} < \delta_{s1}, \theta_{s2} < \delta_{s2} \,|\, y, s), \tag{9.1}$$

where θ_{e1}, θ_{e2}, respectively, are the treatment effect versus placebo or an active comparator for efficacy endpoint 1 and endpoint 2, whereas θ_{s1}, θ_{s2} are the treatment effect versus placebo or an active comparator for safety endpoint 1 and 2, respectively.

For the calculation of POS, suppose the null hypothesis to be tested is H_0: $\theta_{k1} \le \delta_{e1}$ or $\theta_{k2} \le \delta_{e2}$ or $\theta_{s1} \ge \delta_{s2}$, $\vartheta_{s2} \ge \delta_{s2}$. POS for multiple efficacy and safety endpoints can be similarly obtained as

$$\text{POS} = E\{\Pr(\text{reject } H_0) \,|\, y, s\}. \tag{9.2}$$

9.4 Simulations

9.4.1 Joint Models

He et al.[4] provided simulation study results for the joint modeling and joint evaluation framework for one efficacy and one safety endpoint. In this section, we provide computation details for the joint mode and joint evaluation framework for multiple efficacy and safety endpoints and investigate the performance of the model and evaluation framework.

For simplicity, a shared parameter structure was implemented. What it translates into is that all marginal models of efficacy and safety endpoints share a common random term U_i. Specifically, two efficacy endpoints are assumed to follow an additive form

$$y_{kij} = X_i^T \beta_k + D_k U_i + \varepsilon_{ij}, \; k = 1,2, \tag{9.3}$$

where $j = 1,\ldots, m$ is the index of the jth longitudinal measurements; ε_i's are independent and identically distributed, and $\varepsilon_i \sim N(0, \sigma^2)$; random term U_i's are also independent and identically distributed and $U_i \sim N(0, \sigma_u^2)$ with coefficient D_k's are the coefficient of random term; let $D_1 = 1$ for identification purpose of the estimation of variance parameters. For our simulation study, we assume that X is a binary variable for treatment group assignment only.

We assume that the safety endpoint is binary and can be modeled as follows:

$$\log \frac{E(S_{ki})}{1 - E(S_{ki})} = X_i^T \alpha + \gamma_k U_i. \tag{9.4}$$

In this model, the efficacy endpoints and safety endpoints are connected through both the fixed effect and random effect. The parameters that need to be estimated are $\{\beta_k, \alpha_k, D_2, \gamma_k, \sigma^2, \sigma_u^2\}$, where $\{\beta_k, \alpha_k\}$ are parameters of interest and $\{D_2, \gamma_k, \sigma_u^2\}$ are nuisance parameters. We simulated three treatment groups.

9.4.2 Posterior Distribution of the Joint Model Parameters

This section provides details of the posterior distributions along with the prior density of the joint model parameters and their initial values.

Prior density is required for each parameter interested. The following prior densities were considered:

$$\beta_k = \{\beta_{k0}, \beta_{k1}, \beta_{k2}\} \sim N\left(\mu_{\beta_k}, \left(\Sigma_{\beta_k}\right)^{-1}\right),$$

$$\alpha_k = \{\alpha_{k0}, \alpha_{k1}, \alpha_{k2}\} \sim N\left(\mu_{\alpha_k}, \left(\Sigma_{\alpha_k}\right)^{-1}\right),$$

$$\sigma^2 \sim IG(a, b^{-1}),$$

$$\sigma_u^2 \sim IG(a, b^{-1}),$$

$$D_2 \sim N(0, c^{-1}),$$

$$\gamma_k \sim N(0, c^{-1}),$$

where $\mu_{\beta_k} = \left(\mu_{\beta_{k0}}, \mu_{\beta_{k1}}, \mu_{\beta_{k2}}\right)^T$, $\mu_{\alpha_k} = \left(\mu_{\alpha_{k0}}, \mu_{\beta_{\alpha 1}}, \mu_{\beta_{\alpha 2}}\right)^T$ both initialized as $(0, 0, 0)^T$; Σ_{β_k} and Σ_{α_k} are 3×3 variance–covariance matrix with initialization as same dimension matrix with all element 0.01; a, b, c are chosen to be $a = 0.1$, $b = 0.1$, $c = 0.01$. All priors are assumed to be noninformative.

The posterior distribution is

$$f\left(\beta_1,\beta_2,\alpha_1,\alpha_2,D_2,\gamma_1,\gamma_2,\sigma,\sigma_u|y,S\right)$$

$$\propto \int\prod_{k=1}^{2} f_k(y_k|\beta_k,D_2,\sigma,u)f_k(S_k|\alpha_k,\gamma_k,\sigma,u)$$

$$\pi(\beta_k,\alpha_k,D_2,\gamma_k,\sigma,u)f(u|\sigma_u)du$$

$$\propto \int\prod_{k=1}^{2}\prod_{k=1}^{n}\left(\sum_{j=1}^{m}\left[\exp\left\{-\frac{1}{2\sigma^2}\left(y_{ij}-X_i^T\beta_k-D_k u_i\right)^2\right\}(\sigma^2)^{-\frac{1}{2}}\right]\right.$$

$$\left.\frac{\exp\left(X_i^T\alpha_k+\gamma_k u_i\right)}{1+\exp\left(X_i^T\alpha_k+\gamma_k u_i\right)}\right)$$

$$\times\left(\Sigma_{\beta_k}\right)^{-\frac{1}{2}}\exp\left\{-\frac{1}{2}\left(\beta_k-\mu_{\beta_k}\right)^T\left(\Sigma_{\beta_k}\right)^{-1}\left(\beta_k-\mu_{\beta_k}\right)\right\}\left(\Sigma_{\alpha_k}\right)^{-\frac{1}{2}}$$

$$\times\exp\left\{-\frac{1}{2}(\alpha_k-\mu_{\alpha_k})^T\left(\Sigma_{\alpha_k}\right)^{-1}\left(\alpha_k-\mu_{\beta_k}\right)\right\}$$

$$(\sigma^2)^{-(a+1)}\exp\left(-\frac{b}{2\sigma^2}\right)\left(\sigma_u^2\right)^{-(c+1)}\exp\left(-\frac{d}{2\sigma_u^2}\right)$$

$$\times\left(\sigma_{D_2}^2\right)^{-\frac{1}{2}}\exp\left(-\frac{b}{2\sigma_{D_2}^2}\right)\left(\sigma_{\gamma_k}^2\right)^{-\frac{1}{2}}\exp\left(-\frac{b}{2\sigma_{\gamma_k}^2}\right)du.$$

The integration of the posterior distribution might have no explicit mathematic form. We employ the Bayesian MCMC method to obtain parameter estimates on the posterior density. The derivation of posterior distributions for each of the parameters should be straightforward and can be similarly derived as in He et al. Therefore, we will not provide the detailed derivation here.

9.4.3 Joint Evaluation Framework

On the basis of the simplified joint models (Equations 9.3 and 9.4) defined in Section 9.4.1, we calculated POTS and POS comparing each treatment group versus placebo or an active comparator.

Without loss of generality, suppose the treatment differential effect of the test drug k compared with placebo or an active comparator on the efficacy measurement is β_k and the safety event probabilities are p_k and p_0 for test drug group k and placebo (or an active comparator) group, respectively. POTS is obtained as in Equation 9.1 as defined in Section 9.3.3. Note that β_k corresponds to θ_{ek} and $p_k - p_0$ corresponds to θ_{sk} in Equation 9.1 described in Section 9.3.3. δ_{ek} and δ_{sk} are chosen to be clinical meaningful thresholds for the evaluation. In the joint model setting, the POTS calculates the probability that the treatment effect exceeds a clinical meaningful threshold while simultaneously the safety profile corresponding to the test drug is within an acceptable range as compared to placebo or an active comparator. Since the posterior distribution of β_k, p_0, and p_k are not readily available, we use Monte Carlo numerical integration to estimate POTS as

$$\text{POTS}_e = \frac{1}{B}\sum_{b=1}^{B}\prod_{k=1}^{2}\left(I\left[\beta_{kb} > \delta_{ke}|y,s\right]\times I\left[p_{kb} - p_{0b} < \delta_{ks}|y,s\right]\right). \tag{9.5}$$

POTS_e denotes the estimated value of POTS, $I[\cdot]$ is an indicator function, B is the total number of samples drawn from the posterior distribution by MCMC for each parameter, and β_{kb}, p_{kb} and p_{0b} are the bth sample from the posterior distribution for parameters β_k, p_k and p_0, respectively.

For the calculation of POS, suppose $\hat{\beta}_k$ is the estimated treatment effect of the test drug dose k versus placebo and $\hat{p}_k - \hat{p}_0$ is the estimated rate difference between test drug dose k and placebo of the safety incidence of interest. By normal approximation,

$$\hat{\beta}_k \sim N\left(\beta_k, \sigma^2\left(\frac{1}{n_k} + \frac{1}{n_0}\right)\right),\ \hat{p}_k - \hat{p}_0 \sim N\left(p_k - p_0, \frac{p_0(1-p_0)}{n_0} + \frac{p_k(1-p_k)}{n_k}\right),$$

where n_k and n_0 are the sample sizes for test drug group k and placebo group in the planned phase 3 studies, respectively. Controlling the type I error at α level, the power function is

$$\begin{aligned}
&\beta_{power}(\beta_k, p_k, p_0, \sigma)\\
&= \Pr\left[(\hat{\beta}_k - \delta_e)/\sigma\sqrt{m} \ge Z_{1-\alpha},\ (\hat{p}_k - \hat{p}_0 - \delta_s)/\sqrt{\frac{p_0(1-p_0)}{n_0} + \frac{p_k(1-p_k)}{n_k}} \le Z_\alpha |\beta_k, p_k, p_0, \sigma\right]\\
&= \left(1 - \Phi\left(Z_{1-\alpha} - \frac{\beta_k - \delta_e}{\sigma\sqrt{m}}\right)\right)\Phi\left(Z_\alpha - \frac{p_k - p_0 - \delta_s}{\sqrt{p_0(1-p_0)/n_0 + p_k(1-p_k)/n_k}}\right),\ m = \frac{1}{n_k} + \frac{1}{n_0}.
\end{aligned}$$

Here, $\Phi(\cdot)$ is the cumulative distribution function of standard normal distribution. Thus,

$$\begin{aligned}
\text{POS} &= E\{\Pr(\text{reject } H_0)|Y, S\}\\
&= \int\prod_{k=1}^{2}\beta_{power}(\beta_k, p_k, p_0, \sigma) f(\beta_k, p_k, p_0, \sigma|y, s)\, d\beta_k dp_k dp_0 d\sigma,
\end{aligned}$$

and can be estimated through Monte Carlo approximation based on the posterior samples $\{\beta_{kb}, p_{kb}, p_{0b}, \sigma_b\}_{b=1}^{B}$, $k = 1, 2$ from the joint model:

$$\mathrm{POS}_e = \frac{1}{B}\sum_{b=1}^{B}\prod_{k=1}^{2}\beta_{power}(\beta_{kb}, p_{kb}, p_{0b}, \sigma_b), \tag{9.6}$$

where POS_e is the estimated value of POS.

We showed in He et al. that when n_k and n_0 approach infinity, that is, $\sqrt{m} = \sqrt{1/n_k + 1/n_0} \rightarrow 0$, POS approaches POTS.[4]

9.4.4 Simulation Setting

For each simulated data set, three treatment groups, dose 1, dose 2, and placebo, were generated, each having 200 subjects. The trial parameters were set up to resemble a clinical trial with longitudinal repeated measurements for efficacy and binary for safety endpoints. The maximum follow-up time was set to be 12 weeks. The design parameters are listed below:

- Efficacy measurements were collected at weeks 0, 2, 4, 8, and 12.
- Safety endpoints were yes or no for a specific adverse event (AE) of interest.
- Efficacy treatment effect 1 for dose 1 or dose 2 versus placebo is 0.9 and 1.2 units, respectively. Efficacy treatment effect 2 for dose 1 or dose 2 versus placebo is 0.8 and 1.2 units, respectively.
- Safety treatment effect 1 for dose 1 or dose 2 versus placebo, respectively, is 4.4% and 8% in favor of placebo. Safety treatment effect 1 for dose 1 or dose 2 versus placebo, respectively, is 7.5% and 12.4% in favor of placebo.

The data for each treatment group were generated according to the models below, where safety endpoints and efficacy endpoints are correlated through both fixed effects and random effects.

$$y_{kij} = \beta_{k0} + \beta_{k1}I\ (\text{dose 1}) + \beta_{k2}I\ (\text{dose 2}) + D_k u_i + \varepsilon_{kij}$$

$$\log\frac{E(S_{Ki})}{1 - E(S_{Ki})} = \alpha_{k0} + \alpha_{k1}I\ (\text{dose 1}) + \alpha_{k2}I\ (\text{dose 2}) + \gamma_k u_i,$$

where $k = 1,2$, and $D_1 = 1$ for avoiding identification issue. The random effect $u_i \sim N\left(0, \sigma_{u_i}^2\right)$, $\varepsilon_i \sim N\left(0, \sigma_i^2\right)$, for simulation purpose $\sigma_{u_i}^2 = 1$ and $\sigma_i^2 = 1$. Other coefficients were set as $\beta_{10} = 0$, $\beta_{20} = 0$, $\beta_{11} = 0.9$, $\beta_{21} = 0.8$, $\beta_{12} = 1.2$, $\beta_{22} = 1.2$, $\alpha_{10} = -1.6$, $\alpha_{20} = -0.1$, $\alpha_{11} = 0.3$, $\alpha_{21} = 0.3$, $\alpha_{12} = 0.5$, and $\alpha_{22} = 0.4$. The corresponding safety percentages for safety endpoint 1 are $p_{10} =$ 0.170 (placebo), $p_{11} = 0.214$ (dose 1), and $p_{12} = 0.250$ (dose 2), and for safety endpoint 2, they are $p_{20} = 0.475$ (placebo), $p_{21} = 0.550$ (dose 1), and $p_{22} = 0.599$ (dose 2). Association parameters, that is, coefficients of common random effects, are $D_2 = 0.5$, $\gamma_1 = 0.5$, and $\gamma_2 = -0.8$. The random effect is generated from a standard normal distribution.

Simulation results are summarized in Table 9.1. Four statistics (estimation bias, estimated standard deviation, empirical standard deviation, and coverage rate) were provided for each parameter. The estimation bias is calculated by the estimated value (average of all estimates) minus the true value; the estimated standard deviation is the average of all standard deviation estimated; the empirical standard deviation is the standard deviation of all estimated parameter values; and the coverage rate evaluates the proportion of times the confidence interval covers the true value with "nominal coverage probability" 0.95. It can be seen that the biases of the estimates are small, and coverage rate is close to 95% for all parameter estimates.

POTS is calculated following Equation 9.5, and when given efficacy threshold δ_e = (1, 1.5, 2, 2.5, 3) and safety threshold δ_s = (5%, 10%, 15%, 20%), POTS for each treatment is summarized in Tables 9.2 through 9.4 with different combinations of efficacy and safety thresholds. As can be seen in Tables 9.2 through 9.4, when the efficacy threshold is low and easy to achieve, and the safety threshold is high, allowing a higher safety incidence in a test drug as compared to placebo, POTS becomes increasingly higher with lower bars for either efficacy or safety thresholds.

To graphically illustrate the decision criteria, we plotted the POTS versus both δ_{e1} and δ_{s1} while fixing $\delta_{e2} = 0.5$ and $\delta_{s2} = 40\%$ in a contour plot as shown in Figure 9.1. It can be observed that when δ_{e1} increases and δ_{s1} decreases, that is, when the clinical significant thresholds become more stringent, POTS decreases.

POS is calculated following Equation 9.6. Figure 9.2 shows the change in POS when the sample size of a proposed phase 3 trial increases for different combinations of efficacy and safety thresholds, δ_{e1} and δ_{s1}, respectively, when fixing $\delta_{e2} = 0.5$ and $\delta_{s2} = 40\%$. It can be seen that in the case with thresholds ($\delta_{e1} = 1.2$, $\delta_s = 0.2$), POS does not exceed 0.1 even with 1000

TABLE 9.1

Average Value of Posterior Statistics of All Parameters over 1000 Simulations

Parameter	Bias	Estimated SD	Empirical SD	Coverage Rate
β_{10}	0.0002	0.058	0.059	0.950
β_{11}	−0.0027	0.082	0.082	0.949
β_{12}	0.0001	0.081	0.080	0.958
β_{20}	−0.0011	0.044	0.045	0.940
β_{21}	−0.0004	0.063	0.065	0.938
β_{22}	−0.0019	0.063	0.061	0.953
p_{10}	−0.0021	0.032	0.033	0.920
p_{11}	−0.0016	0.036	0.036	0.945
p_{12}	−0.0011	0.038	0.038	0.945
p_{20}	−0.0021	0.045	0.046	0.940
p_{21}	0.0003	0.045	0.045	0.946
p_{22}	−0.0051	0.044	0.043	0.927
D_2	0.0105	0.069	0.068	0.958
γ_1	0.0448	0.035	0.035	0.957
γ_2	−0.0336	0.031	0.031	0.946
σ	0.0002	0.026	0.026	0.952
σ_u	0.0002	0.028	0.028	0.949

Note: Bias = estimated value − true value. Coverage rate = percentage of (2.5%, 97.5%) contains true value. Empirical SD = SD of estimated parameter. Estimated SD = mean of estimated standard deviation.

TABLE 9.2

POTS Based on Various Efficacy Thresholds and Safety Threshold (Safety Endpoint 1 = 20% and Safety Endpoint 2 = 10%)

Test Drug	Efficacy Threshold			
Efficacy endpoint 2	0.75		0.95	
Efficacy endpoint 1	0.75	0.95	0.75	0.95
Dose 1	0.711	0.119	0.003	0.001
Dose 2	0.259	0.258	0.259	0.258

TABLE 9.3

POTS Based on Various Efficacy Thresholds and Safety Threshold (Safety Endpoint 1 = 20% and Safety Endpoint 2 = 15%)

Test Drug	Efficacy Threshold			
Efficacy endpoint 2	0.75		0.95	
Efficacy endpoint 1	0.75	0.95	0.75	0.95
Dose 1	0.717	0.120	0.003	0.001
Dose 2	0.555	0.554	0.554	0.553

TABLE 9.4

POTS Based on Various Efficacy Thresholds and Safety Threshold (Safety Endpoint 1 = 20% and Safety Endpoint 2 = 20%)

Test Drug	Efficacy Threshold			
Efficacy endpoint 2	0.75		0.95	
Efficacy endpoint 1	0.75	0.95	0.75	0.95
Dose 1	0.718	0.120	0.003	0.001
Dose 2	0.828	0.823	0.823	0.821

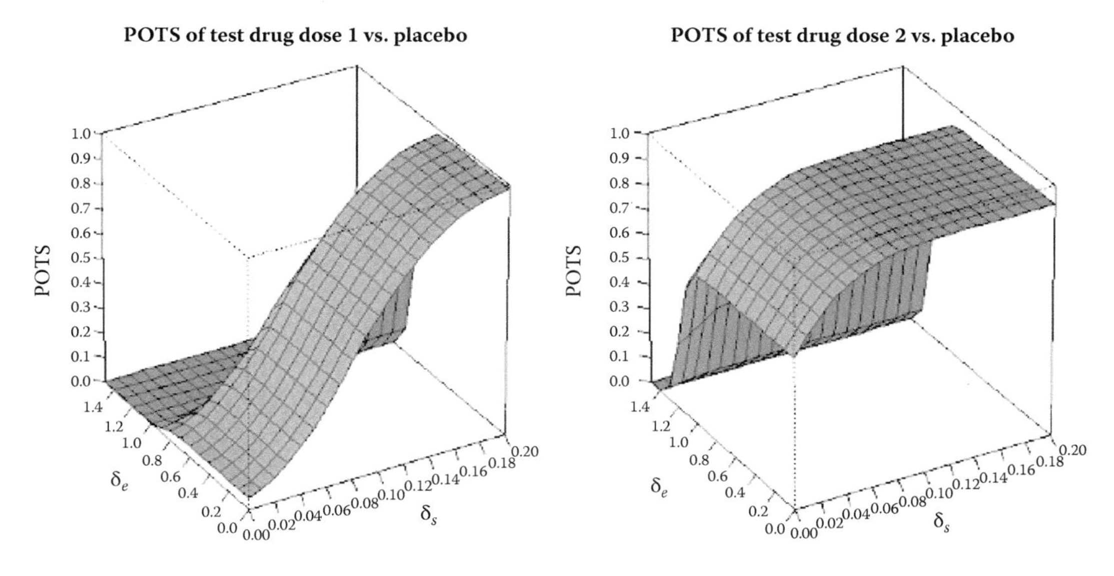

FIGURE 9.1
Contour plots of POTS against δ_{e1} and δ_{s1} for both test drug 1 and test drug 2 versus placebo.

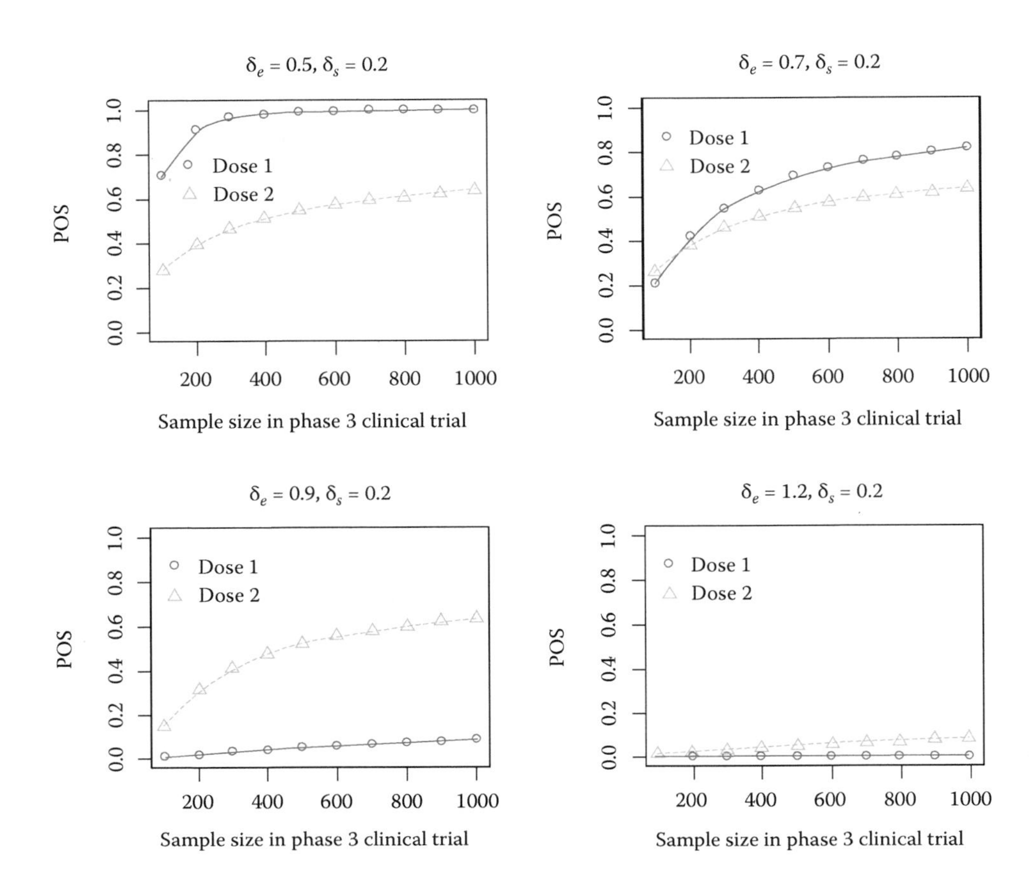

FIGURE 9.2
POS for both active treatments given certain efficacy and safety thresholds.

subjects per treatment group, indicating a very unlikely successful phase 3 clinical trial. On the basis of this threshold, if true, and POS value, the decision makers can then decide whether a phase 3 clinical trial should be conducted at all.

9.5 Real Case Study Application

This section presents a real clinical case study. The study was completed previously. We retrospectively fit our joint model and joint evaluation approach to the completed study to assess and evaluate B–R profile at that time point in the clinical development program. For B–R assessment, we will focus our discussion on POTS results as it represents the best statistic for such an assessment, since the definition and derivation of POTS take into consideration the analysis condition and current treatment options, as well as accounts for inherent uncertainties for the estimates of efficacy and safety endpoints. For confidentiality reasons, the name and details of the study are masked.

This is a case study for the treatment of a disease. The study was an 8-week double-blind, randomized, placebo control study in diseased subjects. The data set contains more than 400 patients randomly assigned to four treatment groups: placebo, test drug dose 1, test drug dose 2, and test drug dose 3. Test drug dose 1 is the lowest dose and test drug dose 3 is the highest. The efficacy endpoints considered are the primary endpoint and a key secondary endpoint, and both are measured as change from on-treatment measurement from baseline to week 8. One of the safety endpoints is defined as mechanism-based AEs, and the second safety endpoint is other AEs during the study (yes or no for each subject). For the primary endpoint, the effect size (vs. placebo) for this particular disease should be at least 0.5 units or above for a dose to be considered clinically meaningful. For the key secondary efficacy point, the effect size (vs. placebo) should be at least 0.3 units or above. For both efficacy endpoints, negative change is indicative of positive efficacy. The mechanism-based AE and other AEs were both considered to be not serious, and if each occurred in no more than 20% of patients at a dose level vs. placebo, this dose level can be considered viable for future trials.

9.5.1 Results for One Efficacy and Safety Endpoints

The application of this case study to the setting of joint model and joint evaluation of one efficacy and one safety endpoints was previously described in He et al.[4] and we provide a brief summary of the key results here.

Table 9.5 presents the results of POTS when δ_e takes different values while holding δ_s as 20%. Clearly, test drug dose 2 is the optimal dose as its POTS value is the highest for all δ_e when fixing δ_s. The disease being treated by the test drug is not a life-threatening disease but can be very bothersome and negatively affects quality of life for patients with the condition. The associated mechanism-based AE is considered not serious. On the basis of previous marketing surveys for the treatment of this disease, both patients and physicians indicated that the patients can tolerate more side effects if a new chemical entity provides better efficacy compared to the treatments on the market. The POTS results showed good B–R profile for both dose 1 and dose 2, if the efficacy threshold is acceptable at 0.5 or 0.7 units while holding the safety threshold at or below 20%.

9.5.2 Results from Multiple Efficacy and Safety Endpoints

The joint modeling and joint evaluation framework for multiple efficacy and safety endpoints as described in Sections 9.2 and 9.3 were applied to the case study data. Table 9.6 summarizes the posterior mean, median, standard deviation, and 95% credible sets. On the basis of the posterior samples, Tables 9.7 and 9.8 presents the results of POTS with various combinations of $\delta_{e1} = -0.5, -0.7$; $\delta_{e2} = -0.3, -0.5$; $\delta_{s1} = 20\%$; and $\delta_{s2} = 15\%, 20\%$, respectively. For completeness, we also present POS against the sample size of the planned phase 3

TABLE 9.5

POTS Based on Various Efficacy Thresholds δ_s (Safety Threshold) = 20%

	δ_e (Efficacy Threshold)		
Test Drug	**−0.5**	**−0.7**	**−1**
Dose 1	0.979	0.861	0.460
Dose 2	1.000	0.986	0.867
Dose 3	0.150	0.149	0.140

TABLE 9.6
Posterior Estimates of Parameters with 95% Credible Sets

Endpoints	Levels	Mean	SD	2.5%	Median	97.5%
Efficacy endpoint 1	Dose 1	−0.418	0.158	−0.732	−0.418	−0.108
	Dose 2	−1.029	0.146	−1.315	−1.029	−0.736
	Dose 3	−1.53	0.182	−1.878	−1.53	−1.174
Efficacy endpoint 2	Dose 1	−0.115	0.233	−0.575	−0.112	0.328
	Dose 2	−0.749	0.226	−1.197	−0.746	−0.305
	Dose 3	−1.485	0.241	−1.958	−1.486	−1.015
Safety endpoint 1	Placebo	0.175	0.037	0.11	0.174	0.253
	Dose 1	0.221	0.04	0.147	0.218	0.306
	Dose 2	0.193	0.038	0.126	0.191	0.275
	Dose 3	0.440	0.047	0.348	0.439	0.534
Safety endpoint 2	Placebo	0.471	0.047	0.376	0.471	0.563
	Dose 1	0.529	0.048	0.433	0.529	0.622
	Dose 2	0.555	0.048	0.462	0.555	0.648
	Dose 3	0.596	0.047	0.504	0.596	0.685
r_1		3.274	0.296	2.765	3.237	3.926
r_2		0.059	0.26	−0.449	0.059	0.573
r_3		0.16	0.23	−0.277	0.154	0.629
σ		0.223	0.041	0.148	0.221	0.311

Note: r_1, r_2, and r_3 are association parameters in the joint model used; σ is the standard deviation of the shared random effect.

TABLE 9.7
POTS Based on Various Efficacy Thresholds and Safety Threshold (Mechanism Based = 20% and Other AE = 15%)

Test Drug	Efficacy Threshold			
Efficacy endpoint 2	−0.3		−0.5	
Efficacy endpoint 1	−0.5	−0.7	−0.5	−0.7
Dose 1	0.102	0.020	0.028	0.007
Dose 2	0.816	0.807	0.807	0.717
Dose 3	0.091	0.091	0.091	0.091

TABLE 9.8
POTS Based on Various Efficacy Thresholds and Safety Threshold (Mechanism Based = 20% and Other AE = 20%)

Test Drug	Efficacy Threshold			
Efficacy endpoint 2	−0.3		−0.5	
Efficacy endpoint 1	−0.5	−0.7	−0.5	−0.7
Dose 1	0.109	0.022	0.030	0.008
Dose 2	0.934	0.924	0.827	0.820
Dose 3	0.122	0.122	0.122	0.122

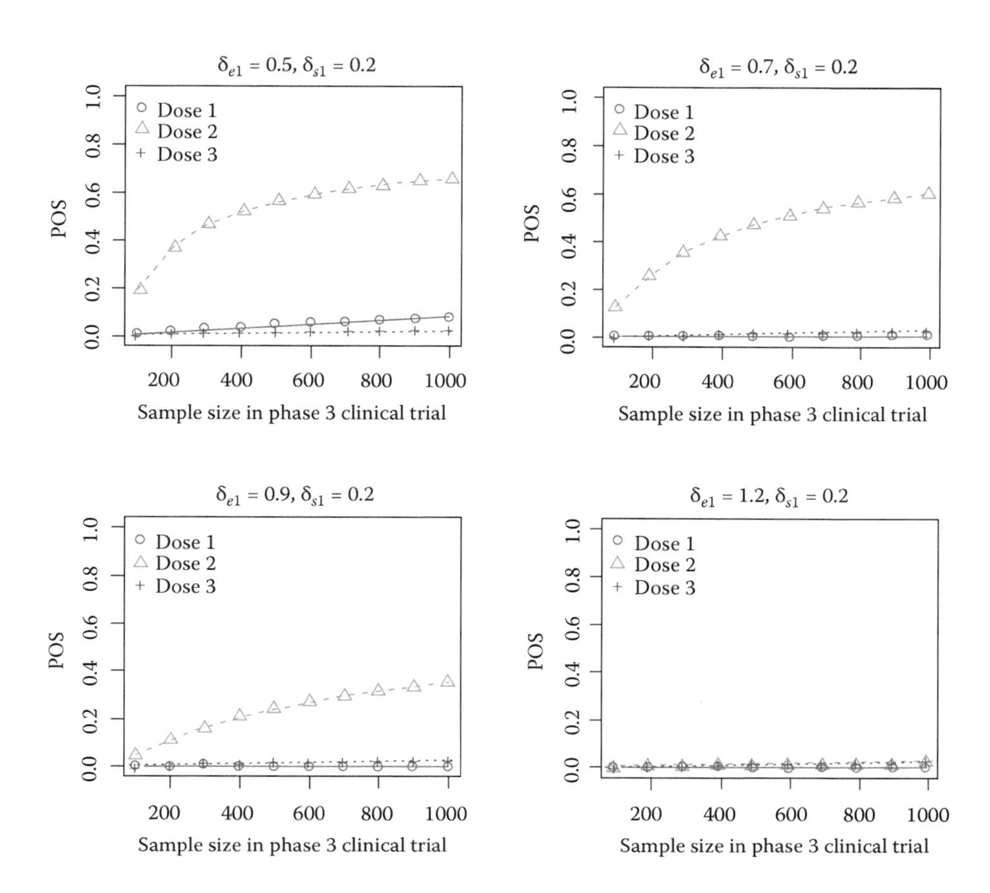

FIGURE 9.3
The POS against the sample size of a planned phase 3 clinical trial at different combinations of the thresholds for case study ($\delta_{e2} = 0$ and $\delta_{s2} = 0.15$).

clinical trial at different combinations of the thresholds of efficacy and safety in Figure 9.3. When considering the likelihood of a dose meeting clinical meaningful thresholds for the two efficacy endpoints and two safety endpoints, it is clear based on Tables 9.7 and 9.8 that test drug dose 2 became the only viable dose to be carried forward for further testing. Hence, a case can be made that if efficacy endpoint 2 was also a key efficacy aspect that needed to be taken into consideration for a full B–R assessment, the proposed framework allows a quantitative assessment to support such decision making.

9.6 Discussions

In this chapter, we extend the joint modeling and joint evaluation framework by He et al. for one efficacy endpoint and one safety endpoint to a framework that allows for multiple efficacy and safety endpoints. Along with the selection of appropriate clinical meaningful thresholds, our proposed approach fits most of the pragmatic criteria for the characteristics of quantitative B–R methods that Phillips[2] described. Our approach separates fact from judgment by distinguishing measured data about favorable and unfavorable effects from the clinical relevance of the effects with the comparison to clinical meaningful thresholds. Further, our approach provides a common unit by quantifying clinical judgments about clinical relevance and trade-offs between the effects by aggregating all effects based on a joint evaluation framework and presenting an overall B–R assessment via a quantity as POTS. Lastly, our approach accommodates uncertainties by quantifying uncertainty about all effects via posterior distributions of the estimated treatment effects. Linking back to the FDA Draft PDUFA V Implementation Plan[7] for a structured B–R evaluation, our approach considers the analysis of condition and current treatment options by comparing the estimated treatment effects and trade-offs with clinical meaningful thresholds that incorporate clinical input and are often common accepted for the disease of interest.

The joint model part of our proposed framework incorporates the intricate relationship between efficacy and safety data, thus providing more accurate depiction of their relationship and inference. This general framework for joint models should be applicable to most clinical trial data. The analysis approaches that were used for the real case study were similar to the approaches specified in the study protocols. For application of the joint modeling approach for an overall risk and benefit evaluation of your clinical trial data, researches should choose models that demonstrate the goodness of fit of your efficacy or safety data. Further, with the choices of appropriate models for the study data, the estimates of model parameters can be extrapolated to doses that were not studied in clinical trials. This may be more suitable for phase 2 to 3 setting. As a result, it is possible to obtain POTS and POS measures for the doses that were not studied in early clinical trials as optimal dose or doses for further testing.

We extend the joint modeling and joint evaluation framework by He et al. to two efficacy and two safety endpoints. Efficiency may not be gained further by incorporating additional efficacy or safety endpoints owing to the increased complexity of the joint models and computational intensity. We recommend that when trialists consider our proposed framework, they first consider the selection of endpoints that are critical for the B–R assessment and decision making.

It is important to differentiate POTS, where the calculation is based primarily on completed study data, from POS, where the calculation is based on early phase data and the intended phase 3 sample size. The authors believe that our proposed framework for B–R assessment could be utilized in various clinical development stages, at the phase 2 stage to inform POC and optimal dose selection, and predict phase 3 POS, and at the phase 3 stage to assess and provide supportive evidence for sufficient and substantial evidence to establish the safety and effectiveness of a drug for regulatory approval.

To make a "Go" decision from phase 2 to phase 3, it should be noted that a high POTS does not necessarily translate into a high POS; conversely, a low POTS cannot be compensated for by a huge phase 3 sample size to hopefully result in a high POS. It should be cautioned that even with high POTS from early clinical trials, a phase 3 clinical program may still face risk of failure if the phase 3 sample size is not adequate or other aspects of phase 3 trial planning are not properly considered and carried out. As noted in Section 9.4.3, POS is bounded by POTS when phase 3 study sample size approaches infinity. Therefore, clinical POC via POTS calculation should be confirmed first before embarking on the planning of phase 3 studies and evaluation of POS.

The magnitude of POTS and POS heavily depends on the clinical meaningful thresholds that are chosen. These clinical meaningful thresholds are specific to disease areas and competitors in the marketplace but can often be chosen with clinical input and a degree of objectivity. Thresholds can be determined based on better efficacy and comparable safety or comparable efficacy but better safety. For efficacy, the determination of a clinical meaningful threshold can be chosen based on effect size reported by claims and labels of drugs in the marketplace for the treatment of the same disease or by a clinical determination of a meaningful improvement of disease status. For safety, the threshold can be determined by the nature and severity of the safety concerns that are associated with the class of new chemical entities or a specific compound. Taken together, the levels of efficacy and safety bars can be set with reference to existing treatments in the market and with consideration of the relative disease severity being treated and the nature of safety concerns.

It should be noted that there is no universal agreed upon cutpoint for POTS. To determine a comfortable POTS cutpoint, a B–R profile is considered favorable, and practitioners should investigate historic information and determine a reasonable cutpoint with input from clinical and commercial colleagues. Based on our own experience, the authors recommend that POTS be at least 80% or higher as sufficient and substantial evidence to establish a favorable B–R profile for regulatory submission or for a "Go" decision to phase 3. Further, POS is obtained on the basis of both early clinical trial data and the planned phase 3 sample size. In the case where POC is considered achieved but the treatment effect is mild to moderate at best, the sample size needed in phase 3 trials can become quite prohibitive to achieve an appreciable level of POS. The feasibility of carrying out large phase 3 trials even when POC is achieved needs to be carefully considered. In considering an acceptable POS, there is again no agreed upon cutpoint among practitioners. However, it should be recognized that the concept of POS, where the average power to achieve clinical meaningful thresholds δ_e and δ_s is derived, is not the same as the concept of the study power, where the power of achieving a statistical significant difference between the test drug versus placebo or active comparator is derived. In this setting, δ_e is set as zero. The authors believe that the evaluation of POS provides clinical trialists a useful additional tool for the assessment of the path forward for their clinical program and that the magnitude of POS to guide a "Go" decision should be judged on a case-by-case basis but should not be less than 50%.

References

1. PROTECT Consortium. Review of methodologies for benefit and risk assessment of medication. http://www.imi-protect.eu/, 2013.
2. Phillips L. Benefit–risk modeling of medicinal products: Methods and applications. In: Sashegyi A, Felli J, Noel R (eds.) *Benefit–Risk Assessment in Pharmaceutical Research and Development*. CRC Press, 59–96, 2014.
3. Franson T, Bonforte P. Policy considerations and strategic issues regarding benefit–risk. In: Sashegyi A, Felli J, Noel R (eds.) *Benefit–Risk Assessment in Pharmaceutical Research and Development*. CRC Press, 113–131, 2014.
4. He W, Cao X, Xu L. A framework for joint modeling and joint assessment of efficacy and safety endpoints for probability of success evaluation and optimal dose selection. *Statistics in Medicine*, 31: 401–419, 2012.
5. Wulfsohn M, Tsiatis A. A joint model for survival and longitudinal data measured with error. *Biometrics*, 53(1): 330–339, 1997.
6. FDA Advisory Committee Meeting, FDA Briefing Document, for the Metabolism and Endocrinology Advisory Committee Meeting, June 13, 2007, http://www.fda.gov/ohrms/dockets/ac/07/briefing/2007-4306b1-fda-backgrounder.pdf.

7. Diecidue E, Van de Ven J. Aspiration level, probability of success and failure and expected utility. *International Economic Review*, 49(2): 683–700, 2008. doi:10.1111/j.1468-2354.2008.00494.x.
8. FDA structured approach to benefit–risk assessment in drug regulatory decision-making draft PDUFA V implementation plan—February 2013, fiscal years 2013–2017. Silver Spring, MD: FDA; February 2013. Available at: http://www.fda.gov/downloads/ForIndustry/UserFees/PrescriptionDrugUserFee/UCM329758.pdf.
9. Chuang-Stein C. Sample size and the probability of a successful trial. *Pharmaceutical Statistics*, 5: 305–309, 2006. doi:10.1002/pst.232.
10. Liu F. An extension of Bayesian expected power and its application in decision. *Journal of Biopharmaceutical Statistics*, 20: 941–953, 2010. doi:10.1080/10543401003618967.

10

Visualization of Benefit–Risk Assessment in Medical Products with Real Examples

Shihua Wen, Weili He, Scott Evans, Haijun Ma, Christy Chuang-Stein, Qi Jiang, Xuefeng Li, George Quartey, and Ramin B. Arani

CONTENTS

ABSTRACT The purpose of graphics or visualization tools for benefit–risk (B–R) assessment and presentation of medicinal products is to illuminate effects and aid decision making among different stakeholders including the patients, clinicians, sponsors, regulatory agencies, and payers. Thoughtful and creative utilization of graphical displays in B–R assessment could often help deliver safe and effective interventions to the patients and enhance the development process. In this chapter, a thorough review of graphical presentations that have appeared in the medical and statistical literature, including peer-review journals, special interest group publications, scientific reports, and Food and Drug

Administration advisory committee meeting materials, is presented. On the basis of the review and with a focus on application to the clinical trial setting, new perspectives and guidance for the application of graphics are presented. Refinements to existing graphics are provided along with illustrative examples to give readers proper context for the appropriate use of various graphics in practice.

10.1 Introduction

In recent years, structured benefit–risk (B–R) assessment has gained increased attention. The draft guidance by the Food and Drug Administration (FDA) released in 2013 (Draft PDUFA V Implementation Plan 2013) described five key components for structured B–R assessment (BRA). The first two components, "Analysis of conditions" and "Current treatment options," set up the clinical context for weighting benefits and risks (often termed *harms*). The other three components, "Benefit," "Risk," and "Risk management," evaluate the critical issues regarding the intervention's efficacy and safety, as well as proposed efforts to address any potential concerns. In the draft guidance, the FDA indicated its belief that a structured BRA can be accomplished by a qualitative descriptive approach for structuring the BRA, while acknowledging that quantification of certain components of the BRA is an important part of the process to support decision making. In this chapter, the definition of qualitative or quantitative BRA follows the same definition as defined in the glossary. In addition, several other proposed structured BRA initiatives developed by the Benefit–Risk Action Team (BRAT) (Coplan et al. 2011), Unified methodology for benefit–risk assessment (UMBRA) Framework by the Centre for Innovation in Regulatory Science (CIRS) organization (Walker et al. 2015), PrOACT-URL framework recommended by the EMA (EMA 2012 Work Package [WP] 4), and Periodic Benefit–Risk Evaluation Report (PBRER) based on International Conference on Harmonization (ICH) Guidance (ICH 2012) have placed a qualitative descriptive approach as a critical part of BRA.

It is said that "a picture is worth a thousand words." Given that the current focus of a structured BRA is mostly on qualitative descriptive approaches, BRA via visual or graphic presentations is even more important in BRA and communication. Although numerous approaches and frameworks have been proposed in recent years, there is no single approach or framework that can be applied and utilized in every setting. This is because BRA is often multifaceted and complex, and the goals of BRA in different settings (e.g., disease areas, clinical development stages) may differ. Therefore, different types of graphics may be needed to support a descriptive depiction of the data for BRA. To that end, graphs and visual tools can facilitate comparisons of groups or variables across multiple settings. Examples may include presenting estimated effects along with variability for different variables, information from different studies, periods, subgroups, and trends. As mentioned in Chapter 4, quantifying uncertainty is an important part of BRA. Graphs depicting point estimates of B–R endpoints along with measures of uncertainty provide an important aspect of BRA.

The Quantitative Sciences in the Pharmaceutical Industry Benefit–Risk Working Group (QSPI BRWG) conducted a thorough review of graphical presentations that have appeared in the medical and statistical literature, including presentations at conferences, peer-review journal articles, special interest group publications, scientific reports, and FDA advisory committee (AdCom) meeting materials. In particular, the WP5 subteam of the Innovative Medicines Initiative Pharmacoepidemiological Research on Outcomes of Therapeutics by a European consortium (PROTECT) presented a useful and comprehensive review of graphs that can be used in B–R Assessment and Presentation (BRAP) (PROTECT Consortium 2013), including forest plot, tree diagram, effects table, bar plot, scatterplot, and area and volume chart. However, the PROTECT review focused more on the philosophical and theoretical aspect of the visualization techniques, and further guidance for application of BRAP in medicinal product development is needed. We provide a summary of these key common graphics that are described in the PROTECT report and other reviews, including presentations at conferences, peer-review journals, special interest group publications, scientific reports, and regulatory submissions. Most of the B–R graphics used in practice are variations of these common graphic types, but we provide relevant clinical settings on the usage with illustration of real examples whenever applicable.

In particular, the QSPI BRWG also conducted an extensive review of recent (2011–2014) FDA AdCom meeting materials in the Center for Drug Evaluation and Research (CDER), Center for Biologics Evaluation and Research (CBER), and Center for Devices and Radiological Health (CDRH) divisions, focusing on the usage of B–R graphics or visual tool presentations in these documents. We found that there is still a need to provide further guidance and case studies on the usages of these graphs in different settings and for different purposes to guide practitioners in their applications. In this chapter, in addition to describing a few commonly used B–R graphs or visual tools, we provide guidance and perspectives for the application and implementation of these graphics and visual tools. We refine existing graphs or visual tools and describe their usages in additional settings where applicable. Illustrative real examples are included to assist the readers with the use of relevant graphs.

This chapter is arranged as follows. In Section 10.2, we illustrate BRAP through the life cycle of a product, focusing on the objectives and clinical setting. Section 10.3 presents a review and elucidation of commonly used B–R graphs we found in literatures. We first describe and explain the graph, provide real examples on the use of the graph in B–R setting, where applicable, discuss the general usage in clinical development, and provide thoughts on the graph generation and software, if applicable. We also suggest refinement of the graphs, as needed. We conclude in Section 10.4.

10.2 BRA through the Life Cycle of Product

Quartey et al. (2012) depicted BRA development and implementation (BRADI) according to the different stages of the product development life cycle in Figure 10.1. This depiction is in line with the stepwise approach that various B–R frameworks are based on, for example, the eight-step PrOACT-URL framework as recommended in the EMA B–R methodology project WP4 report (EMA 2012). Appropriate graphical and visualization techniques together with various qualitative and quantitative BRA methods can be applied throughout the whole product life cycle to aid decision making.

BRA development and implementation should begin early in clinical development. In order to carry out a BRA, it is important to understand the targeted product profile including the intended indication and the availability of alternative treatments, whether the

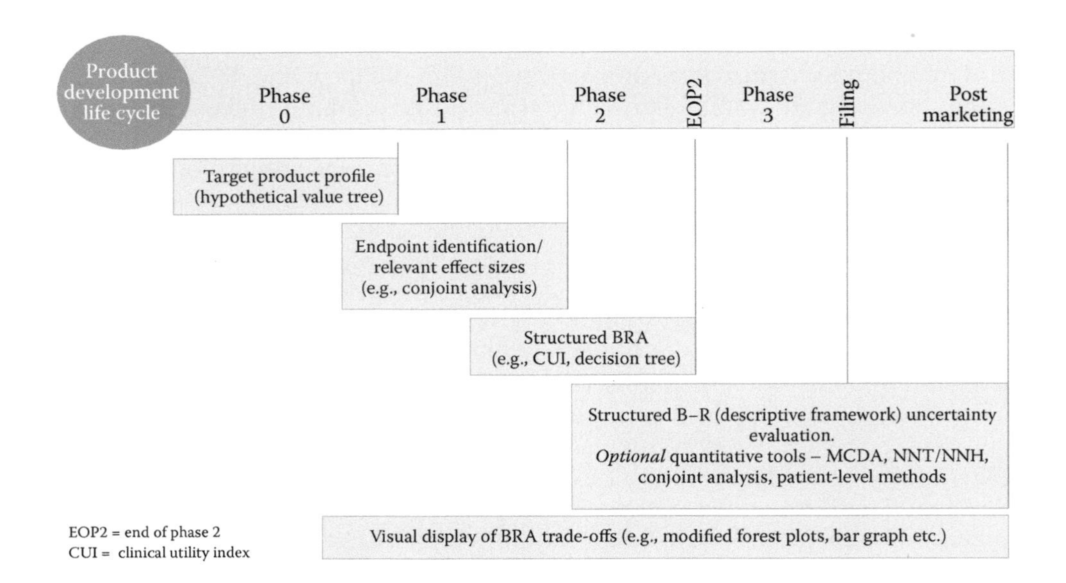

FIGURE 10.1
BRADI according to the different stages of clinical development. (From Quartey, G. EFSPI/FMS/DSBS Joint meeting, Sweden, June 8, 2012.)

treatment meets the criteria for unmet medical need, the severity and morbidity of the condition, the affected population, patients' and physicians' concerns, the time frame for health outcomes, and the decision makers for these considerations. This could be done at the early stage, such as phase 1 of a clinical development program. Next and ideally also in the early development phase, a product team should move to define the BRA problem at hand, including whether the B–R problem is mainly a problem of uncertainty, or of multiple conflicting objectives, or some combination of the two, or something else. The key factors that need to be considered in solving the BRA problem include study design considerations for later stage clinical trials and what sources and adequacy of data that should be collected for a full B–R evaluation. Once a product team obtains a more in-depth understanding of the BRA problem at hand, the team needs to contemplate study designs and sources of data for a full BRA evaluation. This is not a trivial exercise and may require considerable resources and time for deliberation. There have been examples in the past of products that failed to gain regulatory approval because of inadequate study design and data collection. One recent example is the failure of rivaroxaban for the indication of acute coronary syndrome (ATLAS trial), where inadequate study follow-up led to failure in gaining regulatory approval of the product.

Once a product team gains clarity on the target product profile (TPP) and related information in the first two steps, the team could establish objectives that indicate the overall purposes to be achieved, including what constitutes a B–R balance, how to determine what additional information is required, how to assess changes in the B–R balance, and what product restrictions should be recommended. To support the objectives, the team could identify relevant efficacy or safety endpoints for B–R evaluation. In addition, it is important to identify clinically meaningful thresholds that cover the favorable and unfavorable effects on the basis of factors such as available alternative treatments, the severity of the condition, patient preference if available, and other related factors. This exercise can be done in the early phase of a clinical development program and be further refined when phase 2 study data become available. Preferably, when phase 2 data are available and the efficacy of the product for a specific indication has been established, the product team needs to consider the comparators that the test drug should be compared to in BRA.

When a product moves to phase 3 development, it is reasonable to assume that more information on the product with regard to favorable and unfavorable effects has been gained from exploratory phase clinical trials. The team may want to refine and improve on the B–R evaluation plan. For confirmatory trials, factors that may need to be considered at study design stage include endpoints for BRA, weighting strategy, length of follow-up, comparators, criteria to determine a favorable or unfavorable B–R profile, B–R analysis methods for the product, including ways to quantify uncertainty for study endpoints, multiplicity adjustment consideration including interim analysis if appropriate, and subgroups for BRA, to name just a few. After the product gains market approval, BRAP should be continued to be updated on the basis of accumulative data from new clinical trials or real-world data.

10.3 Summary of the Review and Interpretation of B–R Visualizations with Real Examples

In this section, we provide a summary of key common graphics that are described in the PROTECT reports or have appeared in other medical or statistical literatures. In our description of various visual tools, we first provide a general description of the graph, then offer real examples of such visualization in BRA application, discuss high-level potential usage in clinical development setting and make suggestions on further refinement or extension of such visual tools, and lastly describe graph generation and suggestions on any available software for implementation.

A list of visual tools reviewed in this section is categorized into the following groups on the basis of their main usage in BRADI stages from early planning to postmarketing. However, it is also recognized that each individual graph or visual tool may be used in multiple stages and serve multiple purposes. For instance, all the graphs or visual presentations in the B–R subgroup identification category and BRA sensitivity analysis category can also be used for B–R analysis and presentation, given the nature that the subgroup identification or sensitivity analysis is part of the B–R analysis as well as its result presentation.

- BRA Planning and Development
    - Value tree
- B–R Analysis and Presentation (from clinical development stage to postmarket setting)
    - Forest plot
    - Individual response profile (IRP) plot
    - Kaplan–Meier (KM) plot
    - 2-D scatterplot
    - Bar graphs
    - Effects table

- B–R Subgroup Identification
  - Subpopulation treatment effect pattern plot (STEPP)
- BRA Sensitivity Analysis Supporting Decision Making
  - Tornado plot
  - B–R plane
  - 3-D B–R threshold plot
  - B–R contours
  - Likelihood ratio graph
  - Q-TWiST Threshold Utility plot

10.3.1 BRA Planning and Development

10.3.1.1 Value Tree

A value tree in the setting of BRA for medical treatment is a qualitative display that lists out the key clinical outcomes that are critical in evaluating the B–R balance of the treatments in a tree structure. Those key clinical outcomes or criteria in the value tree should reflect the effectiveness, administrative advantage, and potential safety concerns of the new treatment. A value tree diagram greatly enhances communication among different stakeholders and is widely used with various BRA frameworks or methodologies, such as the BRAT (now CIRS-BRAT framework), the PrOACT-URL framework, and multicriteria decision analysis (MCDA) (PROTECT 2013). The value tree also provides the structural foundation to construct the effects table, which provides the main clinical data to conduct a BRA (see details in Section 10.3.2.6).

The EMA Benefit–Risk Methodology Project conducted a few "field tests" (pilot studies) for BRA. One pilot study is to evaluate the B–R profile of Drug X, an add-on therapy for rheumatoid arthritis versus methotrexate alone. Under the PrOACT-URL framework, a value tree as shown in Figure 10.2 was drawn in the "Objective" step (i.e., the "O" in PrOACT-URL) to prepare for the prospective MCDA (EMA 2012 WP3). The key benefits

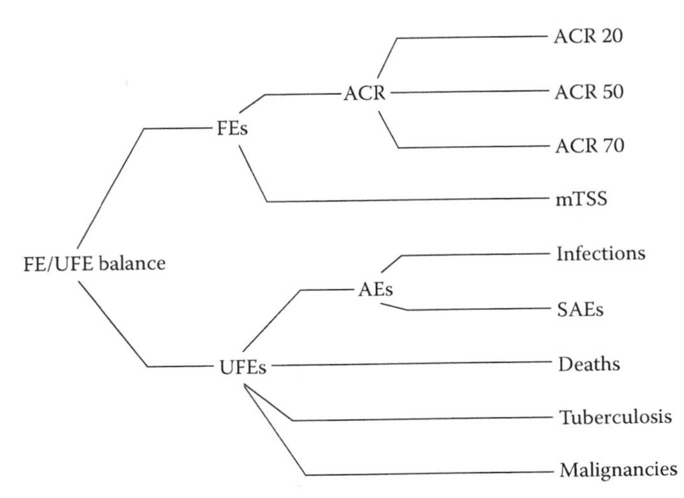

FIGURE 10.2
A value tree diagram for an MCDA analysis. (Extracted from Figure 1 in EMA_WP3.)

or the favorable effects are the two classes of clinical outcomes, one is the ACR (American College of Rheumatology: ACR 20, 50, and 70 each corresponding to a 20%, 50%, and 70% improvement on the patient's ACR score, respectively), and the other is the mTSS (Modified Total Sharp Score). The key risks or the unfavorable effects are five major adverse drug reactions—infections, serious adverse events (AEs), deaths, tuberculosis, and malignancies. Each of the clinical benefit or risk outcome was clearly represented by a branch or subbranch of the tree in the value tree diagram. The B–R category (group of B–R outcomes, i.e., ACR), the individual main (primary) B–R outcomes, and the potential B–R outcomes (not shown) were color coded for better visualization. When the clinical data are available, each individual branch in the value tree may form one row in the effects table. A schematic map of the process from the value tree to effects table is shown in Figure 10.3. Notice that the number of risk outcomes is more than the number of benefits outcomes as shown in this value tree, but it does not imply that the risk is higher than the benefit for the add-on therapy. Moreover, the value tree itself does not provide sufficient details on how it was created and why certain clinical outcomes were selected. Therefore, it is always a good practice to provide a thorough documentation of the rationales and process by which the value tree was created.

The value tree can be used for the study-level or program-level BRA. It can include multiple benefits and risks, or just one benefit and one risk outcome. In addition, the value tree can also be used for patient-level B–R analyses, because the clinical outcomes listed in the value tree form the basis in constructing the decision rule for each individual patient. For a sensitivity analysis purpose, multiple versions of value trees may be created for BRA as well.

The value tree can be used throughout various stages of drug development in any therapeutic area. In the design stage of a new trial or planning a new clinical program, the value

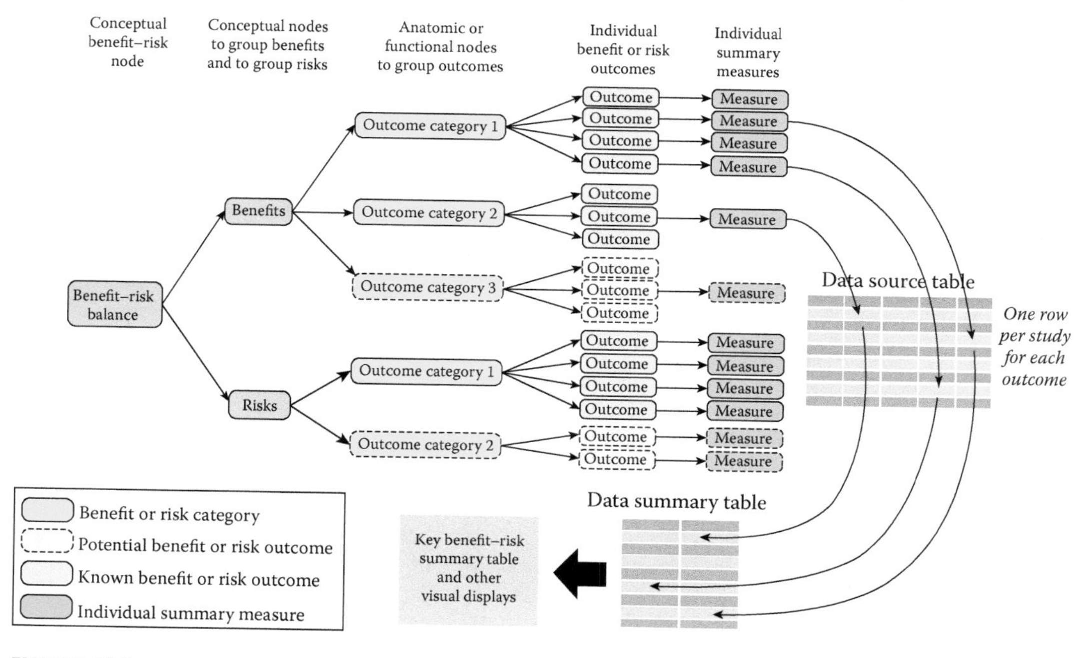

FIGURE 10.3
A schematic map of the process from the value tree to effects table. (Reprinted with permission from CIRS PhRMA BRAT Process Guide, version 1.0, Centre for Innovation in Regulatory Science.)

tree can help establish the TPP since the tree structure clearly lists out the key B–R profile that the product under development needs to demonstrate in order to win the regulatory approval and be commercially viable. During a trial, the value tree may be updated as data accumulate. For instance, an unexpected but important type of adverse drug reaction might be observed during the trial, and it is critical to include such emerging information in the value tree for a more accurate and balanced B–R evaluation. After the trial is finished and the trial data are being analyzed, the value tree could be referenced to construct the effects table, where summary data according to each B–R outcome in the value tree could be tabulated and appropriate analysis and graphic presentation could be generated. After the data have been analyzed for a B–R evaluation and sent for discussion with the regulatory agencies, such as in an end-of-phase 2 meeting or pre-NDA submission meetings, the value tree could serve as an effective visual tool to facilitate an open and transparent B–R discussion around the selection of key information for BRA. In addition, the value tree can be presented to other stakeholders as well, such as payers and patient groups, to convey the key B–R message of the treatment should the product be approved for market access.

Creating a value tree diagram itself is relatively straightforward. A value tree generally has two branches, namely, benefits (favorable effects) and risks (unfavorable effects), stretched out from the base node. For each branch, multiple subbranches may be created with each subbranch corresponding to one benefit or risk outcome. Sometimes, similar classes of clinical outcomes can also be grouped together and become the middle layer. A number of software can help generate the value tree diagram, such as the MCDA software Hiview 3, the CIRS-BRAT framework tool, or simply the MicroSoft Word or PowerPoint, which may take a little bit more effort to plot the tree.

10.3.2 B–R Analysis and Presentation—From Clinical Development to Postmarketing

10.3.2.1 Forest Plot

A forest plot is a graphical display designed to illustrate the relative strength of treatment effects for multiple entities, such as different scientific studies, various subgroups, or different study endpoints (Lalkhen and McCluskey 2008; PROTECT 2013). It has been widely used in medical research, especially in meta-analysis of randomized controlled trials and subgroup analysis, as an efficient way to present the results graphically. Forest plots are commonly presented in a top-down format with two panels side by side. The left-hand panel lists the information of the entities including the name of the studies or clinical variables, sample size, observed number of events by treatment groups, and treatment effects (e.g., odds ratio, mean difference, standardized effect size). The right-hand panel is the plot itself, which is usually composed by a vertical line representing no treatment effect and a set of horizontal lines—the forest of lines produced gives rise to the name *forest plot*—representing the confidence interval (CI) of the treatment effect for each of these entities listed on the left (Lewis and Clarke 2001). A dot (which could be a square or circle) inside each of the intervals on the plot denotes the mean treatment effect, and the area of the dot may be proportional to the information of the entries, for example, the weight of the study or the size of the subgroup. There are some variations of the form of the forest plot as well. For instance, a forest plot can also be plotted in a horizontal format, or the horizontal line in a top-down–formatted forest plot can also be drawn as a horizontal bar (rectangular), and so on.

In the BRA setting, a forest plot is a quantitative display and naturally fits into a B–R framework (e.g., CIRS-BRAT framework) to present the treatment effects of multiple benefits and risks outcomes that are critical in evaluating the B–R balance of the medicinal products. The treatment effects can be either the direct clinical measurements or the various B–R metrics including number needed to treat or harm (NNT or NNH), B–R ratio (BRR), difference of the overall B–R score based on MCDA, difference on the quality-adjusted life years, to name just a few. Besides presenting the treatment effects of the key benefits and risks outcomes, which may be laid out in a value tree, a forest plot can also be used to present the overall B–R measures for different subgroups or clinical studies to visually investigate the impact of the heterogeneity from the various patient groups. The vertical line in the forest plot under the BRA scenario usually represents the neutral line with either side of the vertical line representing results favoring one treatment over the other, and the horizontal lines in the forest plot represent the CIs of the measurements, which could be for an individual clinical B–R outcome or for a particular patient group. If the CI for a certain measure crosses the vertical line, it means that, at the given level of confidence, the corresponding effect size does not demonstrate a statistically significant benefit or harm for that individual benefit or risk outcome (sometimes, p values are also presented in the plot). The ability of summarizing both the mean effects and their corresponding CIs makes the forest plot an excellent method to graphically evaluate the uncertainty in a BRA.

Figure 10.4 shows an example of forest plots created from the Tableau software to present multiple benefits and risks outcomes for natalizumab compared with a comparator for treating multiple sclerosis in a phase 3 study (Nixon et al. 2013). The treatment effect for each benefit and risk outcome is absolute rate difference. In the forest plot, the benefits and risks outcomes are color coded and grouped appropriately. A vertical dash line at $x = 0$ refers to the no-effect line (i.e., rate difference is 0). The left side of the vertical dash line favors the experimental drug (natalizumab). The right side of the vertical dash line favors the control (i.e., the comparator drug). For instance, the number of patients who relapsed in the experimental drug group was approximately 250 subjects lower than that in the comparator group per 1000 patients, and such difference is statistically significant (does not cross the no-effect line), indicating that the experimental drug demonstrated significant benefit on the reduction of relapse rate over the comparator. Similarly for the risk of reactivation of serious herpes infections, the rate in the experimental drug group is slightly higher than that in the comparator. However, the numerical increase of such risk is not statistically significant as the CI across the no-effect line, indicating that the experimental drug might have a potential problem in increasing the risk of reactivation of serious herpes infections, but such risk may not be significantly different from the comparator drug. Forest plots present multiple benefits and risks outcomes in one picture, which greatly help understand the overall B–R profile of the study drug. In addition, the upper portion of Figure 10.4 shows a standard forest plot of the clinical benefits and risks outcomes. When the relative importance among the clinical outcomes needs to be considered in the B–R evaluation, they can be expressed into numerical weights and incorporated into the forest plot as shown in the lower portion of Figure 10.4.

Figure 10.5 shows a forest plot of a cross-study comparison on NNT between rifaximin and control for patients with irritable bowel syndrome (IBS), which was presented at the November 2011 FDA Gastrointestinal Drugs AdCom meeting (Salix Main Presentation 2011). Although the studies, Tegaserod-358 and Tegaserod-307, in the middle of the forest plot have a larger variability, the lower bounds cross the middle vertical line into the "No-Benefit" zone; majority of the studies have a positive NNT around 10 and their CI are away from the No-Benefit zone. This potentially suggests a favorable B–R profile of rifaximin over control.

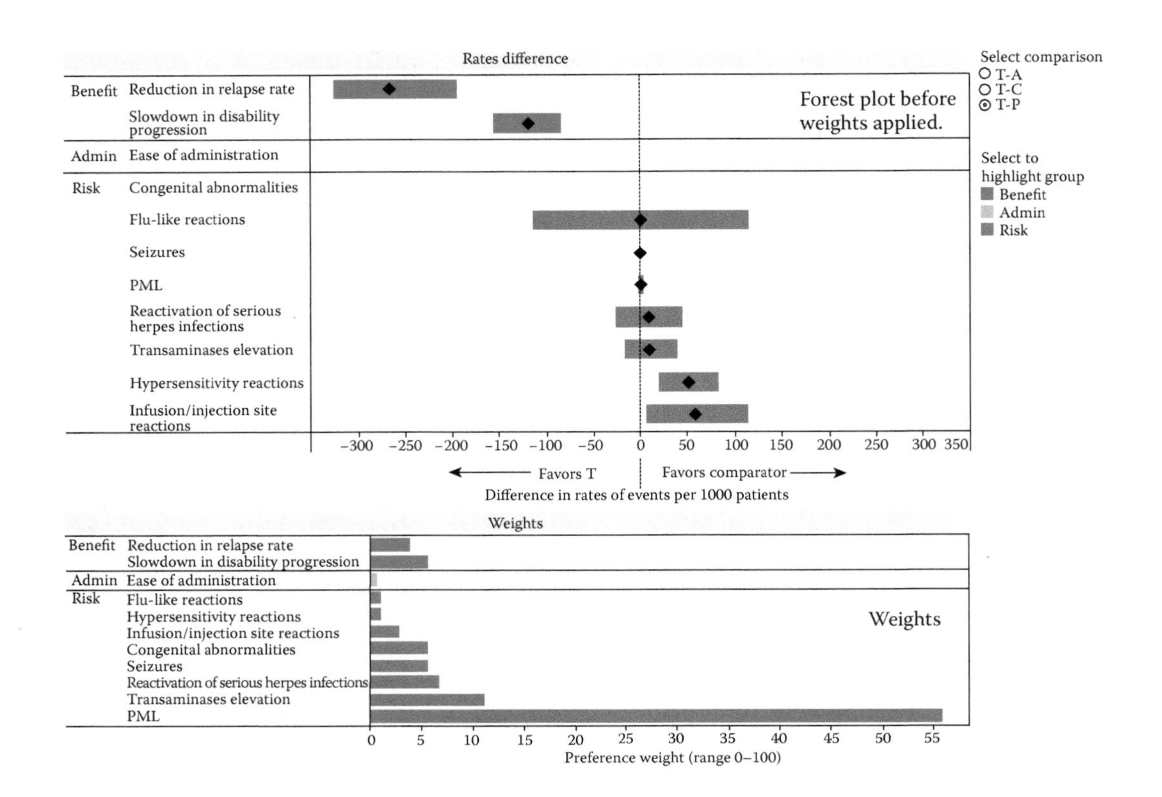

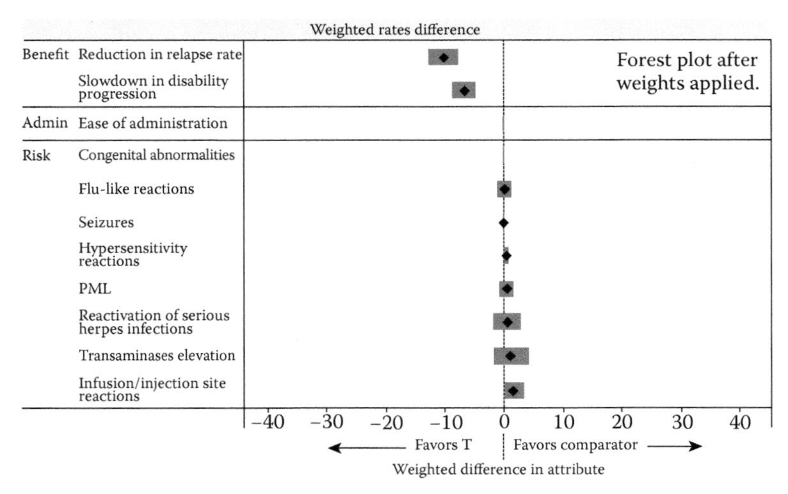

FIGURE 10.4
An example forest plot with or without weighing in relative importance of each benefit or risk outcome. (Extracted from Nixon et al. IMI WP5 Benefit Risk Case Study Report Natalizumab (Wave 1 and Wave 2), 2013.)

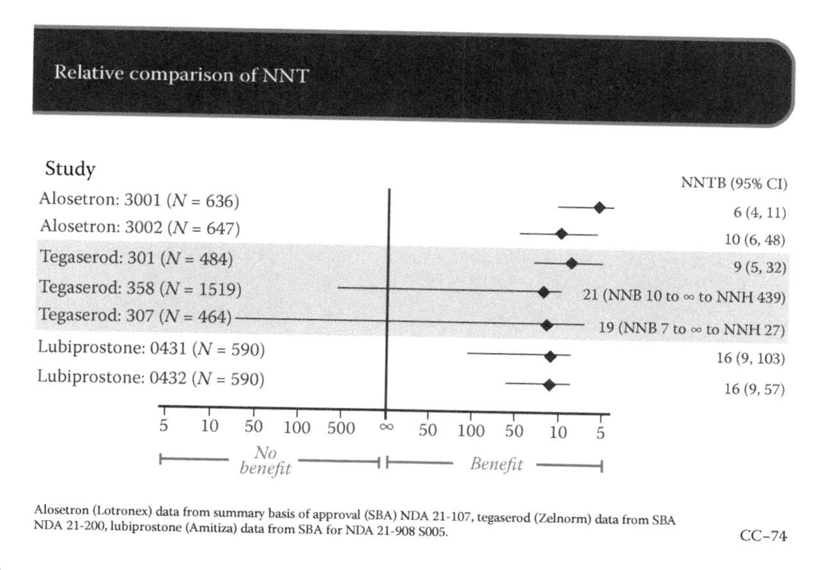

FIGURE 10.5
A forest plot for cross-study comparison on NNT between rifaximin and control for IBS patients. (Extracted from rifaximin sponsor's AdCom slide.)

A forest plot is primarily used in the presentation stage after the clinical results are obtained. Various forest plots have appeared in clinical study reports, scientific publications, briefing documents, and presentations at regulatory meetings. It has been widely used across different therapeutic areas as means of B–R communication to various stakeholders including regulators, physicians, patient groups, and other experts. For instance, the QSPI BRWG conducted a comprehensive review on the usage of B–R graphics or visualization methods in recent years (2011–2014)'s FDA AdCom meeting materials in CDER, CBER, and CDRH divisions. Forest plots are perhaps the most frequently used graphic technique to demonstrate the B–R profile of a product or treatment under review or discussion.

The generation of a forest plot in a B–R setting is no different from creating forest plots under other contexts, for example, meta-analysis. Besides writing customized codes to generate a forest plot, some existing software packages, such as Metafor (a free R package) and comprehensive meta-analysis (commercial software), have built-in functionality to create forest plots. In addition, the CIRS-BRAT framework tool can also generate forest plots without intensive programming, but only for dichotomous outcomes.

10.3.2.2 IRP Plot

The IRP plot (Norton 2011) is a longitudinal display of subject-level responses, where the responses are ordinal data with each category representing a different level of B–R trade-off. It considers B–R as a dynamic process, allowing patients to change state over the course of a trial. It is a nice quantitative tool to examine temporal changes of B–R profile and heterogeneity across subjects. It is most useful in data exploration and analysis stage but can also be used in the presentation stage. At each visit or predefined window, each subject is assigned to one of five categorical outcomes: benefit without an AE, benefit with an AE, neither, AE without benefit, and early withdrawal. Note that the five categories are ordered from the most favorable to the least favorable B–R trade-off. This is an extension of the model introduced by Chuang-Stein et al. (1991) for a summary at the end of study to longitudinal visits. The data for each treatment arm are displayed using a stacked line plot that has the visit windows as x-axis and subject ID as y-axis. The longitudinal responses of a subject are represented by a segmented line where each segment of the line is colored according to which category that response belongs to. These lines are then stacked together and sorted according to the order of the five categories. The stacked line plots for each treatment arm are displayed side by side for a visual comparison, and the sorted lines constitute areas of different responses with each treatment that can be easily visualized for level and magnitude of responses.

In the example extracted from Norton (2011) as in Figure 10.6, B–R response data from each patient are sorted starting from the last period, then the penultimate one, and so on. The thickness of each row is proportional to the number of subjects who had that longitudinal B–R response. The last vertical slice corresponds to the end of study responses. It is apparent that the hydromorphone arm (plot on the left) had more AE-free benefit (green) and fewer dropouts (black) at the end of the study than the placebo group (plot on the right). This pattern started to appear early in the trial and was consistent across visits.

In the BRA setting, the IRP plot visually evaluates the overall B–R profile between treatments through comparing the area of a certain color. It can be used for therapeutic areas where longitudinal responses are of interest. It is particularly appropriate for treatments that provide symptomatic relief for chronic conditions. However, one should be aware of

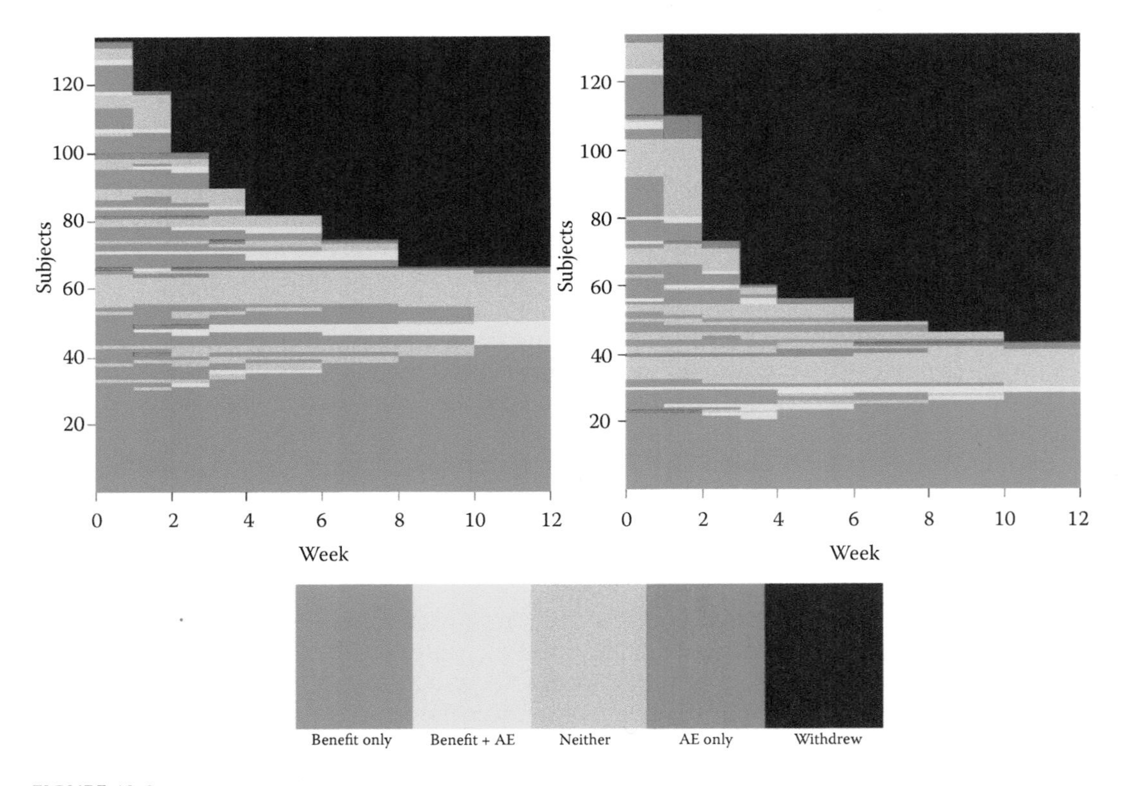

FIGURE 10.6
Example IRP plot. Left plot is for the hydromorphone arm and the right plot is for the placebo group. (Extracted from Norton, J.D., A longitudinal model and graphic for benefit–risk analysis, with case study. *Drug Information Journal*, 45 (2011): 741–747.)

a few issues when producing and reviewing such plots. The plots of each treatment arm should be scaled to have the same total area, especially when sample sizes are different. The x-axis is preferred to be on real time scale. Different coloring schemes and sorting order may give a different impression and thus should be chosen carefully.

Several straightforward extensions could be considered. For example, the five categories could be modified to better reflect the benefits and risks in different therapeutic areas. The number of categories can also be reduced or increased to show the B–R trade-off at coarser or finer scales. The example plot in Figure 10.6 implicitly gives the same weight to all visits. If results of later visits are considered more important, longer line segments could be used for later visits so that it gives more visual weight to later visits, but be aware that the x-axis is not the "real time scale" any more. The input data for the IRP plot often need to be derived from individual responses of study efficacy and safety endpoints, which will require clinical thinking to determine which endpoints and outcomes should be counted in these categories. Imputation of intermittently missing efficacy data and AE start and end dates may be necessary for the calculation of a subject's B–R responses for each visit window. Once input data are prepared, the creation of the plot can be done using basic plotting functions in most statistical software or packages. To the authors' knowledge, the individual response plot has been implemented in JReview; however, some customized coding may still be expected.

10.3.2.3 KM Plot

The KM estimator, also known as the product limit estimator, is widely used to estimate the probability of surviving (or not observing a certain event/endpoint) over a period (Kaplan and Meier 1958). A KM plot is a series of horizontal steps of declining magnitude where each step indicates the occurrence of at least one event. Sometimes 1 – KM (1 – probability of survival or event free) is plotted, which displays the estimated probabilities of death (or observing a certain event).

As shown in Figure 10.7, the KM curves for the efficacy endpoint (a composite endpoint of death, myocardial infarction [MI], ischemia-driven revascularization, stent thrombosis)

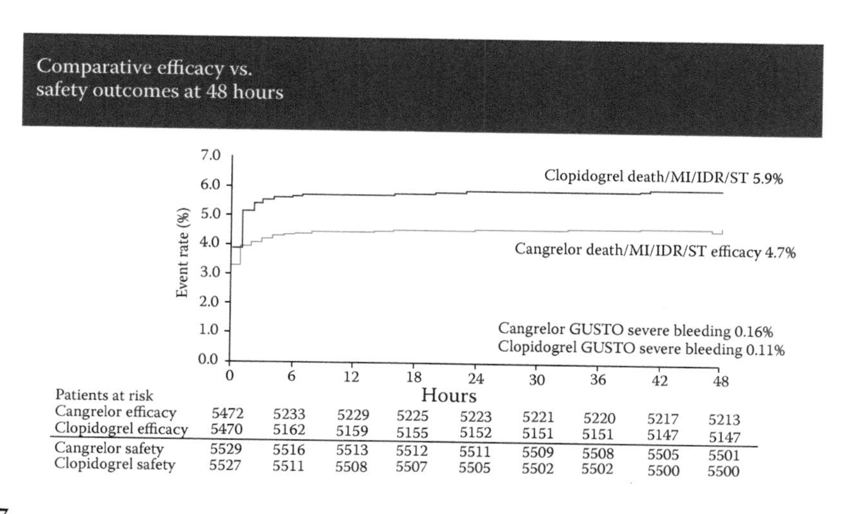

FIGURE 10.7
Comparison of the main B–R profile between cangrelor and clopidogrel. (Extracted from cangrelor sponsor's AdCom slide.)

and the safety endpoint (Global Utilization of Streptokinase and Tissue Plasminogen Activator for Occluded Coronary Arteries severe bleeding) for the development drug cangrelor and the comparator drug clopidogrel are displayed in one plot (TMC Presentations 2014). This provides a visual contrast of large efficacy difference but small safety difference between the two drugs. The efficacy effect was shown shortly after treatment initiation and stayed stable during the whole follow-up period. However, it is worth mentioning that as the efficacy and safety endpoints are displayed on their original scale, it is important that they are of similar clinical importance. Otherwise, the comparison may be visually deceptive.

Alternatively, displaying the difference of the KM estimates between the treatment groups for the efficacy and safety endpoints may be a more direct illustration of the balance between benefit and risk. In Figure 10.8, the excess number of events per 10,000 patients of the efficacy endpoint (the composite of nonbleeding cardiovascular death, MI, and ischemic stroke) and that for the safety endpoint (fatal bleeding and symptomatic ICH) are calculated as the difference of KM estimates between the investigational drug rivaroxaban and placebo over the follow-up (FDA Briefing Document 2012; Janssen Briefing Information 2012). A negative value favors the investigational drug rivaroxaban and a positive value favors placebo. The plot clearly illustrates the trade-off between big gain in benefit (i.e., large risk reduction in the composite efficacy endpoint) and small increase in risk (i.e., small increase in the occurrence of the composite safety endpoint) of the investigational drug compared to placebo. The 95% CI at four different time points were also provided to illustrate the statistical variability of the estimates.

The plot in Figures 10.7 and 10.8 was for one efficacy and one safety endpoint, but it could potentially be extended to account for multiple benefits and risks, but the endpoints need

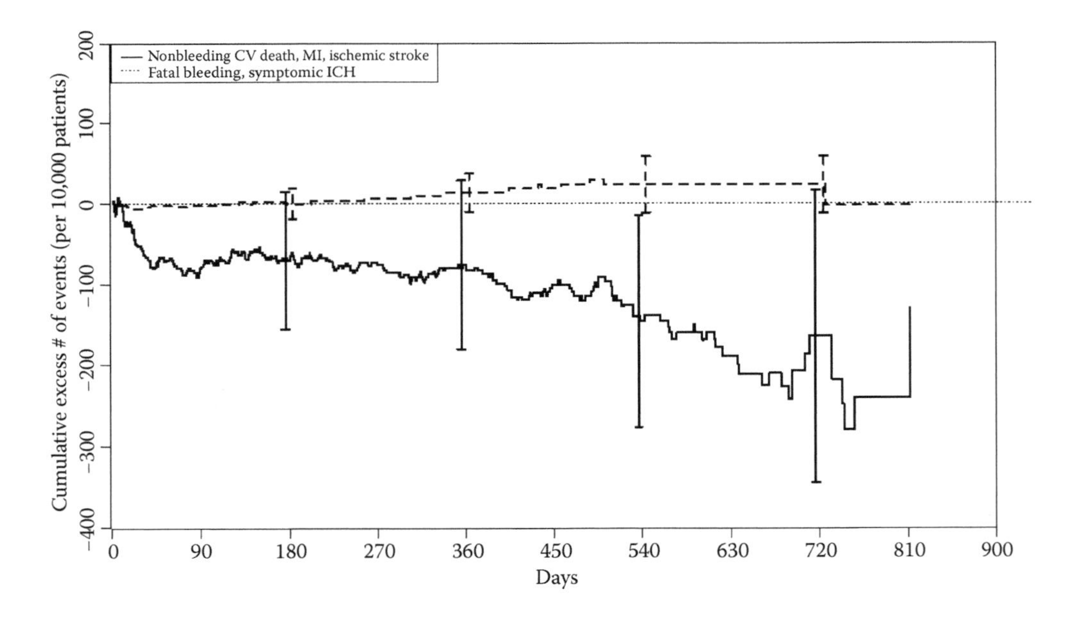

FIGURE 10.8
Cumulative excess number of events based on the KM method for the difference of both the key efficacy and safety measures between rivaroxaban 2.5 mg b.i.d. and placebo. (Extracted from Figure 21 in the Rivaroxaban sponsor's AdCom briefing document.)

to be processed, for example, rederived to be one benefit endpoint and one risk endpoint, synthesized into a net clinical outcome (i.e., a single composite endpoint), or combined into a weighted B–R score. Otherwise, the plot may have too many curves and become too complicated to digest. The abovementioned example of rivaroxaban was actually a rederivation of the original study endpoints. The original efficacy and safety endpoints were decomposed and regrouped to form one benefit and one safety endpoint, which were comparable in clinical importance and mutually exclusive to avoid double counting. Figure 10.9 (Jiang et al. 2013) shows an example of combining differences of KM estimates between treatment groups for multiple benefits and risks into a weighted B–R score. Equal weights were used in Figure 10.9 for illustration but different weighting schemes could have been applied to reflect the relative importance of the endpoints. Factors to consider with regard to weighting are discussed in Chapter 4. Bootstrap method was used in producing the unadjusted 95% CI at two different time points to account for the correlations between the endpoints. The weights were treated as fixed values. Wen et al. (2014) also proposed two statistical approaches, the delta method and the Monte Carlo approach, to calculate the CI for the weighted overall B–R score from MCDA where the correlation between criteria are also taken into account.

The KM plot can be used to aid BRA and is useful at both the analysis and presentation stage. It is especially helpful to demonstrate the temporal change of treatment effect and B–R balance. One efficacy and one safety endpoint can be displayed in one plot to give an easy overview of the B–R profile change over time. KM plots can be produced in most statistical software or packages. Some customized coding may be necessary to prepare data for plotting purposes.

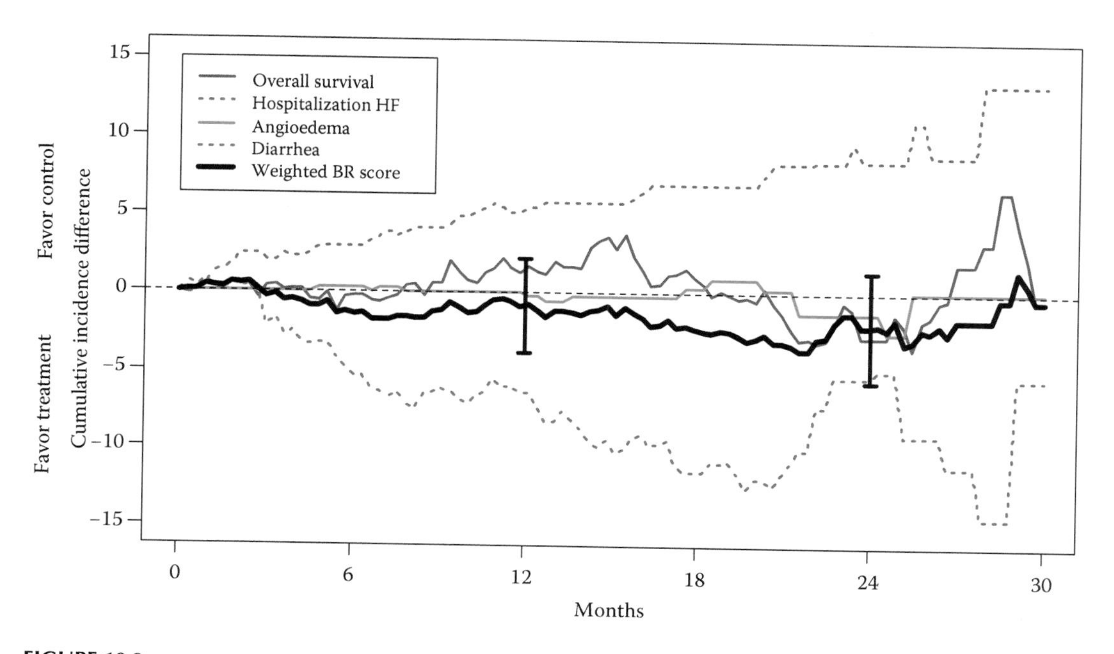

FIGURE 10.9
Overall B–R score weighted based on KM curves from several efficacy and safety endpoints. (Extracted from a slide from Jiang, Q. et al., Susan Shepherd, Benefit–Risk Assessment Methods: A Spectrum from Qualitative to Quantitative. SCT/FDA Benefit:Risk Workshop 2013.)

10.3.2.4 2-D Scatterplot

Assuming that benefits and risks (harms) can each be measured on a continuous scale or can be transformed as such, a scatterplot (benefit vs. harm) of patient scores could then be plotted for one point per patient. If the patient scores congregate in the quadrant with high benefit and low harm, then this would be indicative of an effective intervention. The result for a control group could be plotted using a different color for contrast. The 2-D Scatterplot is particularly useful for visualizing the association between benefits and harms.

Figure 10.10 represents a 2-D scatterplot presented by the FDA at an FDA AdCom meeting on June 6, 2014, for evaluating the B–R profile of "KAMRA Inlay—Model ACI 7000" as part of a PMA Submission by AcuFocus, Inc. (FDA Presentations 2014). At the meeting, the committee reviewed the KAMRA Inlay for the indication of improvement of near and intermediate vision in presbyopic patients who require near or intermediate correction. The inlay is intended to be placed intrastromally in the cornea. The device was designed to improve uncorrected near visual acuity (UCNVA), that is, the "benefit," but could potentially lower the uncorrected distance visual acuity (UCDVA), that is, the "harm."

The FDA asked the applicant to create scatterplots with the horizontal reference line drawn at a change of −5 letters in UCDVA and the vertical line drawn at a change of +10 letters in UCNVA. The FDA chose these reference lines because they considered a change in visual acuity of 5 letters to be within the measurement error and 10 letters change to be significant. With the vertical reference line at +10 letters, 66% (86/130) of subjects fell into the top right (most desirable) quadrant, 12% (15/130) fell into the bottom right, 14% (18/130) fell into the top left, and 8% (11/130) fell into the bottom left (least desirable).

If the continuous scales for benefit and risk are bounded, then a quantitative comparison can be constructed. For any particular patient coordinate (i.e., bivariate score), the (i.e., Euclidian) distance to the "ideal outcome" (i.e., benefit = maximum and risk = minimum)

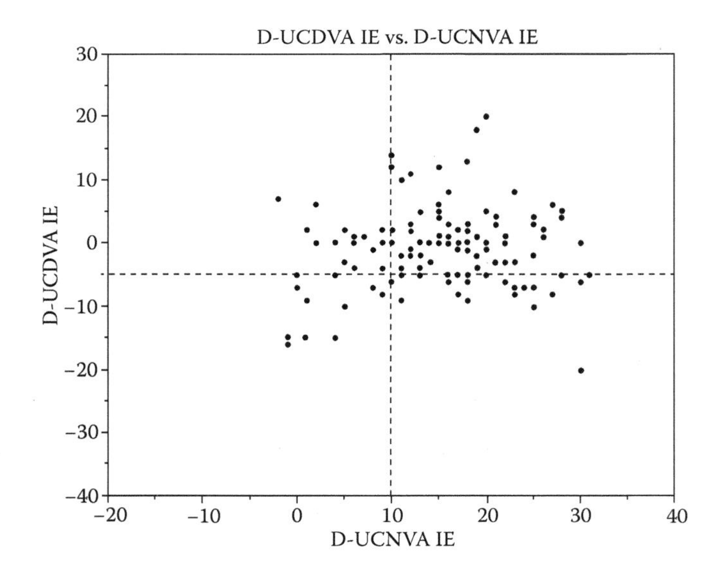

FIGURE 10.10
Example of 2-D scatterplot for the change in UCNVA versus change in UCDVA from Baseline to Month 12 with D-UCNVA = 10, D-UCDVA = −5 as reference lines in a clinical trial. (Extracted from KAMRA Inlay FDA Executive Summary Figure 33.)

could be effectively constructed, reducing the patient outcome to a single dimension. The distances could then be summarized by intervention and compared. An extension to this approach could be made to incorporate the potential imbalance of the importance of one unit on the benefit versus risk scale by using weights. The Euclidian plane could also be separated into ordinal regions of desirability (preferably according to prespecified definitions). Between-intervention comparisons of the proportions of patients that fall into these regions could then be compared using methods that compare ordinal measures. Sensitivity analyses could be performed as definitions of the regions vary.

The 2-D scatterplot is a display for patient-level B–R profiles. It can be created by most statistical software.

10.3.2.5 Bar Graph

In the BRA setting, bar plots are used in presenting treatment effects for important clinical endpoints that are used in evaluating the B–R balance of the medicinal products across treatment arms.

Different variations of bar plots that can be useful for slightly more complex data structures are grouped and stacked bar plots. These are used to explain subtle differences between groups or strata. In the context of quantitative BRA, bar plots may be used to represent the B–R index across treatment arms while grouped or stacked bar plots are used to illustrate the treatment effect of key endpoints that contributed to the calculation of the B–R index. It should be noted that if the number of overall categories is large (e.g., greater than 3) then it becomes hard to distinguish the difference between the groups and subgroups and it becomes harder to compare the sizes of the individual categories.

Figure 10.11 illustrates variations of bar plots. The choice between grouped bar plots (Figure 10.11a) and stacked bar plots (Figure 10.11b and 11c) depends on whether absolute size or relative size of categories is of interest. If the goal is to display relative differences within each category, it is recommended to use stacked percentage bar plot (Figure 10.11c).

Figure 10.12 illustrates the use of both overall bar and stacked bar plots to display the total B–R score and treatment effects on 11 individual endpoints that contribute to the total B–R score for natalizumab against other treatments (placebo, interferon beta-1a, or glatiramer acetate). Positive incremental B–R components (in favor of natalizumab) were stacked vertically above the x-axis, and the negative incremental B–R components were

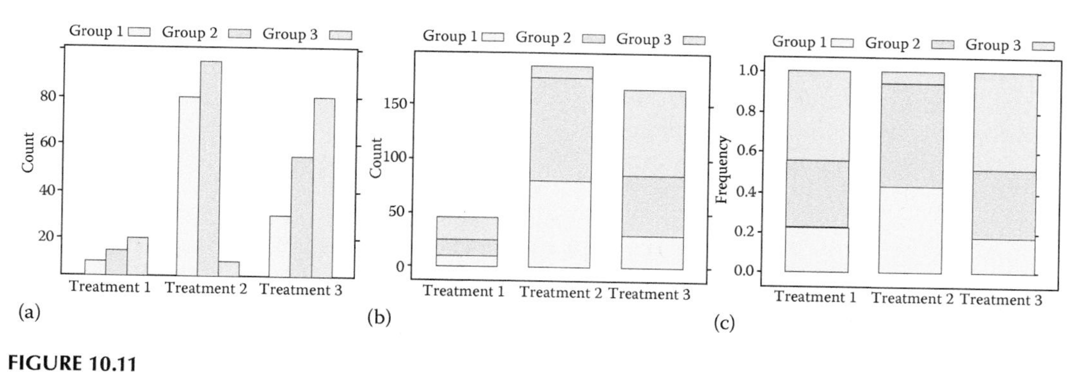

FIGURE 10.11
Variations of bar plots. (a) Grouped bar plot, (b) stacked bar plot using absolute size, and (c) stacked bar plot using relative size.

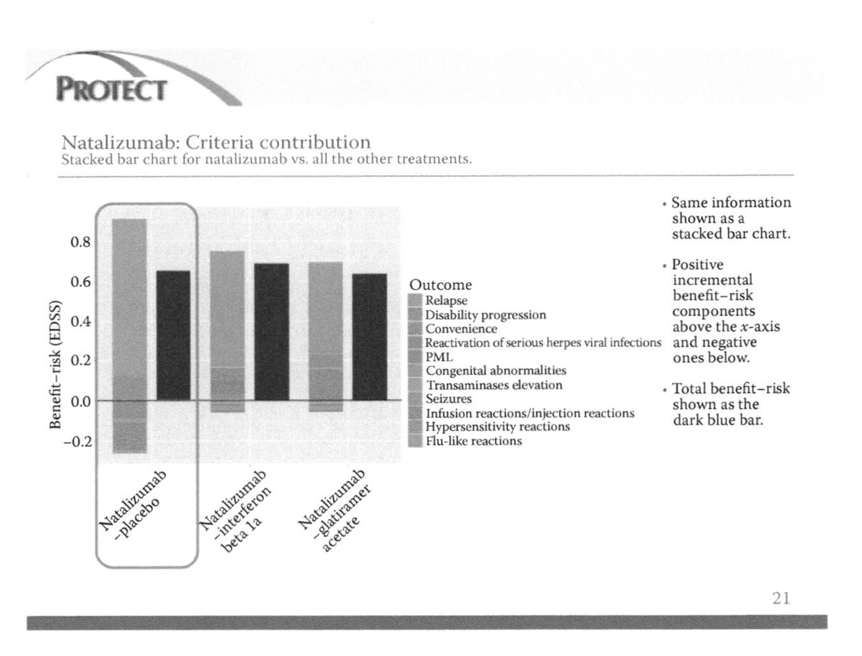

FIGURE 10.12
Stacked bar plot for natalizumab versus other treatments. (From Ashby, D. Visualizing Benefit–Risk for Drug Regulations. Basel PhUSE SDE, July 3, 2014, Basel, CH. http://www.phusewiki.org/docs/Basel%20SDE%20 2014%20presentations/PROF_ASHBY.pdf.)

stacked below the y-axis. The sum of all the components is shown as a blue bar in the plot. Also from Figure 10.12, it can be observed that too many categories per group add visual noise, making it hard to identify patterns in the data. It is noted that if there is a natural increasing or decreasing order to the categories such as increasing dosed arms, then bar plots can be used to identify optimal dose or to compare trend of B–R index across arms.

In summary, bar plots are a simple yet powerful tool to display difference in B–R scores across (sub)categories when the number of (sub)categories is small. Excel and other statistical packages or visualization tools can be used to generate bar plots.

10.3.2.6 Effects Table

The effects table displays all the favorable and unfavorable effects that are important for a BRA. For each of these favorable and unfavorable effects, the table includes definitions of the effects, the unit of measurement for each effect with the plausible range of data, and the measured data for any comparators (which might include more than one dose of the drug). By providing ranges, the relative importance of effects is judged by comparing effect swings from worst to best on these scales, which could be useful for some potential quantitative modeling. The last column in the table offers an opportunity to comment on uncertainties about how effects might influence the BRA (EMA/297405/2012, May 9, 2012). The effects table can help visualize benefit and risk effects that will be included in the BRA. Which endpoints to be included in an effects table need to be discussed. While the selection could be subjective, it typically requires clinical judgment. In general, only the effects that have an appreciable effect on the BRA should be included at the final version of the effects table.

Figure 10.13 is a sample effects table constructed by the following steps (EMA 2012 WP4):

1. **Identify only those favorable and unfavorable effects relevant to the BRA.** For the favorable effects, it may include not only the primary endpoint but also secondary endpoints and the key exploratory endpoints such as the efficacy endpoints and quality of life endpoints. For both the favorable effects and the unfavorable effects, some endpoints may not be prespecified, especially the safety endpoints.
2. **Provide descriptions of the effects.** The descriptions help nonexperts understand how the effects were measured. The scales mentioned in the column "Description" in Figure 10.13 are defined in Grossman and Gordon (2007). SLEDAI (Systemic Lupus Erythematosus Disease Activity Index) is a score that represents disease activity as judged by physicians for 24 items associated with standard weightings that are summed to give an overall score ranging from 1 to 105. BILAG (British Isles Lupus Assessment Group) consists of 86 items that represent a physician's judged or measured activity in eight organ-based systems. A weighted scoring system based on intent to treat provides an overall score ranging from 0 to 72. BILAG A is associated with severe disease, whereas BILAG B is associated with less active disease. In addition, the PGA scale used here is a 0–10 scale with 10 being worst. However, the scale is reported to range from 0 to 3 in some publications.
3. **Define the measurement scales.** The range should encompass measured values that could realistically be expected to extend from worst to best.
4. **Identify the options.** These can include the drug with different doses, a placebo, a comparator, and actions to restrict or limit.
5. **Display the data.** This can be pooled or separate results for each clinical trial.
6. **Comment on effect uncertainties.** It is important to briefly elaborate the reason(s) for different sources of uncertainty.

An effects table is a powerful tool and can provide much increased consistency and clarity to the BRA. While the type of information to include in an effects table is suggested above, there is some flexibility to modify the information in the table based on what may be relevant to an assessment. In addition, one may display an effects table along with a forest plot to further enhance visualization of the B–R effects. Currently, there is no requirement to include an effects table into a Market Authorization Application (EMA WP5/74168/2014). However, EMEA has started to put effects table in the Rapporteurs Day 80 report and update it in a continuous base, and some companies have also put effects table in their submission to adapt such regulatory change.

10.3.3 B–R Subgroup Identification

10.3.3.1 Subgroup Treatment Effect Pattern Plot

Heterogeneity of intervention effects can affect B–R considerations. When there is a desire to evaluate how an intervention effect varies as a function of a single continuous covariate, then a STEPP can be constructed (Bonetti and Gelber 2000, 2004). STEPP is a moving average approach to examine the heterogeneity/homogeneity of an intervention effect as a continuous characteristic varies. Subgroup-specific CIs and global confidence bands

Effects		Name	Description	Best[1]	Worst	Units	Placebo[2]	10 mg[2]	1 mg[2]	Uncertainties (See EPAR ¶2.8)
Favorable Effects (pooled data based on the EPAR)	SLE Responder Index (SRI)	SLEDAI % Improved ≥ 4	Percentage of patients with at least 4 points' reduction in SLEDAI[3]	100	0	%	41	53	48	Approved only for patients with high disease activity. Uncertainties remain about optimal treatment duration, maintenance doses, treatment holidays and rebound phenomenon.
		PGA % no worse	Percentage of patients with no worsening in Physician's Global Assessment[4] (worsening = an increase of less than 0.3 points)	100	0	%	66	75	76	
		PGA Mean score	Overall mean change of PGA score from baseline for the study population	1.0	0	Difference	0.44	0.48	0.45	
		BILAG A/B	Percentage of patients with no new BILAG[3] A/2B	100	0	%	69.0	75.2	70.1	
	Secondary Endpoints	CS Sparing	Percentage of patients that reduced the dose of corticosteroids by more than 25% and to less than 7.5 mg/day	100	0	%	12.3	17.5	20.0	Support from the analyses of the secondary endpoints is weak for the overall population
		Flare rate	Number of new BILAG A cases per patient year	0	5	Number	3.51	2.88	2.90	
		QoL	Mean change in the total score of SF 36 (Short Form)	0	100	Difference	3.5	3.4	3.7	
Unfavorable Effects		Potential SAEs	Potential for developing tumour, opportunistic infections or PML	100	0	Judgement	100	0	90	The mechanism of action could increase potential for developing infections.
		Infections	Proportion of patients with serious infections that are life-threatening	0	10.0	%	5.2	5.2	6.8	
		Sensitivity Reaction	Proportion of patients with hypersensitivity reactions at any time in the study	0	2.0	%	0.10	0.40	0.30	

FIGURE 10.13
Hypothetical example of an effects table for belimumab, treatment of systemic lupus erythematosus, based on the EPAR EMEA/H/C/002015 published on 09/08/2011. (1) Best and worst: For similar scales, the most preferred and least preferred values that would be realistically realizable (e.g., 0 to 100% for both SLEDAI and PGA scales). For dissimilar scales, a range that facilitates comparing the relative importance of the scales (e.g., infections 0%–10%, and sensitivity reaction 0%–2%). (2) Treatment effect estimates. (3) Scales defined in Grossman and Gordon (2007). (4) The PGA scale used here is a 0–10 scale with 10 being worst. However, the scale is reported to range from 0 to 3 in some publications. (Extracted from EMA 2012 WP4 page 12.)

for the intervention effect can be constructed for subgroup-specific and overall inference. Although STEPP does not directly address the BRA, it provides a visual way to examine the impact of the subgroup to the benefit and risk measures and help identify the subgroup(s) with a favorable B–R profile.

STEPP was utilized in the International Breast Cancer Study Group (IBCSG) IX trial of 1715 postmenopausal, node-negative women who were randomized to receive tamoxifen for 5 years versus cyclophosphamide methotrexate fluorouracil (CMF) and tamoxifen for 5 years (IBCSG 2002). Evidence suggested that differences between the treatments depend on estrogen receptor (ER) status (often measured on the log scale), with CMF resulting in higher disease-free survival (DFS) for women with low ER status but not for women with higher scores (Colleoni et al. 2005). STEPPs were constructed displaying the intervention differences in 5-year DFS as a function of ER status (Figure 10.14).

The freely available R code can be found at http://cran.r-project.org/web/packages/stepp/.

10.3.4 BRA Sensitivity Analysis Supporting Decision Making

10.3.4.1 Tornado Plot

The tornado diagram is a common visual tool to evaluate uncertainty and conduct deterministic sensitivity analysis. It is widely used in financial analysis, project planning, and other economic areas. In the setting of assessing the B–R of medical treatments, the tornado diagram is used to evaluate the impact of the uncertainty from each clinical outcome to the overall BRA. Usually, the clinical factors or outcomes with larger impact are put at the top of the graph. Factors or outcomes with smaller impact are placed toward the bottom. The resulting graph resembles a half or complete tornado, thus the name tornado diagram or tornado plot.

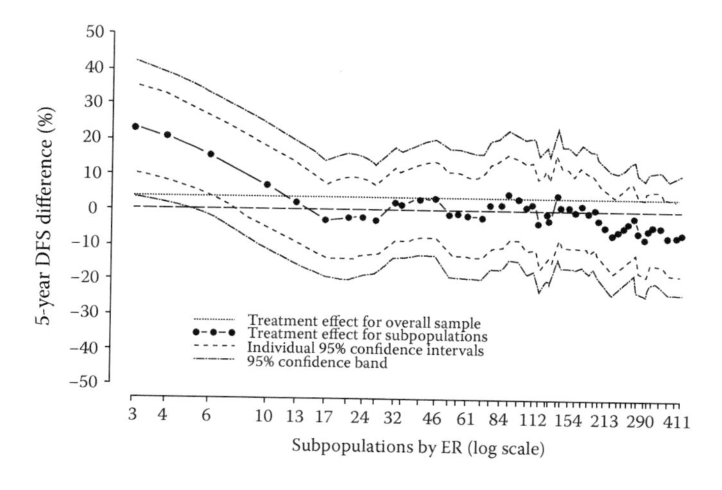

FIGURE 10.14
STEPP plot for IBCSG Trial IX data—ER subgroup for the difference in 5-year DFS as a function of ER status. The horizontal line above zero indicates the difference in DFS in the overall sample. The dots indicate point estimates of the differences in DFS for specific subpopulations defined by the respective ER status. The inner band represents individual CI estimates for the differences in DFS for specific subpopulations defined by the respective ER status. The outer band is a simultaneous 95% confidence band estimate for the differences in DFS for the entire population. There are clear benefits associated with CMF when log(ER) is 6 or smaller but there are no benefits for patients when log(ER) is 13 or greater and thus risks would outweigh benefits for this group of patients.

Figure 10.15 was extracted from a case study report on the BRA of natalizumab (Nixon et al. 2013) on patients with multiple sclerosis. The tornado diagram was employed to determine which among selected key B–R outcomes had more impact on the change of the incremental overall B–R score between natalizumab and the comparator. Figure 10.15 displays results of a sensitivity analysis by varying the relative importance (weights) of each clinical outcome. The range of the weight change for the sensitivity analysis was ±20% of the original weight in the primary analysis. The left part of the graph lists out the selected clinical outcomes that contributed to calculation of the incremental B–R score for natalizumab relative to the comparator. The right part is the plot itself. The *x*-axis on the top and bottom indicate the scale of the incremental overall B–R score between natalizumab and the comparator, which was computed from the MCDA approach. The incremental B–R score from the primary analysis (the base case) was 0.42. By increasing the weight of "Relapse (reduction)" from 8% to 9.6% (20% higher than the original 8%) and keeping the weights unchanged for other outcomes, the incremental B–R score increased to 0.52. When decreasing the weight of "Relapse (reduction)" from 8% to 6.4% (20% lower from 8%) and keeping the weights unchanged for other outcomes, the B–R score decreased to 0.32. Such changes were visually shown in the top bar and color coded with red for cases of increased weight and green for cases of decreased weight, compared to the base case. Similarly, the B–R score increased as the weight of the "Infusion/injection (adverse) reactions" decreased from 3% to 2.4%, because the infusion/injection risk rate in the natalizumab group was higher than the comparator. By downplaying the importance of such risk in the B–R consideration, the overall B–R profile of natalizumab increased. From Figure 10.15, it is easy

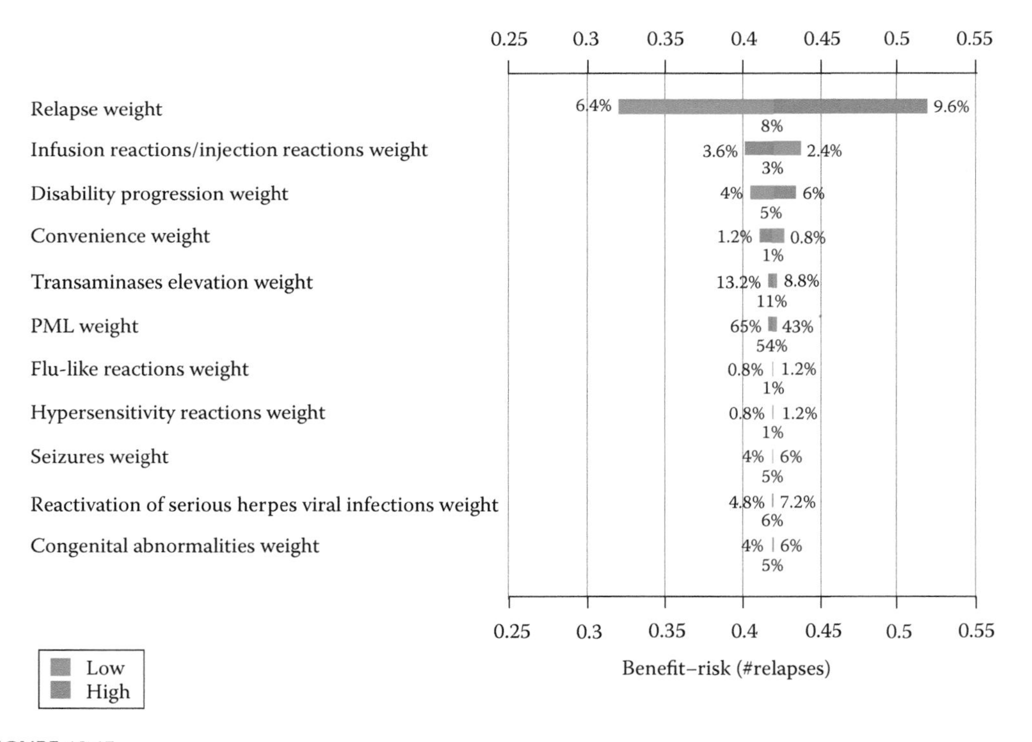

FIGURE 10.15
Tornado diagram to assess the sensitivity of each clinical outcome to the incremental overall B–R score between natalizumab and comparator.

to see that the clinical outcome of relapse reduction played the most important role in the overall B–R evaluation, while the risk of congenital abnormalities played the least. The risk of PML was given the highest weight (54%) in the overall B–R consideration, but the overall B–R change was not very sensitive to PML's weight change.

The tornado diagram is a quantitative display of the robustness of the overall B–R profile with respect to the uncertainty of the key benefits and risks outcomes. The uncertainty could come from the data level, such as the variation of the observed data or the change on the data source. Alternatively, the uncertainty could come from the relative importance assigned to various clinical outcomes (weights). Tornado diagrams are primarily used in the analysis and presentation stage with certain quantitative B–R metrics or methods, such as MCDA, BRR, NNT, or NNH, for sensitivity analysis purposes (Mt-Isa et al. 2013). Because the tornado plot is essentially a special bar plot similar to a forest plot, any statistical or visualization software such as R, SAS, and Microsoft Excel can produce it.

10.3.4.2 B–R Plane

The B–R or risk–benefit (R–B) plane (Lynd and O'Brien 2004) is a two-dimensional plot with the average difference in the probability of achieving a benefit with the new therapy relative to a standard therapy plotted on the *x*-axis (ΔB) and the average difference in the probability of an AE plotted on the *y*-axis (ΔR). Both axes therefore range from −1 to 1, with 0 at the origin. The quadrants of the B–R plane are labeled with points of the compass (NE, SE, NW, SW) (Figure 10.16). Moving from left to right along the *x*-axis indicates increasing benefits attributable to the new therapy. Positive values (to the right of the vertical axis) represent greater benefits with the new treatment, whereas negative values indicate that standard therapy provides greater benefit.

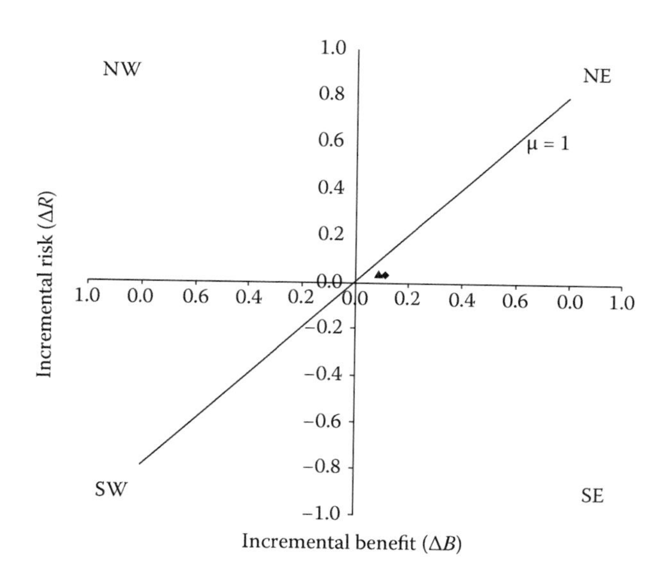

FIGURE 10.16
The R–B plane. Values along each axis are the differences in the probabilities of an event occurring. The ▲ marks the point estimate of the BRR for enoxaparin versus unfractionated heparin for the prevention of proximal DVTs (0.031, 0.085, 0.031); the ◆ marks the point estimate of the BRR for enoxaparin versus unfractionated heparin for the prevention of all DVTs (0.11, 0.031).

Similarly, positive y-coordinates indicate a greater probability of an AE secondary to the new treatment; negative values indicate that standard treatment is more likely to cause adverse effects. The (ΔB, ΔR) coordinates falling in either the SE or the NW quadrant indicate that one strategy is dominant over the other (i.e., one therapy provides greater benefit at lower risk). In the SE quadrant, the new therapy dominates standard therapy, and vice versa in the NW quadrant. Many proposed new treatments lie in the NE quadrant, however, indicating that they are more likely to provide a benefit with a higher probability of AEs. In the NE and SW quadrants, therefore, the decision to use one therapy over another depends on where the (ΔB, ΔR) coordinate falls relative to the R–B acceptability threshold (μ), which is the maximum number of additional AEs the decision maker is willing to accept to realize one additional beneficial outcome.

For the example of low-dose unfractionated heparin versus enoxaparin for the prophylaxis of venous thromboembolism after major trauma (Lynd and O'Brien 2004), if it can be assumed that the incremental risk and the incremental benefit of enoxaparin versus unfractionated heparin are known with certainty, then the true incremental probability of precipitating a major bleed is $P_{\text{bleed}} = 0.031$. The incremental benefit of preventing proximal and all deep vein thrombosis (DVT) is $P_{\text{prox}} = 0.085$ and $P_{\text{all}} = 0.110$, respectively; these points are plotted on the R–B plane in Figure 10.17. Considering that the line with the slope $\mu = 1$ represents a willingness to accept up to one major bleed to avert one DVT, then enoxaparin is the appropriate treatment strategy since the slope of the lines through both (ΔB, ΔR) coordinates is less than $\mu = 1$.

Lynd and O'Brien (2004) also described a limitation of the B–R plane. Although the first-order uncertainty of the random variation in the outcomes of individual patients, contingent on other underlying parameters, is important in any R–B evaluation, the second-order uncertainty, or the imprecision or uncertainty of the estimates of these probabilities, is also of paramount importance, but is not incorporated in the B–R plan as shown in Figure 10.16. Lynd and O'Brien (2004) described a Bayesian approach to modeling R–B data, which involved developing a probabilistic model incorporating the uncertainty around both the risks and

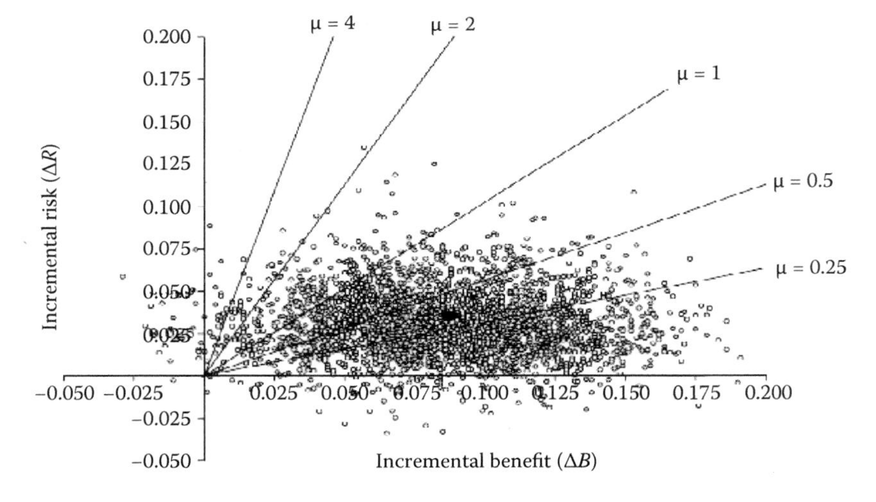

FIGURE 10.17
Results of the second-order Monte Carlo simulation of the DVT trial plotted on the R–B plane: the incremental probability of a DVT (ΔB) versus the incremental probability of major bleed (ΔR). Lines extending from the origin into the NE quadrant represent different R–B threshold values (μ). The ● marks the point estimate of the R–B ratio.

benefits simultaneously by specifying probability distributions for each model parameter to represent their uncertainty. Then, they employed a second-order Monte Carlo simulation in which randomly selected values from each specified distribution are considered, along with the joint uncertainty of the risks and benefits. Thus, within the Bayesian framework, ΔR and ΔB are considered random variables with values that follow specific distributions.

Lynd and O'Brien (2004) indicated that there are two potential methods for quantifying the joint density of the uncertainty around the risks and benefits, depending on whether one has access to patient-level data. If data are available, a nonparametric bootstrap sample of the data can be selected repeatedly; if original data are not available, a simulation can be run using information on the distributions fit to the data. From these simulations or bootstrap estimates, the incremental R–B pairs can be plotted on the R–B plane and the proportion of that estimate falling below a line with a slope equal to μ can be determined as μ is varied from 0 to ∞. Figure 10.17 shows the simulation results from Lynd and O'Brien. Plotted on the R–B plane are lines representing B–R acceptability thresholds ranging from 0.25 to 4 included in the NE quadrant. Only 24 of the 3000 points fell in the NW quadrant, indicating only a 0.8% chance that heparin is dominant in preventing proximal DVTs (i.e., more effective and lower risk).

The R–B plane along with the Bayesian approach to quantify the uncertainty in the estimates of probabilities is a very useful approach in B–R evaluation. The concept of R–B thresholds incorporates clinical input along with the understanding of the analysis of condition and current treatment for an intervention. The B–R plane has the ability to present B–R trade-offs under various R–B thresholds in one setting.

The R–B plane is primarily used to illustrate 1-benefit versus 1-risk trade-off based on either group-level or patient-level information, comparing to clinically meaningful and acceptable thresholds. It can be used throughout various stages of drug development in any therapeutic areas but primarily at major decision points. When early phase data become available, the graph and its associated approach can be used to illustrate B–R trade-off for key clinical endpoints for a go/no-go decision for further clinical development. When confirmatory trial data become available, it can be used to provide supportive evidence on B–R trade-offs. The B–R plane is nothing but a type of line and dot plot that could be generated by any statistical computing software, such as SAS, R, and so on. To the authors' knowledge, there is no commercially available software to generate the B–R plane in particular.

10.3.4.3 3-D B–R Threshold Plot

He and Fu (Chapter 9) proposed a joint evaluation framework, via the Bayesian method, that assesses B–R by comparing efficacy and safety data with clinical meaningful thresholds that are chosen with the consideration of medical condition and current treatment options. Assuming that the posterior distributions for the estimated treatment effect for efficacy and safety endpoints had been derived, He and Fu (in press) developed a measure, called probability of technical success (POTS), as follows:

$$\text{POTS} = \Pr(\theta_e > \delta_e \text{ and } \theta_s > \delta_s \mid Y, S),$$

where θ_e denotes the treatment effect for an efficacy endpoint, θ_s denotes the treatment effect for a particular safety endpoint of interest, δ_e denotes a clinically meaningful threshold for efficacy of which treatment is deemed efficacious and marketable if $\theta_e > \delta_e$, and δ_s denotes a safety threshold of which the safety of the treatment is considered acceptable if $\theta_s < \delta_s$. Y and S represent efficacy or safety data from a clinical trial. They used Monte Carlo numerical integration to derive the POTS. It should be noted that the concept of

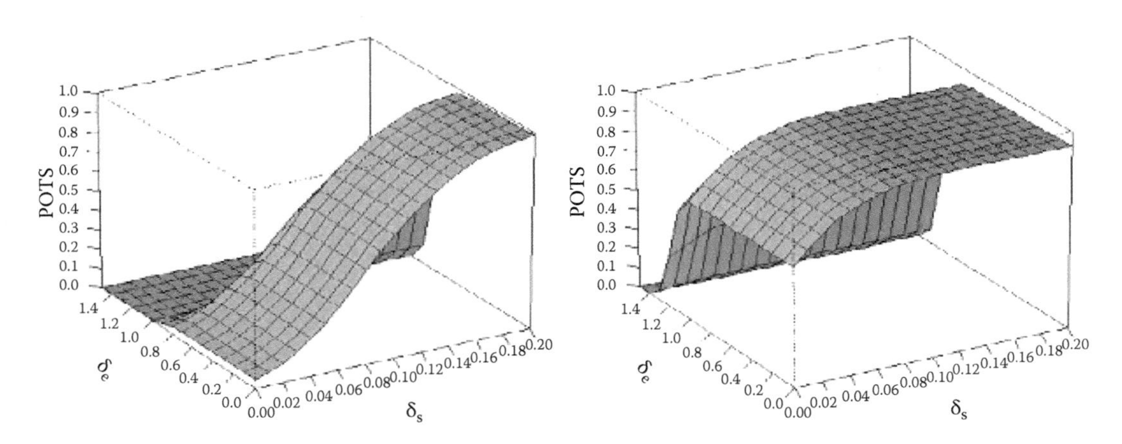

FIGURE 10.18
POTS for drug dose 1 versus placebo (left) and drug dose 2 versus placebo (right).

clinically meaningful thresholds He and Fu (in press) employed is very similar to the R–B acceptability thresholds that Lynd and O'Brien (2004) utilized.

To graphically illustrate the decision criteria, POTS is plotted against different δ_e and δ_s values for a set of B–R profiles based on data from a clinical trial. Figure 10.18 presents POTS for drug dose 1 versus placebo (left plot) and drug dose 2 versus placebo (right plot) for the example described in He and Fu in Chapter 9. It can be observed that when δ_e increases and δ_s decreases, that is, when the clinical significant thresholds become more stringent, POTS decreases. The decision on whether benefit outweighs risk can be made if POTS is relatively high, say at 0.8 or above, given relevant efficacy and safety thresholds.

The 3-D B–R threshold plot is another useful way in B–R evaluation, as it clearly shows the B–R trade-offs on the basis of clinical study data. Although the POTS measure itself is not quantified with uncertainty measure, Lynd and O'Brien's approach with a Monte Carlo simulation approach can be utilized to provide that additional measure of uncertainty. Similar to the B–R plane, the 3D B–R threshold plot is also primarily used to illustrate 1-benefit versus 1-risk trade-off on the basis of either group-level or patient-level information, comparing to clinically meaningful and acceptable thresholds. This graph and the associated approach can be used in clinical development, and the setting is similar to that of the B–R plane. There is no commercially available software to generate the graph, and the authors developed R code to generate the graph.

10.3.4.4 R–B Contours

The R–B contour (RBC) is a two-dimensional graph showing a set of nonlinear curves that join equal levels of confidence (or probability) associated with the risks and benefits of one intervention when compared with another (Shakespeare et al. 2001). This method provides a view of the confidence levels of benefit and risk pairs. The x-axis represents the degree of benefit, and the y-axis represents the degree of risk. For each specified benefit increment and each risk increment, the confidence level is calculated (as the probability that a specified size of benefit or risk exists) and the product of benefit confidence and risk confidence is taken as the confidence level of the pair. As the authors of the method suggested, this method can help physicians or clinicians to choose between competitive therapies. The benefit and risk are not integrated in this method. Actually, this method is just about the presentation of benefit and risk with confidence information. The RBC can be generated easily by use of standard statistical packages, by calculating and plotting the confidence level for every possible size of benefit and risk of one intervention over the other. RBCs can be generated for any outcome, whether for absolute or relative benefit or detriment, recurrence rates, or toxicity, that is, for any outcome that can be analyzed by means of CIs. The curve allows an independent assessment of the probability associated with a benefit of clinical relevance to the clinician and patient.

Figure 10.19 shows an example of RBC for absolute 3-year survival benefit and absolute 99.95% probability that chemo-radiotherapy, compared with radiotherapy alone, was associated with more grade 3 and grade 4 acute toxicity (Shakespeare et al. 2001). In this example, the authors assumed independence between acute toxicity and survival. Therefore, the RBC is simply a product of the two confidence levels. Each contour (identified with a percentage probability) connects identical probabilities for various R–B scenarios. For example, the RBC shows whether clinician A is willing to accept a 30% probability of acute toxicity as long as there is a 10% improvement in the chance of survival, respectively (Shakespeare et al. 2001). These two lines intercept on the 70% RBC. Thus, there is 70% confidence (or probability) that the criteria set by clinician A are met (and 30% probability that they are not) (Shakespeare et al. 2001). On the other hand, clinician B decides that she will change practice only if the following criteria are met: chemoradiotherapy must improve survival by at least 5%, but must not increase acute toxicity by more than 40%. Clinician B also refers to the RBCs in Figure 10.19 and draws her scenario. The two lines intercept very close to the 97% contour. Thus, there is 97% probability that her criteria are met, and only

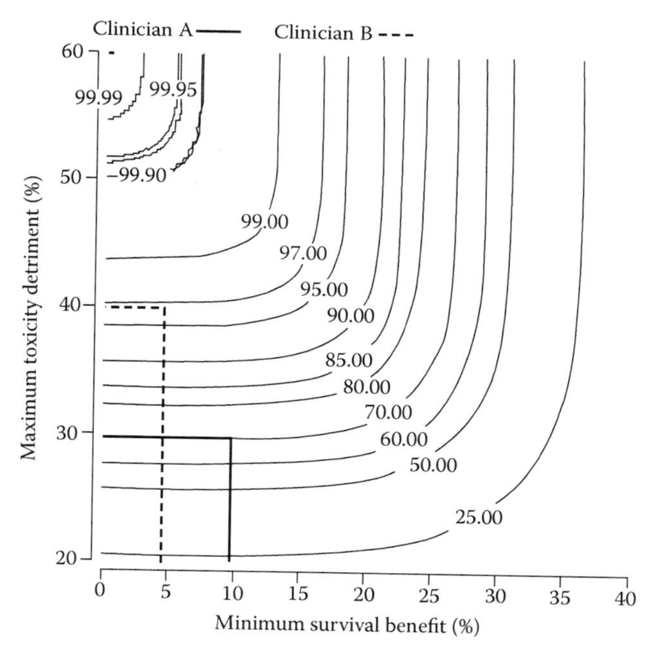

FIGURE 10.19
Confidence associated with absolute 3-year survival benefit increase and absolute toxicity detriment for chemoradiotherapy compared with radiotherapy alone in Intergroup study 0099 (Al-Sarraf et al. 1998). Solid line, clinician A; dashed line, clinician B.

a 3% probability that the criteria are not met. Therefore, clinician B decides that she can confidently change her practice on the basis of this study (Shakespeare et al. 2001).

The RBC plot can be used to represent benefit and risk information throughout the life cycle of drug development in any therapeutic area. Information from various stages of drug development can be extracted and R–B trade-off can be represented visually by this method. RBC can be constructed to represent BRA information at the population level as well as at the individual patient level. This can be achieved by finding out from each patient or physician the amount of risk he or she is willing to accept to obtain a certain benefit, and a set of individual RBC R–B can be determined. The RBC plot only deals with one benefit criterion and one risk criterion for the comparison of two options and does not allow for multiple risks and multiple benefits from a drug therapy. Also, the benefit and risk are not integrated in this method. Additionally, RBC plots provide stakeholders (e.g., clinicians) with a mechanism of translating the results of studies into treatment for individual patients, thus improving the clinical decision-making process. Any statistical or visualization tool can be used to plot the contour lines in the plot.

10.3.4.5 Likelihood Ratio Graph

The likelihood ratio graph (Biggerstaff 2000) is a two-dimensional plot to compare the sensitivity (true positive rate, the rate of reporting positive when it is truly positive) and specificity (true negative rate, the rate of reporting negative when it is truly negative) simultaneously between two tests or diagnostic algorithms. When we compare the performance of two algorithms by sensitivity and specificity estimates, it may at times be difficult to decide which algorithm is preferable. When both the sensitivity and specificity of one algorithm are higher than the other, it is clear that the one with higher sensitivity and specificity is better; however, if sensitivity of one algorithm is higher than the other but the specificity is lower, it is not clear which algorithm is better. Biggerstaff (2000) proposed a graphical display, shown in Figure 10.20, to help visualize when a decrease in specificity is offset by an increase in sensitivity to yield improvement in both positive and negative predictive values for a given algorithm.

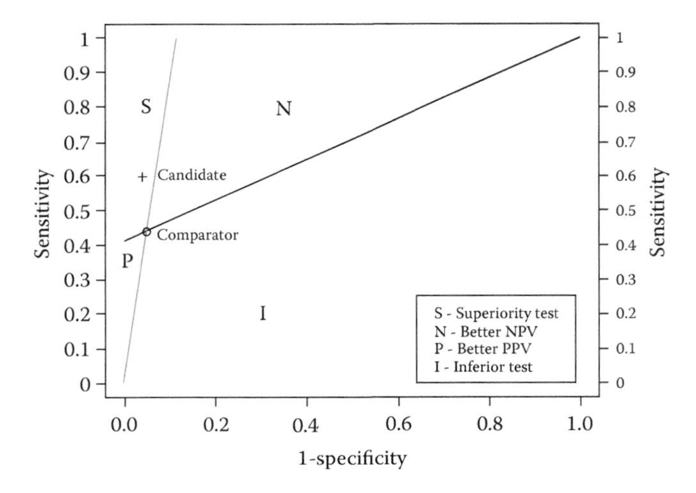

FIGURE 10.20
Example of likelihood ratio graph extracted from Biggerstaff (2000).

The reference point (small circle) represents the sensitivity and specificity of the comparator or the reference algorithm. The slope (sensitivity/(1 − specificity)) of the black line joining the reference point to (0, 0) point represents the positive likelihood ratio (PLR) of the comparator algorithm. Since the PLR and positive predictive value (PPV) are highly correlated, a higher PLR implies a higher PPV. A point above this line means that it is better than the comparator for confirming the presence of disease. The slope (1 − sensitivity/specificity) of the (gray) line joining the reference point to the (1, 1) point represents the negative likelihood ratio (NLR) of the comparator algorithm. Similarly, since the NLR and negative predictive value (NPV) are highly correlated, a lower NLR represents a higher NPV. A point above the NLR line means that it is better than the comparator for confirming the absence of disease.

The PLR and NLR lines divide the plane into four areas. An algorithm with sensitivity and specificity in the upper left corner (as represented by S) of the graph would have a PLR higher than the comparator algorithm and an NLR lower than the comparator algorithm, implying that it is superior to the comparator algorithm. Similarly, an algorithm with sensitivity and specificity in the lower right corner (as represented by I) of the graph would have lower PLR and higher NLR than the comparator algorithm, thereby implying both predictive values lower than the comparator algorithm, implying inferiority. An algorithm with sensitivity and specificity in the lower left corner (as represented by P) of the graph would have a higher PLR and a higher NLR than the comparator algorithm, thereby implying higher PPV and lower NPV. This algorithm will be better at detecting the presence of disease compared to the comparator algorithm. An algorithm with sensitivity and specificity in the upper right corner (as represented by N) of the graph would have a lower PLR and a lower NLR than the comparator algorithm, thereby implying lower PPV and higher NPV. This algorithm will be better at detecting the absence of disease compared to the comparator algorithm.

As an example, Figure 10.21 compares the candidate, an alternative (ATRI NM ≥ 30), and comparator algorithms for screening human papillomavirus cervical cancer (Roche

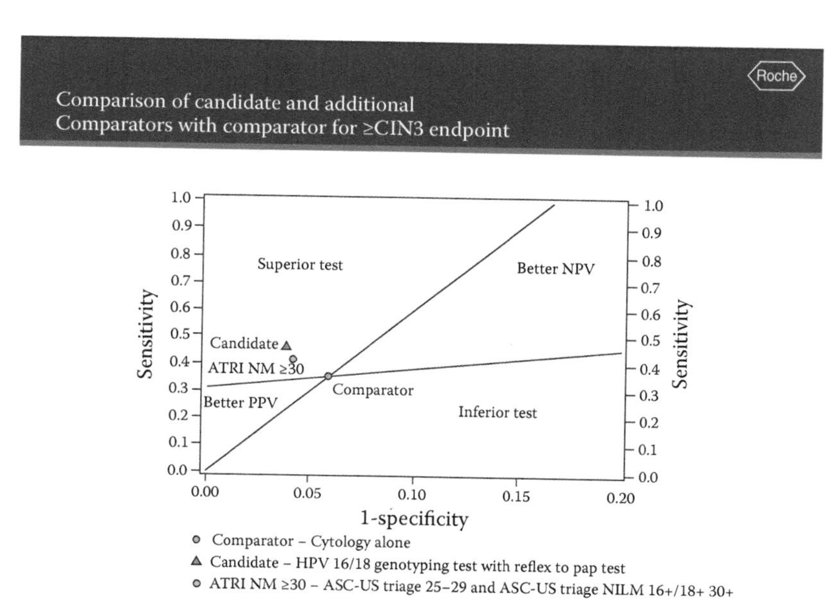

FIGURE 10.21
Example of likelihood ratio graph extracted from Roche Adcom presentation 2014.

Presentation 2014, page 32). The figure shows that the candidate is closer to the top left corner of the graph, which suggests that the candidate is superior, as both sensitivity and specificity are higher when compared with the comparator.

Biggerstaff (2000) pointed that in this graph he had implicitly assumed that the sensitivity and specificity pairs for tests are known without error. In particular, the likelihood ratios graph does not incorporate any measures of variability for the estimates of sensitivity and specificity used in constructing the graph in practice. Indeed, he urged that a formal comparison be made, where appropriate, by computing CIs for either the individual sensitivities and specificities or the likelihood ratios or comparative measures of these. Incorporation of CIs for the likelihood ratios or sensitivities and specificities into the likelihood ratios graph can be made in a natural way to allow a more formal, yet still graphical, comparison of two independent tests' characteristics. The determination of which diagnostic test to use in practice depends upon more than the raw diagnostic abilities of the competing tests. Costs and other more qualitative issues may factor into the determination, and this graph does not attempt to incorporate these. Comprehensive decision theoretic methods could be employed to fully analyze the structure of complex situations.

The likelihood ratio graph is primarily used to display the performance of diagnostic tests. It can be deemed as a special case of the B–R plane when two value functions need to be compared simultaneously. The Bayesian approach can be used to quantify the uncertainty in estimating the sensitivity and specificity. There is no commercially available statistical software to generate this graph. It can be generated using the general graphing capability of SAS or R.

10.3.4.6 Q-TWiST Utility Threshold Plot

Q-TWiST (Quality-adjusted time without symptoms of disease or toxicity) was used by Gelber et al. (1993) to compare cancer therapies. The idea behind Q-TWiST is to first divide the overall survival time of each individual into three clinical health states: (1) Toxicity (TOX): time spent with severe or life-threatening AEs before disease progression; (2) TWiST: time without toxicity of treatment or symptoms of disease progression; and (3) Progression or relapse (REL): period after disease progression until death or censoring. See Figure 10.22 for an illustration of Q-TWiST (Mt-Isa et al. 2013). Under this classification,

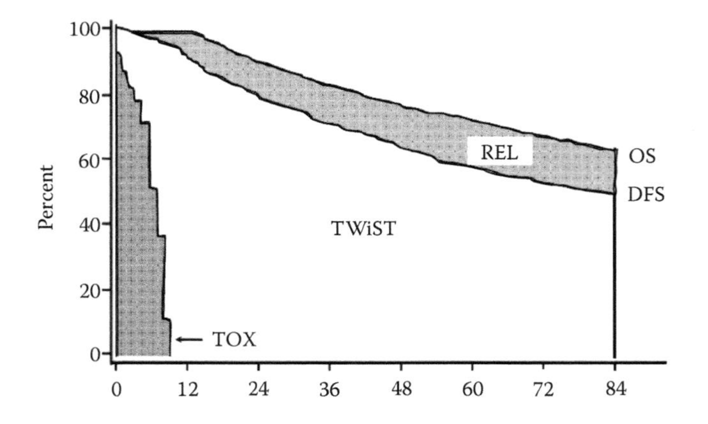

FIGURE 10.22
Area graph showing partitioned survival curve for one treatment in a Q-TWiST analysis. (Extracted from Mt-Isa et al. Review of visualization methods for the representation of benefit risk assessment of medication, 2013, page 35.)

TWiST is time to progression subtracted by time spent in the TOX state. Quality of life can be incorporated into the three clinical health states by introducing a utility to each state. Assuming that the utility of the TWiST state is 1 (the highest utility), we will use u_T and u_R, both between 0 and 1, to denote utilities assigned to the states of TOX and REL. Using these utilities, one can derive Q-TWiST as

$$\text{Q-TWiST} = u_T \times \text{TOX} + \text{TWiST} + u_R \times \text{REL}.$$

Two treatments can be compared based on the mean Q-TWiST for patients receiving the treatments. Mean Q-TWiST for each group is a weighted average of mean TOX, mean TWiST, and mean REL for that group. Gelber et al. (1993) proposed to calculate the mean amount of time spent in each of the three health states using the KM method constructed for each health state individually.

Instead of selecting specific values for u_T and u_R to compare between two treatments, one can vary the utilities for TOX and REL across the full range of their possible values and see how the treatments compare. If a new treatment has a higher mean Q-TWiST than the standard care in nearly all areas of the region defined by [0, 1] × [0, 1], this will suggest that new treatment has a more favorable B–R profile. One way to display such results without resorting to a three-dimensional plot is to use a utility threshold plot as shown in Figure 10.23, which was constructed using data from Irish et al. (2005) with TOX defined by severe AEs. In Figure 10.23, the y-axis represents u_T and the x-axis represents u_R. Lines are drawn to show combinations of (u_T, u_R) that will give a constant difference in mean Q-TWiST between two treatments.

The reason why contours of constant difference in mean Q-TWiST are linear is because Q-TWiST is a linear function of u_T and u_R. To see this, let Δ(mean TOX) denote the difference in mean TOX, Δ(mean TWiST) represent the difference in mean TWiST, and Δ(mean REL) indicate the difference in mean REL, between two groups (new treatment – standard care).

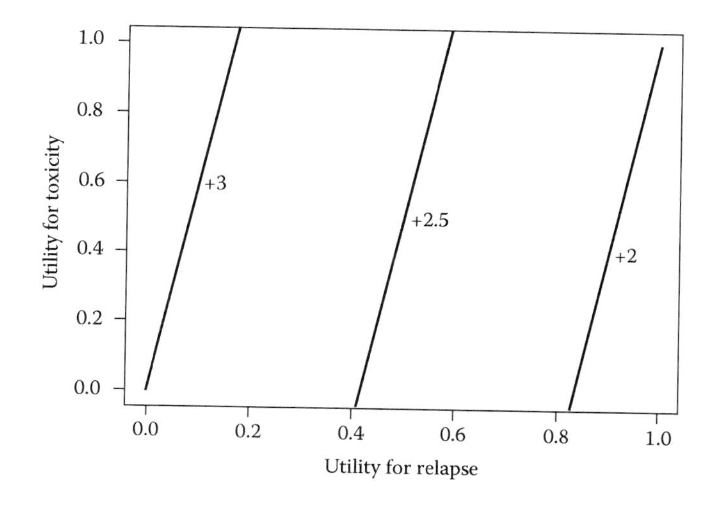

FIGURE 10.23
Utility threshold plot for Q-TWiST where the y-axis represents utility associated with TOX while the x-axis represents utility associated with REL. (Based on data from Irish W. et al. Quality-adjusted survival in a crossover trial of letrozole versus tamoxifen in postmenopausal women with advanced breast cancer. *Annals of Oncology* 16 (2005): 1458–1462.)

The difference in mean Q-TWiST between the new treatment and the standard of care can be expressed as

$$\text{Diff in mean Q-TWiST} = u_T \times \Delta(\text{mean TOX}) + \Delta(\text{mean TWiST}) + u_R \times \Delta(\text{mean REL}) \quad (10.1)$$

Setting the left hand side in Equation 10.1 equal to a constant C, we can derive the relationship in Equation 10.2.

$$u_T = -\frac{\Delta(\text{mean REL})}{\Delta(\text{mean TOX})} u_R + \frac{C - \Delta(\text{mean TWiST})}{\Delta(\text{mean TOX})} \quad (10.2)$$

Therefore, points (u_T, u_R) that define a constant difference in mean Q-TWiST lie on the line defined by Equation 10.2.

The Q-TWiST utility threshold plot can be viewed as a sensitivity analysis for how the comparison between the treatment groups varies as a function of the utilities associated with different health states. The concept of a utility threshold plot could be applied in other situations where benefit and risk endpoints are combined in a different manner than linearly. When benefit and risk are combined in a multiplicative fashion, contours that provide a constant value for the comparative B–R measure will take a different form from linear. The plot could also be used in a health technology assessment (HTA). For an HTA, factors such as cost and patient's quality of life play an important role. Any statistical software, such as R or SAS, can produce the graph.

10.4 Discussions and Conclusion

In this chapter, we have presented 14 different types of graphs or visualizations for BRA. More than 20 figures have been illustrated, most with real examples. We believe that the graphs or visual tools described in this chapter will give the audience a good overview of the most frequently used graphical techniques in the BRA area. Table 10.1 summarizes the utility of various B–R graphs. Although they are generally categorized into four different application categories, the majority of the graphs and their variations/derivatives are cross-category and can be applied in different clinical stages and serve multiple purposes.

In the "BRA planning and development" category, which is relatively the early stage for a BRA, visual tools such as value tree, effects table, and B–R contours can be used to construct the scope and the data foundation for the perspective BRA. In the "B–R Analysis and Presentation (pre- to postmarket)" category, all the graphs or visual tools mentioned in this chapter can be applied except some of them may have focus on certain utility such as for primary analysis or for sensitivity analysis. Moreover, depending on the specific B–R analysis, these graphs can be generated using either clinical trial data in the premarket clinical development stage or the real-world evidence data collected in the postmarket setting. For instance, an effects table can summarize key benefit and risk data for regulatory submission seeking market approval. The key B–R information in the effects table can certainly be updated by new safety data from real practice after the product is on the market. Similarly, the B–R contour is used in the planning stage to set the initial B–R trade-off for a BRA. Such B–R trade-off might be changing as more clinical data come in. After the

TABLE 10.1

Utility for Different B–R Graphs

Graphical Methods/ Characteristics	BRA Planning and Development	B–R Analysis and Presentation (Pre- to Postmarket)	B–R Subgroup Identification	BRA Sensitivity Analysis Supporting Decision Making
Value tree	X	X		X
Forest plot		X	X	X
IRP plot		X		
KM plot		X		
2-D scatterplot		X		X
Bar graphs		X	X	X
Effects table	X	X		
STEPP		X	X	
Tornado plot		X		X
B–R plane		X		X
B–R contours	X	X		X
3-D B–R threshold plot		X		X
Likelihood ratio graph		X		X
Q-TWiST utility threshold plot		X		X

product is on the market and more patient preference data are collected, the B–R contour might be updated as well to reflect the latest trade-off from patients' points of view.

In the "B–R Subgroup Identification" category, the STEPP is specially developed to visually examine the heterogeneity of the B–R profiles among subgroups in response to the study treatment. However, a forest plot or a bar plot can also be used to plot out and evaluate the B–R balance within each subgroup. Besides a tornado plot and other plots that are categorized in the category of "BRA Sensitivity Analysis Supporting Decision Making" as shown in Section 10.3, value trees, forest plots, bar plots, and scatterplots can certainly be used for sensitivity analysis as well. For instance, multiple value trees could be used to evaluate the robustness of the B–R profile owing to different sets of selection of the key B–R outcomes. Multiple versions of forest plots or bar plots can be plotted based on data from different data sources. The 2-D scatterplot can be used to depict how the patients are distributed regarding their key benefit and risk measure as shown in Figure 10.10, but it can also be used to demonstrate a joint distribution of incremental harm and incremental benefit in a probabilistic simulation (Figure 31 of Mt-Isa et al. 2013). Therefore, flexible adoption and creative utilization of various visual presentations are always needed in order to apply the right graphical techniques in the appropriate situations.

There are certainly additional graphical types that are used for BRA but are not covered in this chapter. However, we believe that the general principle of using the graphical techniques is more important than covering all possible graph types for our purpose, although we have attempted to cover the most frequently used ones. When illustrating a graph, one needs to keep in mind that the graph should be easy to understand, should be able to integrate benefits and risks in a direct and natural way and preferably in the same unit, and should be practical and easy to generate. It should also be noted that in most situations, the discussions on B–R analysis methods and metrics should have been determined when it arrives at the point of graphic presentations. Throughout this chapter, we assume that information on B–R methods, B–R metrics, and endpoint selections along with weighting and quantification of uncertainty have been considered and addressed. Readers are referred to the relevant chapters in this book for discussions on these topics.

References

Al-Sarraf M et al. "Chemoradiotherapy versus radiotherapy in patients with advanced nasopharyngeal cancer: Phase III randomized Intergroup study 0099." *Journal of Clinical Oncology* 16 (1998): 1310–1317.

Ashby D. "Visualizing Benefit–Risk for Drug Regulations." Basel PhUSE SDE, 3rd July 2014, Basel, CH. http://www.phusewiki.org/docs/Basel%20SDE%202014%20presentations/PROF_ASHBY.pdf.

Biggerstaff BJ. "Comparing diagnostic tests: A simple graphic using likelihood ratios." *Statistics in Medicine* Vol. 19 No. 5 (2000): 649–663.

Bonetti M and Gelber RD. "A graphical method to assess treatment—Covariate interactions using the Cox model on subsets of the data." *Statistics in Medicine* Vol. 19 No. 19 (2000): 2595–2609.

Bonetti M and Gelber RD. "Patterns of treatment effects in subsets of patients in clinical trials." *Biostatistics* Vol. 5 No. 3 (2004): 465–481.

Chuang-Stein C, Mohberg NR, Sinkula MS. "Three measures for simultaneously evaluating benefits and risks using categorical data from clinical trials." *Statistics in Medicine* Vol. 10 No. 9 (1991): 1349–1359.

Colleoni M et al. "Timing of CMF chemotherapy in combination with tamoxifen in postmenopausal women with breast cancer: Role of endocrine responsiveness of the tumor." *Annals of Oncology* Vol. 16 No. 5 (2005): 716–725.

Coplan PM, Noel RA, Levitan BA et al. "Development of a Framework for Enhancing the Transparency, Reproducibility, and Communication of the Benefit–Risk Balance of Medicines." *Clinical Pharmacology & Therapeutics* Vol. 89 No. 2 (2011): 312–315.

European Medicines Agency (EMA). "The Benefit–risk methodology project documents: Work Packages (WP) 1 to 5 (2011–2014)" currently available on EMA website at: http://www.ema.europa.eu/ema/index.jsp?curl=pages/special_topics/document_listing/document_listing_000314.jsp&mid=WC0b01ac0580223ed6

FDA Briefing document, rivaroxaban, for the May 22, 2012 Meeting of the FDA/CDER Cardiovascular and Renal Drugs Advisory Committee. http://www.fda.gov/AdvisoryCommittees/CommitteesMeetingMaterials/Drugs/CardiovascularandRenalDrugsAdvisoryCommittee/ucm304754.htm.

FDA Presentations, KAMRA™ Inlay, for the June 6, 2014 Meeting of the FDA/CDER Ophthalmic Devices Panel Advisory Committee (Medical Devices). http://www.fda.gov/downloads/AdvisoryCommittees/CommitteesMeetingMaterials/MedicalDevices/MedicalDevicesAdvisoryCommittee/OphthalmicDevicesPanel/UCM400433.pdf.

Gelber RD, Goldhirsch A, Cole BF. "Evaluation of effectiveness: Q-TWiST." *Cancer Treatment Review* 19 (Supplement A) (1993): 73–84.

Grossman J and Gordon CP. "Clinical Indices in the Assessment of Lupus." In: *Dubois' Lupus Erythematosus*, 7th Ed. D. J. Wallace and B. H. Hahn. Philadelphia, PA, Lippincott Williams & Wilkins (2007): 920–932.

He W and Fu B. "Benefit–Risk Evaluation using a framework of joint modeling and joint evaluations of multiple efficacy and safety endpoints." In: Jiang Q, He W (eds.) *Benefit–Risk Assessment Methods in Drug Development: Bridging Qualitative and Quantitative Assessments*. CRC Press, in press.

International Breast Cancer Study Group (Castiglione et al.). "Endocrine responsiveness and tailoring adjuvant therapy for postmenopausal lymph node-negative breast cancer: A randomized trial." *Journal of National Cancer Institute* 94 (2002): 1054–1065.

International Conference on Harmonization Guideline: Periodic Benefit–Risk Evaluation Report (PBRER) E2C(R2), 2012.

Irish W, Sherrill B, Cole B, Gard C, Glendenning GA, Mouridsen H. "Quality-adjusted survival in a crossover trial of letrozole versus tamoxifen in postmenopausal women with advanced breast cancer." *Annals of Oncology* 16 (2005): 1458–1462.

Janssen Briefing Information, Rivaroxaban, for the May 23, 2012 Meeting of the FDA/CDER Cardiovascular and Renal Drugs Advisory Committee. http://www.fda.gov/downloads/AdvisoryCommittees/CommitteesMeetingMaterials/Drugs/CardiovascularandRenalDrugsAdvisoryCommittee/UCM304757.pdf.

Jiang Q, Ke C, Ma H. "Susan Shepherd, Benefit–Risk Assessment Methods: A Spectrum from Qualitative to Quantitative." SCT/FDA Benefit: Risk Workshop, December 2013.

Kaplan EL and Meier P. "Nonparametric estimation from incomplete observations." *Journal of the American Statistical Association* Vol. 53 No. 282 (1958): 457–481.

Lalkhen AG and McCluskey, A. "Statistics V: Introduction to clinical trials and systematic reviews." *Continuing Education in Anesthesia, Critical Care & Pain* Vol. 8 No. 4 (2008): 143–146.

Lewis S and Clarke M. "Forest plots: Trying to see the wood and the trees." *BMJ* 322 (2001): 1479–1480.

Lynd L and O'Brien B. "Advances in risk-benefit evaluation using probabilistic simulation methods: An application to the prophylaxis of deep vein thrombosis." *Journal of Clinical Epidemiology* Vol. 57 No. 8 (2004): 795–803.

Mt-Isa et al., "Review of visualization methods for the representation of benefit risk assessment of medication." Available at: http://protectbenefitrisk.eu/documents/ShahruletalReviewofvisualisationmethodsfortherepresentationofBRassessmentofmedicationStage1F.pdf. Accesed February 15, 2013.

Nixon et al., "IMI WP5 Benefit Risk Case Study Report Natalizumab (Wave 1 and Wave 2)." 2013.

Norton JD, "A Longitudinal Model and Graphic for Benefit–risk Analysis, With Case Study." *Drug Information Journal* Vol. 45 (2011): 741–747.

PROTECT Consortium. "Review of methodologies for benefit and risk assessment of medication 2013" available at: http://www.imi-protect.eu/documents/ShahruletalReviewofmethodologiesforbenefitandriskassessmentofmedicationMay2013.pdf.

Quartey G, EFSPI/FMS/DSBS Joint Meeting, June 2012, Sweden.

Roche Presentations, cobas® HPV Test, for the March 12, 2014 Meeting of the FDA/CDRH Materials of the Microbiology Devices Panel Advisory Committee (Medical Devices). http://www.fda.gov/downloads/AdvisoryCommittees/CommitteesMeetingMaterials/MedicalDevices/MedicalDevicesAdvisoryCommittee/MicrobiologyDevicesPanel/UCM389491.pdf.

Salix Main Presentation, Xifaxan (rifaximin), for the November 16, 2011 Meeting of the FDA/CDER Gastrointestinal Drugs Advisory Committee. http://www.fda.gov/downloads/AdvisoryCommittees/CommitteesMeetingMaterials/Drugs/GastrointestinalDrugsAdvisoryCommittee/UCM281497.pdf.

Shakespeare TP, Gebski VJ, Veness MJ, Simes J. "Improving interpretation of clinical studies by use of confidence levels, clinical significance curves, and risk–benefit contours." *Lancet* 357 (2001): 1349–1353.

Structured Approach to Benefit–Risk Assessment in Drug Regulatory Decision-Making Draft PDUFA V Implementation Plan-Fiscal Years 2013-2017, http://www.fda.gov/downloads/ForIndustry/UserFees/PrescriptionDrugUserFee/UCM329758.pdf.

TMC Presentations, Cangrelor, for the February 12, 2014 Meeting of the FDA/CDER Cardiovascular and Renal Drugs Advisory Committee. http://www.fda.gov/downloads/AdvisoryCommittees/CommitteesMeetingMaterials/Drugs/CardiovascularandRenalDrugsAdvisoryCommittee/UCM386780.pdf.

Walker S, McAuslane N, Liberti L, Leong J, Salek S. "A Universal Framework for the Benefit–Risk Assessment of Medicines: Is This the Way Forward?" *Therapeutic Innovation & Regulatory Science* Vol. 49 No. 1 (2015): 17–25.

Wen S, Zhang L, Yang B. "Two Approaches to Incorporate Clinical Data Uncertainty into Multiple Criteria Decision Analysis for Benefit–Risk Assessment of Medicinal Products." *Value in Health* 17 (2014): 619–628.

Section V

Benefit–Risk Assessment Case Studies and Lessons Learned

11

Practical Considerations for Benefit–Risk Assessment and Implementation: Vorapaxar TRA-2°P TIMI 50 Case Study

Weili He, Daniel Bloomfield, Yabing Mai, and Scott Evans

CONTENTS

ABSTRACT The benefits of a medicine can only be understood in the context of the risks or harms associated with that medicine, and vice versa. In recent years, health authorities and industry-wide working groups have actively pursued structured benefit–risk (B–R) assessment efforts. Despite these efforts, a paucity of published B–R case studies that utilized a structured B–R framework remains. In this chapter, we describe a case study for the development and implementation of a structured B–R framework in the vorapaxar TRA-2°P TIMI 50 (Thrombin Receptor Antagonist in Secondary Prevention of Atherothrombotic Ischemic Events) study, along with key considerations that went into the evaluation.

11.1 Introduction

Secondary prevention of cardiovascular (CV) events in patients with atherosclerosis remains a significant medical and societal problem despite available therapies. Despite medicines for secondary prevention, patients with atherosclerotic CV disease are at substantial risk of recurrent thrombotic events. Platelets have a central role in atherothrombosis and are an important target for drug treatment. Inhibition of platelets with P2Y12 inhibitors added to aspirin for up to a year after myocardial infarction (MI) reduces recurrent thrombotic events but increases bleeding. In patients with atherosclerosis in the peripheral arteries, the benefits of P2Y12 inhibitors and aspirin are less clear. There are no known medications with an acceptable B–R profile in patients with a history of ischemic stroke. Additional therapeutic options are being evaluated on top of standard of care (with aspirin or a P2Y12 inhibitor) for long-term secondary prevention of CV events.

Evaluation of such therapies for long-term secondary prevention requires a B–R assessment in order to balance the beneficial reduction in the risk of CV events with the risk of bleeding in these patients.

11.1.1 Clinical Background of Vorapaxar and TRA-2°P TIMI 50 Trial Design and Key Results

Vorapaxar is a selective antagonist of the protease-activated receptor-1 (PAR-1), the primary thrombin receptor on human platelets, which mediates the downstream effects of thrombin, a critical coagulation factor in hemostasis and thrombosis (Coughlin 2005). Thrombin-induced platelet activation has been implicated in a variety of CV disorders including thrombosis, atherosclerosis, and restenosis after percutaneous coronary intervention. As an antagonist of PAR-1, vorapaxar blocks thrombin-mediated platelet activation and thereby has the potential to reduce the risk of atherothrombotic complications of coronary disease (Chackalamannil et al. 2008).

The Thrombin Receptor Antagonist in Secondary Prevention of Atherothrombotic Ischemic Events (TRA-2°P TIMI 50) study was an outcome trial that evaluated the safety and efficacy of vorapaxar for the secondary prevention of CV events. The study was conducted in 1032 study sites in 32 countries, and the study period was from September 26, 2007, to December 23, 2011. The study randomized 26,449 patients who had a history of atherosclerotic CV disease who underwent a hierarchical randomization into one of three strata based on their presentation: (1) history of recent spontaneous MI within the previous 2 weeks to 12 months, (2) history of recent ischemic stroke, or (3) symptomatic peripheral arterial disease. Patients were randomized to receive vorapaxar (2.5 mg daily) or matching placebo on top of standard of care, which included aspirin in all patients and the combination of aspirin and a P2Y12 inhibitor in approximately 75% of patients. Patients were followed for a median of 30 months.

The primary efficacy endpoint was a composite of death from CV causes, MI, stroke, and urgent coronary revascularization (UCR). The secondary composite efficacy endpoint included only "hard events" including death from CV causes, MI, and stroke. The key safety endpoints with regard to bleeding assessment included the Global Use of Strategies to Open Occluded Coronary Arteries (GUSTO) classification system with GUSTO moderate or severe bleeding defined as the safety endpoint of primary interest. GUSTO severe bleeding was defined as fatal, intracranial, or bleeding with hemodynamic compromise requiring intervention. GUSTO moderate bleeding was defined as bleeding requiring transfusion of whole blood or packed red blood cells without hemodynamic compromise.

A clinical-events committee whose members were unaware of the study-group assignments adjudicated all components of the primary and major secondary efficacy endpoints and bleeding episodes. The primary efficacy analysis was conducted on an intention-to-treat (ITT) basis among all patients who underwent randomization, and safety analyses were performed on an as-treated basis among patients who were randomized and received one or more doses of a study drug. The primary efficacy and safety analyses were performed with the use of a Cox proportional hazards (PH) model, with the study group and stratification factors at randomization as covariates. Cumulative event rates at 3 years were calculated with the use of the Kaplan–Meier (KM) method.

In January 2011, as a result of an increased number of intracranial hemorrhages (ICHs) observed in patients with a history of stroke randomized to vorapaxar, the independent Data Safety Monitoring Board (DSMB) recommended that subjects with any stroke pre- or postrandomization should discontinue study treatment but that the study should continue to its completion. In response to the DSMB recommendations, the Sponsor amended the Statistical Analysis Plan (SAP) to include additional subpopulations of subjects without a prior history of stroke (Morrow et al. 2012).

The primary analysis of the overall study that included all patients randomized in an ITT analysis was robustly positive and demonstrated a clear benefit of vorapaxar compared to placebo on top of standard of care. The primary composite endpoint occurred in 1259 patients (11.2%) in the vorapaxar group and in 1417 patients (12.4%) in the placebo group (hazard ratio [HR] for the vorapaxar group vs. placebo group, 0.88; 95% confidence interval [CI], 0.82 to 0.95; $P = 0.001$). The key secondary endpoint occurred in 1028 patients (9.3%) in the vorapaxar group and 1176 patients (10.5%) in the placebo group (HR, 0.87; 95% CI, 0.80 to 0.94; $P < 0.001$). GUSTO moderate or severe bleeding occurred in 4.2% of patients who received vorapaxar and 2.5% of those who received placebo (HR, 1.66; 95% CI, 1.43 to 1.93; $P < 0.001$). There was an increase in the rate of ICH with 109 patients (0.8%) in the vorapaxar group, as compared with 64 patients (0.5%) in the placebo group (HR, 1.70; 95% CI, 1.25 to 2.32; $P < 0.001$) (Morrow et al. 2012).

11.1.2 Rationale for the US Label Population

The decision to contraindicate vorapaxar in patients with a history of stroke or transient ischemic attack (TIA) represents an unstructured B–R analysis by the DSMB. On January 8, 2011, a DSMB meeting was convened, triggered by an increased number of ICH events reported since the last DSMB meeting in October 2010. The DSMB observed that in the TRA-2°P TIMI 50 study, the difference in ICH events was widening and there was a nearly twofold increase in HR compared to what they saw in October 2010. In addition, subjects in the study arm had an increased number of events in all bleeding categories but within the range of what was expected. On the basis of the data available at that time, the DSMB believed that the efficacy data showed a clear clinical benefit of the study drug especially in the reduction of MI. There was also a reduction in overall stroke in the study arm even with the excessive ICH, suggesting that the study drug may have provided protection against ischemic stroke at the cost of excessive hemorrhagic stroke. Additional analyses revealed that among the patients with a history of stroke where the risk of ICH was the highest, there was no evidence of an efficacy benefit to compensate for the substantially increased risk of ICH and other serious bleeding events and no reduction in mortality. As a contrast, among the subjects without a history of stroke, the ICH rate was only slightly higher in the study arm compared to placebo, but there are also compensating benefits with significant reductions in both the primary and key secondary endpoints that are on par with the targets estimated by the study protocol. The DSMB concluded that subjects with any stroke before or after randomization shall discontinue receiving randomized treatment and recommended continuing the trial to completion.

At the same DSMB meeting, the TRACER (thrombin receptor antagonist for clinical event reduction in acute coronary syndrome) study, which was a multicenter, randomized, double-blind, placebo-controlled study aimed at evaluating the safety and efficacy of vorapaxar in addition to standard of care in subjects with acute coronary syndrome, was also reviewed. The study results were reported by Tricoci et al. (2011). In TRACER, the DSMB observed an excess of ICH events in the study arm, but in contrast to TRA-2°P, the benefit in terms of efficacy was marginal and the reduction in the primary and key secondary efficacy endpoints of the trial was less than the expected 15% specified in the protocol. The DSMB believed that it was highly unlikely that the study would demonstrate a significant reduction in ischemic events if the study continued. Furthermore, the study had nearly reached the number of primary and key secondary endpoint events for which the study was powered. Therefore, the DSMB determined that patients in the trial should no longer be exposed to the substantially increased risk of bleeding given the marginal benefit in efficacy observed. The Board voted unanimously to discontinue the study drug in all patients and to close out the trial.

TRA-2°P TIMI 50, assessed in its entirety, is a robustly positive trial ($P = 0.001$ for the primary endpoint and $P < 0.001$ for the secondary endpoint). However, as observed by the DSMB, the risk of ICH associated with vorapaxar was substantially higher in patients with a history of stroke (2.4% in the vorapaxar group vs. 0.9% in the placebo group; HR, 2.55; 95% CI, 1.52 to 4.28) compared to patients without a history of stroke (0.6% in the vorapaxar group vs. 0.4% in the placebo group; HR, 1.55; 95% CI, 1.00 to 2.41) (Morrow et al. 2012). In addition, in patients randomized into the stroke stratum, there was no evidence of efficacy (HR, 1.03; 95% CI, 0.85 to 1.25) (FDA Adversary Committee 2014). Given that patients with a prior history of stroke were at an increased risk of ICH that was not offset by sufficient benefit, the Sponsor recommended that vorapaxar should be contraindicated in patients with a history of stroke. Furthermore, because of the clinical imprecision in distinguishing between stroke and TIA, contraindication was extended to those patients with a history of stroke or a history of TIA.

In order to preserve the integrity of the clinical trial after the positive results in the overall population, subsequent analyses included all patients who met the inclusion criteria for the trial based on atherosclerotic vascular disease in the coronary and peripheral arteries but excluded patients with a history of a stroke or TIA for whom vorapaxar is contraindicated because of the increased risk of ICH. Of note, some of these patients had a recent MI only (within 12 months), some had symptomatic peripheral arterial disease with or without a distant MI (<12 months), and others had both peripheral artery disease (PAD) and a recent MI.

The rest of this chapter will discuss a more nuanced B–R analysis that balances the benefit of vorapaxar in reducing major CV events with the risk of bleeding. We focus on the US label population or the post-MI/PAD population that represents an ITT sample of 20,170 subjects for efficacy evaluation and an as-treated sample of 20,108 subjects for safety evaluation.

11.1.3 Key TRA-2°P TIMI 50 Study Results in the US Label Population

When added on top of standard of care, vorapaxar resulted in 17% reduction in the primary efficacy endpoint (first occurrence of CV death, MI, stroke or UCR; HR, 0.83; 95% CI, 0.76 to 0.90; $P < 0.001$) in the US label population. The treatment effect of vorapaxar on the key efficacy endpoints persisted throughout the entire trial duration as evidenced by the continued separation of the KM estimates of the cumulative hazard rates of key clinical events over time. A similar significant and durable reduction of 20% was observed in the key secondary efficacy composite endpoint (CV death, MI, or stroke; HR, 0.80; 95% CI, 0.73 to 0.89; $P < 0.001$) (ZONTIVITY US label, 2014). Figure 11.1 presents the KM estimate of time to the first occurrence of the primary efficacy endpoint event in the US label population. The rates of all components of the composite endpoints (first event in the case of multiple events) were also reduced. Clinical benefit was demonstrated across all prespecified subpopulations. Table 11.1 presents the key efficacy results for the US label population.

Treatment with vorapaxar was associated with an increased risk of bleeding. Table 11.2 shows the key bleeding outcomes of the US label population that excluded subjects with a history of stroke or TIA. Having excluded patients with a history of stroke or TIA, the incidences of ICH and of GUSTO severe bleeding associated with vorapaxar were reduced compared to the overall population. The rates of GUSTO severe bleeding were similar in the vorapaxar and placebo groups. In the US label population, the 3-year KM estimates for GUSTO severe or moderate bleeding endpoints were 3.7% in the vorapaxar group and 2.4% in the placebo group (HR, 1.55; 95% CI, 1.30 to 1.86). This increase in GUSTO severe or moderate bleeding over placebo was driven largely by an increase in GUSTO moderate bleeding. The 3-year KM event rate for fatal bleeding was 0.2% for both the vorapaxar and placebo groups (HR, 1.15; 95% CI, 0.56 to 2.36).

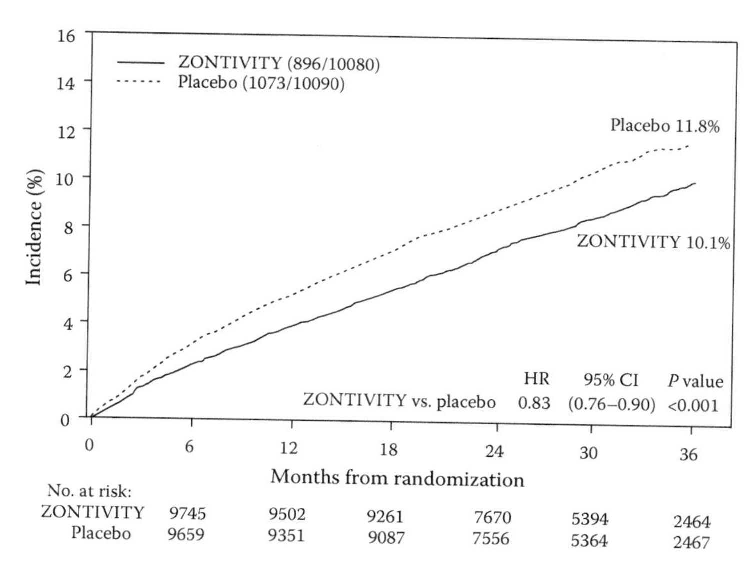

FIGURE 11.1
Time to first occurrence of the composite endpoint of CV death, MI, stroke, or UCR in post-MI/PAD patients without a history of stroke or TIA in TRA-2°P.

TABLE 11.1

TRA-2°P: Time to First Event in Post-MI/PAD Patients without a History of Stroke or TIA (Event Accrual Period: Randomization to Last Visit)

	Placebo (n = 10,090)		ZONTIVITY (n = 10,080)			
Endpoints	**Patients with Events[c] (%)**	**KM%[d]**	**Patients with Events[c] (%)**	**KM%[d]**	**HR[a,b] (95% CI)**	***P* Value[b]**
Primary composite efficacy endpoint (CV death/MI/stroke/UCR)[b,c]	1073 (10.6%)	11.8%	896 (8.9%)	10.1%	0.83 (0.76–0.90)	<0.001
Secondary composite efficacy endpoint (CV death/MI/stroke)[b,c]	851 (8.4%)	9.5%	688 (6.8%)	7.9%	0.80 (0.73–0.89)	<0.001
Other Secondary Efficacy Endpoints (First Occurrences of Specified Event at Any Time)[e]						
CV death	239 (2.4%)	2.8%	205 (2.0%)	2.4%	0.86 (0.71–1.03)	
MI	569 (5.6%)	6.4%	470 (4.7%)	5.4%	0.82 (0.73–0.93)	
Stroke	145 (1.4%)	1.6%	98 (1.0%)	1.2%	0.67 (0.52–0.87)	
UCR	283 (2.8%)	3.0%	249 (2.5%)	2.8%	0.88 (0.74–1.04)	

[a] HR is ZONTIVITY group versus placebo group.
[b] Cox PH model with covariates treatment and stratification factors (qualifying atherosclerotic disease and planned thienopyridine use).
[c] Each patient was counted only once (first component event) in the component summary that contributed to the primary efficacy endpoint.
[d] KM estimate at 1080 days.
[e] Including patients who could have had other nonfatal events or subsequently died.

TABLE 11.2

Non–CABG-Related Bleeds in Post-MI/PAD Patients without a History of Stroke or TIA (First Dose to Last Dose + 30 Days) in the TRA-2°P Study

	Placebo (n = 10,049)		ZONTIVITY (n = 10,059)		
Endpoints	**Patients with Events (%)**	**KM%[c]**	**Patients with Events (%)**	**KM%[c]**	**HR[a,b] (95% CI)**
GUSTO Bleeding Categories					
Severe	82 (0.8%)	1.0%	100 (1.0%)	1.3%	1.24 (0.92–1.66)
Moderate or severe	199 (2.0%)	2.4%	303 (3.0%)	3.7%	1.55 (1.30–1.86)
Any GUSTO bleeding (severe/moderate/mild)	1769 (17.6%)	19.8%	2518 (25.0%)	27.7%	1.52 (1.43–1.61)
Fatal bleeding	14 (0.1%)	0.2%	16 (0.2%)	0.2%	1.15 (0.56–2.36)
ICH	31 (0.3%)	0.4%	45 (0.4%)	0.6%	1.46 (0.92–2.31)
Clinically significant bleeding[a]	950 (9.5%)	10.9%	1349 (13.4%)	15.5%	1.47 (1.35–1.60)
Gastrointestinal bleeding	297 (3.0%)	3.5%	400 (4.0%)	4.7%	1.37 (1.18–1.59)

[a] Clinically significant bleeding includes any bleeding requiring medical attention including ICH, or clinically significant overt signs of hemorrhage associated with a drop in hemoglobin (Hgb) of ≥3 g/dL (or, when Hgb is not available, an absolute drop in hematocrit (Hct) of ≥15% or a fall in Hct of 9% to <15%).
[b] HR is ZONTIVITY group versus placebo group.
[c] KM estimate at 1080 days.

11.1.4 Rationale for B–R Assessment in TRA-2°P TIMI 50

The use of antiplatelet or anticoagulant agents to prevent CV events requires a B–R assessment in order to balance the beneficial reduction in the risk of CV events with the risk of bleeding in appropriate patients. The TRA-2°P TIMI 50 study was designed to assess the effectiveness of vorapaxar on top of contemporary standard of care versus standard of care alone in a secondary prevention high-risk population. In this study, patients were extremely well treated with aspirin, P2Y12 inhibitors, statins, beta blockers, and anti-hypertensive medications, all of which have shown to improve outcomes in patients with or at risk for atherosclerotic CV disease. Despite this comprehensive approach to secondary prevention, the rate of CV death, MI, or stroke remained high in the post-MI/PAD population with no history of stroke or the TIA population. This residual risk is clearly evident in the placebo arm of the study, which had a 3-year KM rate of CV death, MI, or stroke as high as 9.5% in the US label population. Ultimately, this assessment depends on weighing the risks of recurrent CV events and bleeding.

In Section 11.2, we describe the key elements and considerations for the TRA-2°P TIMI 50 B–R assessment (BRA). We present the results of TRA-2°P TIMI 50 study BRA in Section 11.3. The final section summarizes the key points of this case study.

11.2 Key Elements of TRA-2°P TIMI 50 B–R Assessment

As mentioned in Chapter 8, many BRA frameworks have been proposed, but to date, there are no universally accepted BRA methods. It is thus reasonable to use multiple approaches for BRA to provide a comprehensive assessment. In this section, we discuss a few key considerations that went into the BRA and implementation in the TRA-2°P TIMI 50 study.

As mentioned in Section 11.1, the decision to contraindicate patients with a prior history of stroke or TIA represents a BRA that was initially suggested by the DSMB during the course of the trial when the DSMB recommended that patients with a history of stroke discontinue study medication. We will not discuss this particular B–R assessment but will focus on the more nuanced BRA of patients who are eligible for treatment with vorapaxar in the context of the US label population that was closely shaped by this specific BRA. We discuss the key considerations that went into the BRA and implementation in the TRA-2°P TIMI 50 study in this section.

11.2.1 Endpoint Selections and Weighting Considerations

When defining a quantitative assessment of the trade-off between benefits and risks, careful consideration must be given to the endpoints chosen for the assessment. It is difficult to weigh effects on different endpoints when the endpoints have differing levels of importance. The TRA-2°P TIMI 50 study protocol prespecified primary and key secondary efficacy endpoints as the composite of CV death, MI, stroke, and UCR, and the composite of CV death, MI, and stroke, respectively. The protocol defined the key safety endpoints related to bleeding risk using the composite of moderate and severe bleeding events according to the GUSTO classification. The focus of the SAP was on prespecified distinct and independent assessments of efficacy and bleeding, but not on a structured and integrated BRA.

It is important to note that the components of the composite endpoints for primary efficacy and safety were not chosen on the basis of their clinical impact. For example, GUSTO moderate bleeds and UCR do not have the same impact as CV death, MI, stroke, or GUSTO severe bleeds; these events should not be treated equally. A patient with a gastrointestinal bleed that requires a transfusion of red blood cells can recover completely without any meaningful consequences. This does not represent the same clinical impact as an ICH, an MI, an ischemic stroke, or death. Similarly, a UCR can occur in the setting of unstable angina where an MI is prevented and there is no damage to the myocardium.

It has been suggested that contemporary B–R assessments in CV areas utilize endpoints that represent benefits and risks that are associated with irreversible tissue damage or death (Unger 2009). Considering the mechanism of action of vorapaxar and the clinical setting in which B–R was assessed, the benefits of vorapaxar would be expected to produce reductions in CV death, MI, and stroke, all of which result in irreversible tissue damage with acute and chronic functional limitations. The benefit created by reducing the risks of irreversible tissue damage would need to be balanced by increases in rates of events of irreversible harm. Indicators of the risk of irreversible harm would include life-threatening or fatal bleeding events, specifically GUSTO severe bleeding including fatal bleeding and ICH.

In designing B–R analyses, it is important to identify whether one outcome endpoint event might be double counted by including it in more than one efficacy or safety endpoint. For example, a procedure performed for a confirmed coronary ischemic event that led to fatal bleeding would be recorded as both a CV death and fatal bleed. A hemorrhagic stroke event would be recorded as both a stroke and a GUSTO severe bleed (ICH). In the TRA-2°P TIMI 50 study, double-counting events were avoided by assigning events to only one mutually exclusive category. Therefore, benefit is assessed by the rates of CV death excluding fatal bleed, MI excluding CV death, and ischemic stroke excluding CV death. Risk is assessed with the endpoints of fatal bleed, nonfatal ICH, and other (nonfatal, non-ICH) GUSTO severe bleeding. Alternatively, a composite endpoint of all-cause death (i.e., one that includes CV death and fatal bleed) may be used to assess B–R trade-off directly for fatal events such as these.

11.2.2 Composite Endpoints for B–R Assessment: Net Clinical Benefit

Net clinical benefit (NCB) is a term that incorporates the benefits and risks of a treatment into a single summary composite endpoint. In the TRA-2°P TIMI 50 study, the NCB of vorapaxar was compared to placebo using a single composite endpoint that included both efficacy and safety outcome events. The TRA-2°P TIMI 50 study protocol prespecified an NCB endpoint that is a composite endpoint of CV death, MI, stroke, and GUSTO moderate or severe bleeding. This NCB endpoint was not intended to be sufficient for a full BRA and it has two important limitations that need to be considered. First, this NCB composite assumes that each of the individual components of the composite have a similar clinical impact; the same weight is assigned to each endpoint event. When the individual endpoints within the composite do not have a similar clinical impact, then large differences in events of less severity may dominate the endpoint even if there are important differences in events of greater severity. For example, as discussed above, GUSTO moderate bleeds do not have the same impact as CV death, MI, stroke, or GUSTO severe bleeds, and yet these events are all treated equally. A more appropriate NCB composite endpoint would include the efficacy endpoints of CV death, MI, and stroke and the safety endpoints of GUSTO severe bleeding (which includes ICH and fatal bleeding). This composite endpoint balances the benefits associated with reducing the risks of irreversible tissue damage and risks associated with events that lead to irreversible harm.

A second important limitation with NCB analysis is that it is highly dependent on the absolute baseline rates of each of the individual endpoints in the composite. In this case, the baseline rates of the efficacy endpoint (CV death, MI, and stroke) are much greater than the baseline rates of GUSTO severe bleeding and ICH. Even significant relative increases in severe bleeding will not have an impact on the NCB analysis, which, on the basis of the unequal baseline rates, is heavily biased as the outset to reflect efficacy rather than safety (this is discussed further below). One way to approach these two biases is to assign unequal weights to each endpoint in the NCB composite. However, determining the different weights is extremely complex (IMI PROTECT 2012).

The statistical analysis of NCB utilized a time to first event analysis via the Cox PH model, assuming independence of the components of the composite endpoints. It should be noted that it is important that the components of NCB should have a similar clinical impact when using this analysis approach; otherwise, if a component endpoint with lesser clinical impact occurred earlier than a more serious component endpoint for a patient, the analysis would have been censored at the earlier time point for this patient and the more serious component would have no impact in the NCB analysis.

11.2.3 Exposure-Adjusted Risk Analysis

The primary analytical approach used to assess the balance between benefit and risk in the TRA-2°P TIMI 50 study was focused on evaluation of risk differences (RDs) based on exposure-adjusted event rates for the first occurrences of the endpoint events. The RD of vorapaxar versus placebo is defined as the absolute difference in incidence rates of the two treatment groups calculated as the number of events per 10,000 patient-years of exposure and was calculated as follows:

$$\text{Exposure-adjusted event rate} = 10{,}000 \times (\text{total number of patients with} \geq 1 \text{ event postrandomization} \div \text{total patient-years of exposure}).$$

For subjects with one or more events, the exposure was calculated based on the time from the randomization to the date of the first event. For subjects without an event, the exposure was calculated based on the time from the randomization to the date of the last visit. The 95% CI for RD was based on the method by Miettinen and Nurminen (1985). The exposure-adjusted event rate, introduced into this study as an additional B–R metric to other time-to-event analysis approaches such as HRs and KM estimates, offers a simple and straightforward way to demonstrate the risk by averaging all qualified events on an overall "at-risk" period throughout the study. This method focuses more on the average, which could vary with respect to different study follow-ups when the assumption of constant risk does not hold. Therefore, one should take caution to use this method for between-study comparisons.

Chapter 8 provides definitions and an in-depth discussion of the pros and cons of numbers needed to treat (NNT) and numbers needed to harm (NNH). We used NNT and NNH as a BRA metric in the TRA-2°P TIMI 50 study, as the metric is easy to understand, allows a simple trade-off between the main benefit and risks, and is commonly included in published study results of similar treatment and patient populations. However, there are a number of limitations to using NNT and NNH that are important to note. While physicians often use NNT and NNH as a way to compare the effectiveness of the class of antiplatelet or anticoagulant therapies across studies, this is problematic for a number of reasons. Cross-study comparisons of the estimates of NNT and NNH are complicated by differences in patient populations, the baseline risk of the populations being studied, study designs, the comparator (e.g., background therapy, active control, placebo control), and differential follow-up. In addition, when the RD between two treatment groups for a given endpoint is very small, the uncertainty with regard to estimates of NNT or NNH is extremely difficult to interpret. NNT/NNH analyses have poor statistical properties, numerous other potential biases, unreliable CIs, and are ineffective in excluding the possibility of no difference between two treatments or groups (Hutton 2010). Despite these important limitations, the use of RDs or NNT/NNH is a common method of weighing benefits and risk in the context of single study and needs to be interpreted with caution. A ratio of the RDs for benefit to the RDs for risk can be used to summarize in a single term the balance of benefit and risk. Chapter 8 provides further discussions on properties of NNT and NNH.

Exposure-adjusted risk analysis can utilize composite endpoints or can allow a comparison of individual endpoints. In the context of the TRA-2°P TIMI 50 study, for the reasons mentioned above, the most appropriate composite endpoints would be CV death, MI, and stroke versus GUSTO severe bleeding. However, RDs can be calculated and graphically displayed for any endpoint including the components of these composite endpoints. This allows the reader to see the trade-off of the types of events that are prevented and that cause harm.

For the TRA-2°P TIMI 50 study, the primary analysis approach focused on the first event. Depending on disease and type of endpoints in a study, recurrent events data are common and contain important clinical information for making assessments of investigational drugs in clinical studies. For the TRA-2°P TIMI 50 study, recurrent events either of the same type or multiple occurrences of different components of a composite endpoint may occur. Recurrent events were incorporated in the calculation of exposure-adjusted risk analysis, where, for patients with multiple events, the exposure was counted as the time from randomization to the time of the last event of interest. The use of first and recurrent events for BRA (or for key efficacy and/or safety analysis) is complicated by the differential opportunity to have a subsequent event based on the first event. In the TRA-2°P TIMI 50 study, an analysis of first and recurrent events was used as a sensitivity analysis in addition to the standard time to first event analysis. However, there were recurrent key efficacy endpoints but recurrent GUSTO severe bleeds occurred rarely. Whether or not to place emphasis on first or recurrent events for BRA or for key efficacy or safety analysis, the complexity of differential opportunity to have a subsequent event should be recognized and well understood in the context of clinical perspective and study designs, and dealt with accordingly as many studies, such as TRA-2°P TIMI 50 study, were not designed to eliminate the biases inherent in the analysis of recurrent events. A detailed discussion of these issues is beyond the scope of this chapter.

11.2.4 Relative Risk versus Absolute Risk

When considering a B–R analysis, a comparison of relative risks (or HRs) is not appropriate in the absence of the absolute risk of an event. This point is illustrated in this study if one compares the relative 20% reduction of CV death, MI, and stroke with an estimated 46% relative increase in ICH. The absolute risk of CV death, MI, and stroke is more than 15-fold higher than the risk of ICH in some patient populations. The 3-year KM rates of the composite endpoint of CV death, MI, and stroke were 9.5% and 7.9% compared to the 3-year KM rates of ICH, which were 0.4% and 0.6% in the placebo and vorapaxar groups, respectively (Tables 11.1 and 11.2), in the US label population. Placing emphasis on the HR, which is a relative risk assessment, can be misleading. In this trial, 46% relative risk increase in ICH in the vorapaxar group may generate a concern without considering the absolute risk of ICH and how rare these events occur. Given that primary efficacy endpoints occur much more frequently than ICH, the relative risk in terms of HR needs to be considered in conjunction with the absolute risk for a full BRA.

11.3 Implementation of TRA-2°P TIMI 50 B–R Assessment

Having discussed the key B–R elements in Section 11.2, this section presents the analysis results utilizing the key elements discussed in Section 11.2.

11.3.1 Net Clinical Benefit

As discussed above, the most appropriate composite endpoint to assess NCB would include benefits associated with reducing the risks of irreversible tissue damage, and risks associated with events that lead to irreversible harm. In the context of the TRA-2°P TIMI 50 study, this would include CV death, MI, stroke, and GUSTO severe bleeding. The 3-year KM rate for this composite endpoint was 9.1% versus 7.5% for placebo versus vorapaxar, respectively. The NCB of vorapaxar was 18% (95% CI, 0.74 to 0.90) estimated by a Cox PH model (see Table 11.3). The NCB was chosen based on biological plausibility: vorapaxar would not be expected to have an impact on noncardiac deaths (such as deaths from cancer, infection, etc.) with the exception of fatal bleeding. An alternative definition of NCB might include all-cause death rather than CV death to avoid important issues associated with informative censoring. When the composite endpoint was defined as all-cause death, MI, stroke, and GUSTO severe bleeding, more events are included and the 3-year KM rate for this composite endpoint was 10.5% versus 9.0% for placebo versus vorapaxar, respectively. It would be hard to argue that the additional events, noncardiac deaths, have less clinical impact than CV death. The HR for NCB using this endpoint was improved by 15% (95% CI, 0.78 to 0.93).

The prespecified composite endpoint for NCB includes UCR and GUSTO moderate bleeding in addition to CV death, MI, stroke, and GUSTO severe bleeding. Inclusion of these more common but less severe events with less clinical impact increases the event rate. An additional 314 events were added to the placebo arm and 359 events were added to the vorapaxar arm. This resulted in a 3-year KM rate of 12.2% versus 11.1% for placebo

TABLE 11.3

Time-to-Event Analyses of the NCB in the Intended Label Population: As-Treated Population-Event Accrual Period: Randomization to Last Visit

	Subjects with Events (%)				
Net Clinical Outcome Endpoints	**Placebo (n = 10,049)**		**Vorapaxar (n = 10,059)**		**HR[a,b] (95% CI)[b]**
CV death/MI/stroke/GUSTO severe	914/10,049	(9.1%)	753/10,059	(7.5%)	0.82 (0.74–0.90)
All-cause death/MI/stroke/GUSTO severe	1052/10,049	(10.5%)	905/10,059	(9.0%)	0.85 (0.78–0.93)
CV death/MI/stroke/UCR/GUSTO severe/GUSTO moderate	1226/10,049	(12.2%)	1112/10,059	(11.1%)	0.90 (0.83–0.98)
All-cause death/MI/stroke/GUSTO severe/GUSTO moderate	1140/10,049	(11.3%)	1067/10,059	(10.6%)	0.93 (0.66–1.02)

Note: Reference data on file.

[a] Hazard ratio is ZONTIVITY group versus placebo group.

[b] Ratio was calculated based on Cox PH model with covariates treatment and stratification factors.

versus vorapaxar, respectively. By adding these additional less severe events, the reduction of NCB is reduced to 10% compared to placebo (95% CI, 0.83 to 0.98) (Table 11.3).

11.3.2 Exposure-Adjusted Risk Analysis

The initial exposure-adjusted risk analysis utilizes the composite endpoints of CV death, MI, and stroke to represent efficacy and GUSTO severe bleeding to represent safety. Computed per 10,000 patient-years, or 10,000 patients treated for 1 year, the exposure-adjusted RD for CV death, MI, or stroke events between the vorapaxar-treated group and placebo groups is −68 (95% CI, −99 to −37) (Figure 11.2). In other words, there were 68 excess events in placebo-treated subjects per patient-year. The NNT, the inverse of the RD, to prevent one CV death, MI, or stroke is 146. This indicates that you would have to treat 146 patients in order to prevent one CV death, MI, or stroke in 1 year. With regard to safety, the RD for GUSTO severe bleeding events (including ICH and fatal bleed events) in the vorapaxar group as compared to the placebo group is 4 (95% CI, −8 to 15), and the NNH is 2602 (note that some numbers in the figure were rounded off). Using these endpoints (CV death, MI, or stroke to GUSTO severe), the ratio of benefit to risk is 68:4, a 17-fold benefit to risk.

For fatal ICH events, the RD is 1 (95% CI, −3 to 5) for the difference between vorapaxar and placebo, and NNH is 8605. The ratio of benefit to risk is 68:4 (CV death, MI, or stroke to GUSTO severe) and 68:1 (CV death, MI, or stroke to fatal ICH) (Figure 11.2). Figure 11.2 also includes additional efficacy or safety endpoints of various clinical impacts to illustrate a full spectrum of BRA.

These data can be translated into graphical summaries in a number of different formats. Figure 11.2 presents the RDs and 95% CI in a forest plot–like format. Another graphical display of the data allows for an immediate visual comparison of benefits and risks (Figure 11.3). Figure 11.3 shows RDs standardized by 10,000 patient-years. On the basis of

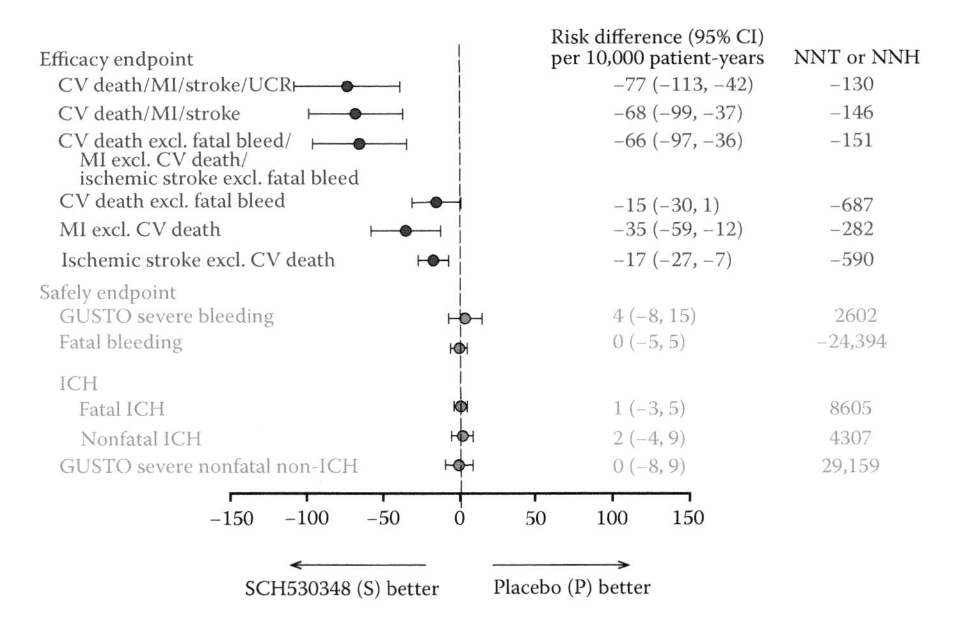

FIGURE 11.2
RDs and NNT or NNH of main efficacy and safety endpoints in the US label population: ITT/as-treated populations.

the approach described above where events of similar clinical impact are compared, for every 10,000 patient-years, treatment with vorapaxar resulted in 68 fewer major CV events (CV death, MI, or stroke), at the cost of two nonfatal ICHs.

Another method of visualizing the assessment of benefit and risk over time utilizes the KM method. In Figure 11.4, the RDs in terms of the cumulative excess number of events between vorapaxar and placebo are displayed over time. In this assessment, the temporal course of benefits of vorapaxar over placebo were measured by the accumulation of the

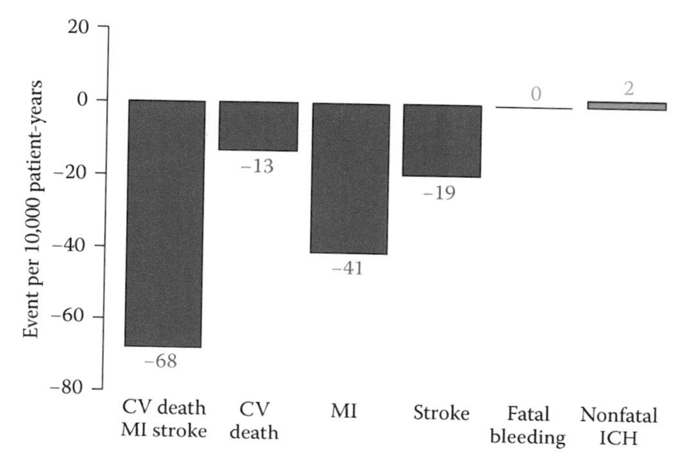

FIGURE 11.3
RD for serious (irreversible) events per 10,000 patient-years, vorapaxar versus placebo.

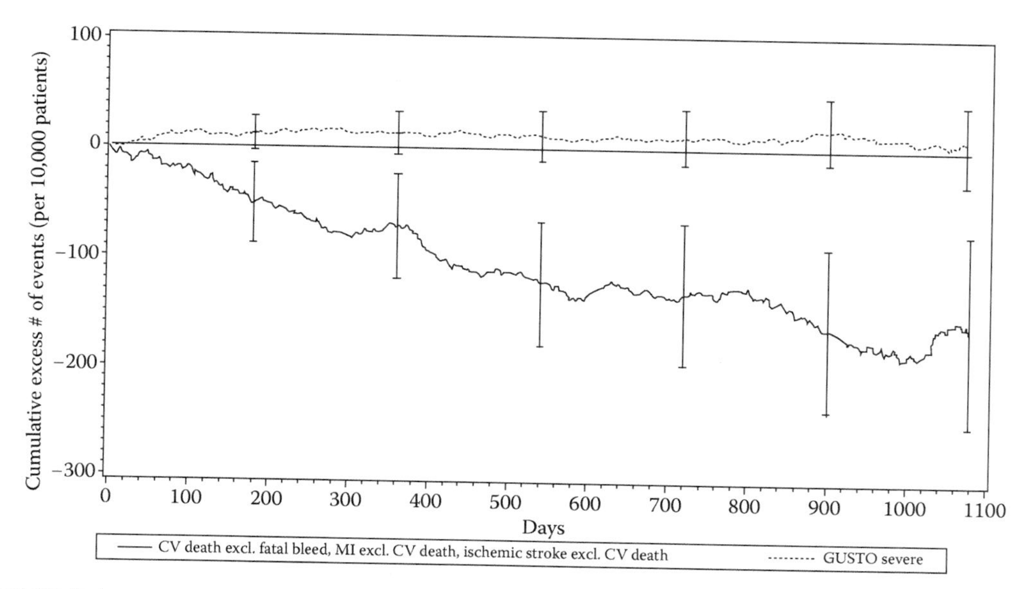

FIGURE 11.4
Cumulative excess number of benefit and harm events. Benefits are the composite of CV death excluding fatal bleed, MI excluding CV death, and ischemic stroke excluding CV death versus risk of GUSTO severe bleeding. Vorapaxar versus placebo: intended label population: ITT and as-treated populations-event accrual period: randomization to last visit.

excess number of events of the composite of the mutually exclusive efficacy endpoints CV deaths excluding fatal bleed, MI excluding CV death, and ischemic stroke excluding CV death, expressed per 10,000 patients, between the two arms of the study. The temporal course of risk was assessed by assessing the cumulative excess number of events over time between vorapaxar and placebo groups of GUSTO severe events per 10,000 patients. Vorapaxar, compared to placebo, was associated with an early and durable effect between benefit and risk trade-off (Figure 11.4). The cumulative excess number of benefit events versus placebo has a time course that indicated a cumulative RD in favor of vorapaxar compared to placebo over time. The cumulative excess number of harm events (GUSTO severe) are positive but flat over time, suggesting a short-term increased risk of this event compared to placebo that equalizes over time. The risk of GUSTO severe bleeding remained low over time. In summary, the magnitude of the benefit compared to risk increased steadily over time, without any apparent loss of effectiveness. This assessment reflects a favorable balance of benefit to risk (Figure 11.4).

11.4 Discussion

This chapter summarizes a multifaceted approach to the assessment of balance of the benefits and risks of vorapaxar secondary prevention of CV events in patients with a history of MI. There was a clear increased risk of ICH in patients with a history of stroke (in the absence of clear benefit), which resulted in a black box warning and a contraindication for patients with a history of stroke or TIA. In the remaining patients with a history of MI or PAD for whom vorapaxar is currently indicated, the balance of benefit and risk was assessed with the exposure-adjusted risk different along with NNT/NNH, the cumulative benefit compared to risk, and the net clinical outcome. Taken together and using all of these methods, vorapaxar results in benefits that outweigh risks compared to placebo. The increased risk of bleeding associated with the use of vorapaxar compared to placebo is sufficiently offset by the observed magnitude of benefit. Vorapaxar was associated with robust early and durable benefits by reducing the rates of CV death, MI, or stroke compared to placebo. In comparison, the absolute risk of severe bleeding is small and stable over time. The use of multiple methods of assessing the balance of benefit and risk and the consistency of these analyses were important to the successful review and approval of the product.

This case study highlights a number of critical issues that need to be considered in a B–R assessment. Regardless of which method of B–R assessment is used, the choice of endpoints that is used to assess benefit and risk is extremely important. In this case study, the relevant endpoints for benefit include the reduction of CV death, MI, and stroke and the relevant endpoints for bleeding risk include fatal bleeding and nonfatal ICH (GUSTO severe bleeding). All of these endpoints represent events that would be associated with irreversible tissue damage or death. The inclusion of events with lesser clinical impact clouds the B–R assessment. This case study also illustrates the importance of absolute risk and highlights potentially misleading interpretations when comparing relative risks (or HRs) of events associated with ischemic events or bleeding. Taken together, this case demonstrates the importance of assessing B–R in the relevant clinical contexts.

The process of developing and implementing the B–R framework and analyses required a close collaboration of a cross-functional team, especially between clinical and statistics. The input from clinical on endpoint selection and their clinical impacts played an important role in the development of the BRA framework. The insight from clinicians on the common use of NNT and NNH in the medical community facilitated the use of these metrics in the TRA-2°P TIMI 50 study B–R evaluation. Further, statistics provided expertise from the analysis perspectives on the use of aforementioned analysis metrics and methods and cautioned the study team on the caveats of the BRA metrics and methods that were important for the interpretation of the BRA results.

Unfortunately, there is still a paucity of B–R case studies in literature using the existing B–R frameworks and analysis methods that have been described. The maturation of quantitative B–R assessments with easy-to-understand graphical presentations of that assessment will be extraordinarily helpful in helping physicians improve patient outcomes. Vorapaxar is an example of a drug where multiple quantitative analyses of the balance of benefit and risk support its use in reducing the burden of CV disease.

References

Chackalamannil, S., Wang, Y., Greenlee, W. J., Hu, Z., Xia, Y., Ahn, H. S. et al., Discovery of a novel, orally active himbacine-based thrombin receptor antagonist (SCH 530348) with potent antiplatelet activity. *J. Med. Chem.* 2008; 51: 3061–3064.

Coughlin, S. R., Protease-activated receptors in hemostasis, thrombosis and vascular biology. *J. Thromb. Haemost.* 2005; 3: 1800–1814.

FDA Adversary Committee meeting, *MSD Briefing Information for the January 15, 2014 Meeting of the Cardiovascular and Renal Drugs Advisory Committee*, http://www.fda.gov/AdvisoryCommittees/CommitteesMeetingMaterials/Drugs/CardiovascularandRenalDrugsAdvisoryCommittee/ucm381326.htm.

FDA ZONTIVITY US Label Rev 05/2014: https://www.merck.com/product/usa/pi_circulars/z/zontivity/zontivity_pi.pdf.

Hutton, J. L., Misleading statistics: The problems surrounding number needed to treat and number needed to harm. *Pharm. Med.* 2010; 24(3): 145–149. doi:10.2165/11536680-000000000-00000.

IMI Pharmacoepidemiological Research on Outcomes of Therapeutics by European ConsorTium (PROTECT). 2012. WP5: Benefit–risk integration and representation. http://www.imi-protect.eu/wp5.html.

Miettinen, O., Nurminen, M., Comparative analysis of two rates. *Stat. Med.* 1985; 4: 213–226.

Morrow, D., Braunwald, E., Bonaca, M., Ameriso, S., Dalby, A., Fish, M. et al., Vorapaxar in the secondary prevention of atherothrombotic events. *N. Engl. J. Med.* 2012; 366: 1404–1413.

Tricoci, P., Huang, Z., Held, C., Moliterno, D., Armstrong, P., Van de Werf, F. et al., Thrombin-receptor antagonist vorapaxar in acute coronary syndromes. *N. Engl. J. Med.* 2011; 366(1): 20–33.

Unger, E., Weighing benefits and risks—The FDA's review of prasugrel. *N. Engl. J. Med.* 2009; 361(10): 942–944.

12

A Quantitative Benefit and Risk Assessment to Determine Optimal Retrieval Time for Inferior Vena Cava Filters in Patients without Pulmonary Embolism

Xuefeng Li, Telba Irony, and Jose Pablo Morales

CONTENTS

ABSTRACT Retrievable inferior vena cava (IVC) filters are increasingly implanted prophylactically in patients who may be at transient risk of pulmonary embolism (PE).

In 2009, the Agency detected an increased trend in the number of adverse events (AEs) related to implanted IVC filters, which was considered a possible safety signal. To properly address the total product life cycle of these devices, an internal multidisciplinary working group was developed with representation from all offices involved in the review and surveillance of these devices with the intent to investigate further these findings and decide as to whether or not regulatory actions should be taken to mitigate any potential risks.

Since the majority of these IVC filters are not removed after the risk of PE has diminished and the true risks of developing a device-related complication after successful placement of an IVC filter is unknown, but such risks would be expected to increase with the duration of implantation as with any chronic implant, the Agency developed a quantitative decision analysis model to assess the benefits and risks associated with these devices to elucidate whether implanted filters should be removed once the risk of PE starts to decrease (Morales et al. 2013).

This chapter discusses the benefit–risk assessment that employed a quantitative decision analysis model to address this issue in the absence of well-controlled clinical studies. On the basis of literature review and expert opinion, the model weighs the risks against the benefits of retrievable IVC filter use as a function of the filter's time in situ so that the optimal time to remove the filters can be easily identified.

The analysis showed that the optimal time to remove the IVC filters from patients without PE and who may be at transient risk of PE is between 1 and 2 months after implantation.

As a result of this analysis, the Center for Devices and Radiological Health at the Food and Drug Administration (FDA) issued two Public Health Notifications, one in 2010 and another in 2012, recommending removing retrievable IVC filters as soon as protection from PE is no longer needed. Our analysis provided supportive evidence to FDA's recommendations.

At the end of this chapter, we discussed practical issues and future applications of similar quantitative models.

12.1 Introduction

As part of the total product life cycle of medical devices, the Center for Devices and Radiological Health (CDRH) at the Food and Drug Administration (FDA) continues to monitor the safety of medical devices after they reached the US market. Whenever a safety signal is detected, a benefit–risk assessment is made to further investigate those findings and decide as to whether or not regulatory actions should be taken to mitigate any potential risks. Although benefits and risks are not weighted against each other quantitatively in most instances, full quantitative benefit–risk analysis models have shown to be increasingly useful. For premarket applications, decisions are usually based on prospectively designed clinical trials to test prespecified hypotheses. However, this is not the case for most postmarket issues that arise in a setting in which there is usually no well-designed clinical trials available to inform regulatory decisions in a timely manner.

In this chapter, we will introduce a case study that employs a quantitative benefit–risk model developed with the intent to address a postmarket safety signal. The devices of interest are retrievable inferior vena cava (IVC) filters.

12.2 Background

IVC filters are small, cage-like devices that are inserted into the IVC (the main vessel returning blood from the lower half of the body to the heart) to capture blood clots and prevent them from reaching the lungs. The first IVC filter intended to prevent the occurrence of pulmonary embolism (PE) was introduced in the US market in 1967.

Venous thromboembolism (VTE), which includes both PE and deep vein thrombosis (DVT), is a major cause of morbidity and mortality in all age groups. VTE is a common disorder with an estimated annual incidence of 5–12 persons per 10,000 (FDA 2011; Kaufman et al. 2009; Stein et al. 2011). The estimated incidence of nonfatal PE ranges between 400,000 and 630,000 cases per year with 50,000 to 200,000 deaths per year directly attributable to PE (Aujesky et al. 2005). Approximately 10% of all hospital deaths can be attributed to PE (Janne et al. 2008). IVC filters play an important role in the prevention of PE.

The first IVC filter with retrieval indications was cleared by the FDA in 2003, and there are now eight retrievable IVC filters currently marketed in the United States. All IVC filters on the market in the United States have the following indications for use: for the prevention of recurrent PE via placement in the vena cava in certain conditions (Kaufman et al. 2009). In addition, all retrievable filters contain the following statement in the indications: the filter may be retrieved in patients who no longer require a filter. Importantly, all retrievable filters are cleared as permanent devices as well. Any use outside the above FDA-labeled indications is considered off-label use of the device.

In 2008, more than half of IVC filter placements utilized retrievable IVC filters and their use continues to rise. Also, it is unknown how many retrievable filters are placed with the intention to be retrieved, that is, filters that are expected to be retrieved after the risk of PE is diminished as is the case in most trauma victims and bariatric and orthopedic surgery patients. According to an IVC filter consensus panel in 2009 (Kaufman et al. 2009), 50% or fewer of retrievable IVC filters are ever removed. Although it is unknown whether they were implanted for transient high risk of PE or for permanent use, this raises significant safety concerns as there are many AEs associated with IVC filters when being left in situ, including IVC thrombosis, DVT, access site thrombosis, filter migration, IVC penetration, filter fracture, and filter embolization to the heart and lungs.

In 2009, the Agency noted a safety signal from postmarket AE reports, suggesting that the number of filter-related events had risen over the past years. CDRH formed an internal multidisciplinary working group with representation from all offices involved in the review and surveillance of these devices with the intent to further investigate these findings and decide as to whether or not regulatory actions should be taken to mitigate any potential risks. As part of these efforts, the working group noted that there were very few clinical studies that had evaluated the off-label use of IVC filters and that there was absence of robust clinical data to inform the balance of benefits and risks over time of off-label IVC filter use in patients for whom the device was inserted with the intent to be used temporarily (not permanently). In addition, since the majority of these IVC filters are not removed after the risk of PE has diminished and the true risks of developing a device-related complication after successful placement of an IVC filter is unknown, but such risks would be expected to increase with the duration of implantation as with any chronic implant, the Agency developed a quantitative decision analysis model to assess the benefits and risks associated with these devices to elucidate whether implanted filters should be removed once the risk of PE starts to decrease (Morales et al. 2013).

The working group explored both a qualitative and quantitative model to address the issue and both approaches provided consistent conclusions. The Agency released an initial public health communication on August 9, 2010, recommending that implanting physicians and clinicians responsible for the ongoing care of patients with retrievable IVC filters consider removing such filters as soon as protection from PE was no longer needed (Decousus et al. 1998). The Agency believed that increased retrieval rates of these devices from patients who no longer require filtration might reduce the associated long-term complications and risks from these devices.

In this chapter, we describe the mathematical model that was developed using data publicly available in the medical literature to determine whether there is a period during which the risk of having the device in situ is expected to outweigh the benefits. We conclude the chapter by discussing the strengths and limitations of this model, practical issues, and future applications of similar quantitative models.

12.3 Analysis Model

The objective of this benefit–risk assessment is to determine when the IVC filters implanted for temporary use should be removed. A quantitative decision analysis model was developed to analyze how the relative benefits provided by the implant and the risks posed by its retrieval or continued implantation vary as a function of time for patients implanted with the device. Quantitative decision analysis is the use of mathematical models to describe, inform, and analyze decision-making problems in the presence of uncertainty. This method of analysis tackles the problem by explicating the values that drive decisions, such as treatment objectives or preferences (Clemen 2012; Raiffa 2012; Schwartz and Bergus 2012), and accounting for uncertain information based on all available data.

To develop the model, we first consulted several experts to identify risks and benefits associated with the use of the IVC filters. In addition, data were collected from the medical literature between 2000 and 2009 to assess the rates of relevant AEs at different times after implantation using the following search terms: vena cava filter, IVC filter, IVCF, caval interruption, and caval filtration. A total of 18 publications were identified and included in the analysis (Antevil et al. 2006; Bovyn et al. 2006; Cherry et al. 2008; Gargiulo et al. 2006; Greenfield et al. 2000; Hoppe et al. 2006; Imberti et al. 2005; Johnson et al. 2009; Kardys et al. 2007; Karmy-Jones et al. 2007; Oliva et al. 2005; Overby et al. 2009; Piano et al. 2007; Rosenthal et al. 2007; Schuster et al. 2007; Toro et al. 2008; Vaziri et al. 2009; Velmahos et al. 2000).

Patients described in the literature with the short-term need for filtration were heterogeneous and encompassed different comorbidities, demographics, and anticoagulation regimens. Because patient-level data were lacking, patients were assumed to have similar risk profiles and prognostic characteristics (i.e., patient subgroups were assumed to be exchangeable), although we recognize that the risks and benefits for individual patients may vary.

Ten significant types of AEs associated with IVC filters were identified based on the signals received by the FDA and on the literature search. These AEs were categorized using qualitative assessment by the FDA clinicians and divided as severe, moderate, or mild. Table 12.1 presents the device risks and their severity scores.

These AEs were classified into three categories: (1) Risk without the filters: this includes death and PE that the device is intended to prevent. It is actually the *benefit* of having the filter in place. (2) Risk in situ: this includes device occlusion, filter embolization, DVT, device penetration, migration, and fracture. (3) Risk of removal: this risk is just a one-time retrieval complication.

To understand the decision analysis model, the influence diagram (Figure 12.1) shows the relationship among benefits, AEs, and risks. The risks are combined under continuous time frame to yield the net risk score that was used for making decisions.

AEs were assigned numerical weights based on a scale developed from independent rankings by three physicians: two vascular surgeons and one interventional radiologist

TABLE 12.1

Device-Related AEs and Relative Severity Scores

Risk	Severity Score
Death	Severe
Recurrent PE	Severe
DVT	Moderate
Filter embolization	Severe
IVC occlusion	Moderate
IVC penetration	Moderate
Filter fracture	Moderate
Filter migration	Mild
Retrieval complications	Mild

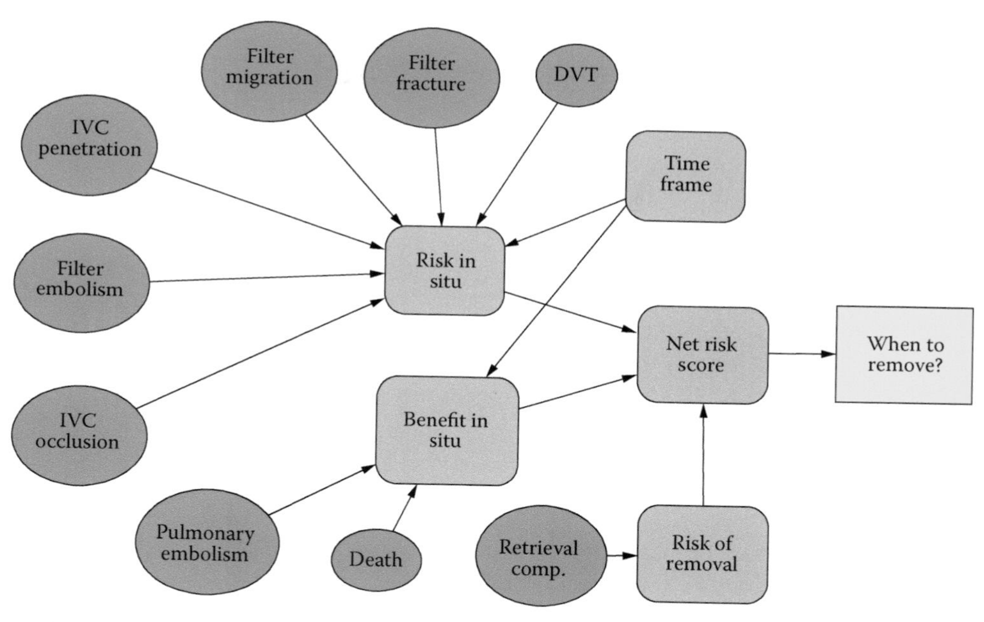

FIGURE 12.1
Influence diagram showing the relationships among AEs and the three different types of risks.

(Table 12.2). The scale ranges from 0 (least severe) to 10 (most severe [i.e., death]). The intervals provided in the table reflect uncertainty about the weights and the variability in clinical significance of individual AEs. Later, the intervals will be used for a sensitivity analysis. The occurrence rates in published studies were usually reported within several time intervals after filter implantation: from 0 to 30 days, from 31 to 180 days, and from 181 days to 2 years.

TABLE 12.2
Weights of Severity and Occurrence Rates of AEs (Estimates from Literature)

AE	Weight	Risk Classification	0 to 30 Days	1 to 6 Months	6 Months to 2 Years	Estimating Method
Death	10	Risk without filters	0%	0%	0%	Relative differences comparing to the no-filter group (which is why some rates are negative)
PE	8 7–9		–4%	–1%	0%	
DVT	5 4–6	Risk in situ	0.27%	1.35%	4.86%	
Filter emboli	8 7–9		0.11%	0.55%	1.98%	A constant monthly rate was assumed
IVC penetration	6 5–7		0.06%	0.30%	1.08%	
IVC occlusion	5 4–6		0.15%	0.75%	2.70%	
Filter fracture	4 3–5		0.02%	0.1%	0.36%	
Filter migration	3 2–4		0.15%	0.75%	2.70%	
Retrieval complications	3 2–4	Risk of removal	3%	3%	4%	One-time risk, which increases slightly over time

Next, we define the risk score functions as follows. Risk score at time t for a specific AE is defined as the cumulative occurrence rate from time 0 to t.

$$\mathrm{RS}_{\mathrm{AE}}(t) = \mathrm{Weight}_{\mathrm{AE}} \int_{s=0}^{t} \mathrm{OR}_{\mathrm{AE}}(s)\,\mathrm{d}s,$$

where $\mathrm{Weight}_{\mathrm{AE}}$ is the weight for AE and $\mathrm{OR}_{\mathrm{AE}}(s)$ is the density function of the occurrence rate for AE. The risk score combines the frequency and severity for each type of AE. The risk score is unitless and is relative because the weights are measured on a relative scale that compares the severity of different AEs. The weight ranges from 0 (no harm) to 10 (most severe [i.e., death]). The occurrence rate is the proportion of patients who experienced the given AE per unit of time (day).

The value function of this decision model gives the overall risk score at time t. It combines the following risks:

1. Risk score in situ (t) equals the sum of risk score from occlusion, filter emboli, migration, penetration, fracture, and DVT.

$$\mathrm{RS}_{\mathrm{in\ situ}}(t) = \mathrm{RS}_{\mathrm{occlusion}}(t) + \mathrm{RS}_{\mathrm{emboli}}(t) + \mathrm{RS}_{\mathrm{migration}}(t) + \mathrm{RS}_{\mathrm{penetration}}(t) + \mathrm{RS}_{\mathrm{fracture}}(t) + \mathrm{RS}_{\mathrm{DVT}}(t)$$

2. Risk score of removal (t)

$$\mathrm{RS}_{\mathrm{removal}}(t) = \begin{cases} 0 & t \neq t_{\mathrm{removal}} \\ \mathrm{RR}(t) & t = t_{\mathrm{removal}} \end{cases}$$

where t_{removal} is the time of removal and RR(t) is the one-time removal risk at time t.

3. Relative risk score without the filter (death and PE).

$$\mathrm{RS}_{\mathrm{no\ filter}}(t) = \mathrm{RS}_{\mathrm{death}}(t) + \mathrm{RS}_{\mathrm{PE}}(t)$$

"Risk without filter" is the benefit gained by having the filter in place. For a filter that has been implanted, the net risk score for keeping the filter in the body is defined as the risk score in situ minus the risk score without the filter, minus the risk score of removal.

$$\mathrm{NRS}(t) = \mathrm{RS}_{\mathrm{in\ situ}}(t) - \mathrm{RS}_{\mathrm{no\ filter}}(t) - \mathrm{RS}_{\mathrm{removal}}(t)$$

An increasing trend of the net risk score indicates that the expected harm of keeping the filter in place outweighs the expected benefits. The turning point is the time when the risk of having the filter in place starts to outweigh the benefit (i.e., the cumulative net risk stops to decrease and starts to increase). It is the earliest day when removal of the filter should be considered.

To better understand the problem and the model, a hypothetical plot (Figure 12.2) provides the basic idea behind the model. The light blue line stands for the risk without this device. In other words, this is the benefit of having the device implanted. It provides great benefit at the beginning but the benefit starts to decrease as time goes by. The green dotted

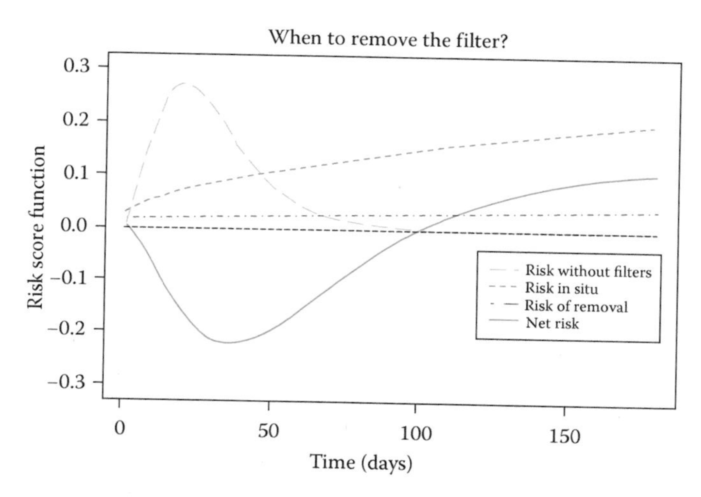

FIGURE 12.2
Hypothetical plot showing the idea behind the decision analysis model.

line stands for the Risk in situ. It is increasing over time. The blue line is the retrieval risk. It is a one-time risk but it may increase slightly over time. The red line is the net risk, which is the Risk in situ minus the Risk without device minus the Risk of removal. It is the net risk of keeping the device in the body. Once the net risk reaches the minimum, the device should be taken out. It should be noted that the top two curves are density functions of occurrence rates while the bottom red curve is the total accumulative risk.

Cumulative AE rates were estimated based on the available literature for the following intervals after filter implantation: 0 to 30 days, 31 days to 6 months, and 6 months to 2 years. These intervals were chosen as they were the most common intervals used in the literature for reporting AEs for IVC filters. Rates for death, PE, and DVT are relative differences comparing the "filter" group with a "no-filter" group. For PE, the event rate was higher in the no-filter group, resulting in a negative point estimate. Since the model focuses on the prophylactic use of filters, that is, filters to be used in patients with a temporary (up to 6 months) need, the rate of PE after 6 months was assumed to be zero (Arcelus et al. 2008; Carmody et al. 2006; Owings et al. 1997). Retrieval complication was considered a one-time risk that occurs at the time of retrieval and includes any associated access site complications. Table 12.2 provides point estimates of occurrence rates used in calculating the risk scores. We used the time-adjusted average method to estimate the occurrence rates.

We assumed continuous density functions for the occurrence rates of all AEs except for "retrieval complication," which can occur only at the time of the retrieval procedure. Specifically, we assume that the PE occurrence rate follows gamma and triangular density functions (Figure 12.3) in which the accumulated PE occurrence rate in 180 days is equal to 5%, the total PE occurrence rate based on observed data. For the occurrence rates, we used 95% confidence intervals since they were estimated through meta-analysis. The occurrence rates for occlusion, embolization, migration, penetration, fracture, and DVT were assumed to follow three different functions: constant, slightly increasing, and slightly decreasing over time. These functions were chosen in a way that each AE has the same cumulative rate at day 180 estimated from literature, as shown in Table 12.2. We believe that these assumptions encompass a wide range of plausible variations on the AE rates, including the unlikely possibility that they may decrease with time. With these assumptions, the net risk score functions and the turning points can be obtained.

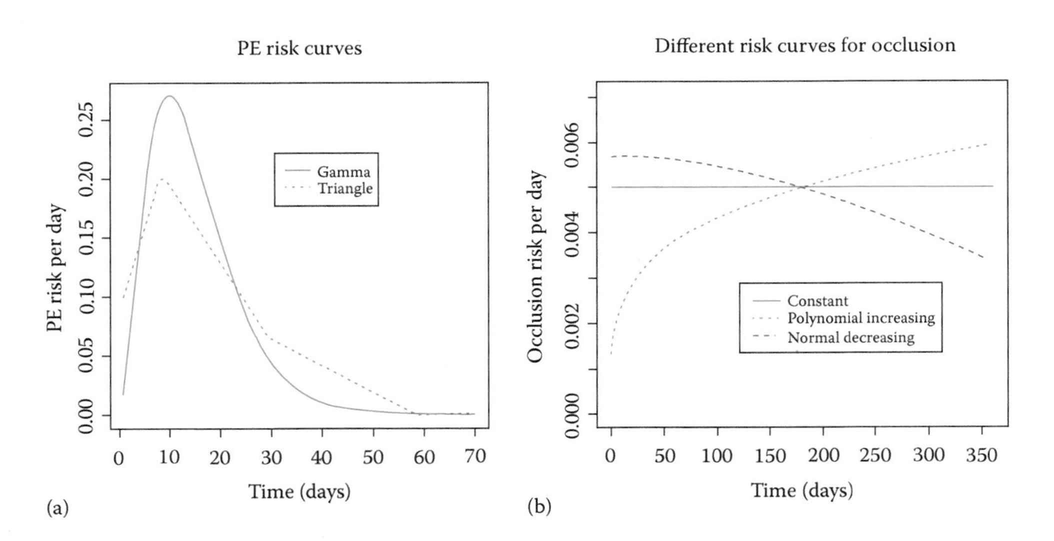

FIGURE 12.3
Assumed occurrence rate functions for PE (a) and other AEs (b).

Once the weights and occurrence function over time are known for each AE, it becomes straightforward to calculate the net risk score function over time. Commercially available decision analysis software (DPL 7, Syncopation Software, Inc., and a free statistical software R) were used to conduct the analysis based on the weights assigned to each AE and its occurrence rate over time.

To assess the impact of variability in obtaining the weights and uncertainty on the occurrence rates, sensitivity analyses were performed for a range of weights and for a range of occurrence rates for each AE. Resulting uncertainty associated with the net risk was reported via the 95% confidence intervals of turning points.

12.4 Results

Figure 12.4 presents the net risk score curves under six different scenarios. The net risk score decreases at the beginning and starts to increase after 5 to 8 weeks.

Table 12.3 presents the numerical results of turning points calculated under different assumptions. If a Gamma occurrence rate is assumed for the PE and constant rates are assumed for other filter-related AEs, the model shows that the risks of complications start to outweigh the protective benefits of the filter at day 35 after implantation. Other scenarios show that the turning point is between 36 and 53 days. Please note that the turning point is the day the cumulative risk stops to decrease and starts to increase.

The intervals in Table 12.3 originated from sensitivity analyses that were performed to assess the variability of the calculated net risk score when the weights and the AE occurrence rates vary within plausible ranges, as shown in Table 12.4. The time interval from 6 months to 2 years is no longer relevant according to the previous results so it is ignored here. The intervals for the weights were based on the minimum and maximum weights assigned by three physician scorers. The intervals for the occurrence rates were estimated based on the literature review. Specifically, the sensitivity analyses were conducted via the Monte Carlo

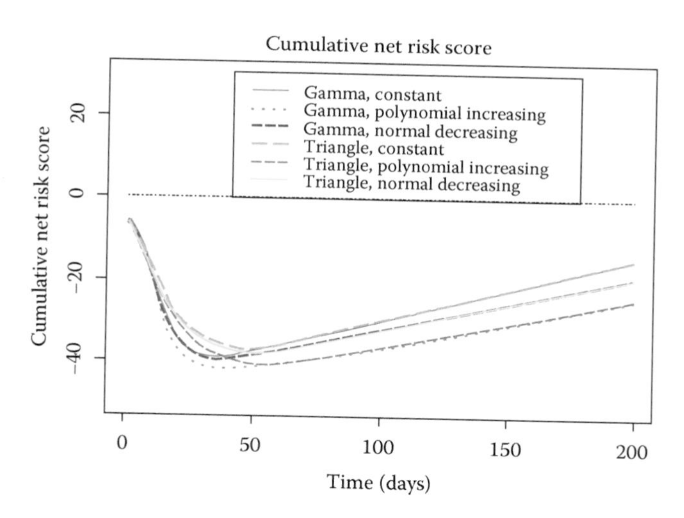

FIGURE 12.4
Net risk score curves under various assumptions. Here, Gamma and Triangular labels mean that the PE occurrence rate follows either Gamma or Triangular density functions as shown in Figure 12.3.

TABLE 12.3
Turning Points and Sensitivity Analyses under Different Function Assumptions

Function for Occurrence Rate of PE	Function for Occurrence Rate of Other AEs	Turning Point and 95% Confidence Intervals (in Days)		
		Original Raters	**Anticonservative Rater**	**Conservative Rater**
Gamma	Constant	35 (30, 40)	30 (22, 36)	38 (33, 42)
	Polynomial increasing	39 (33, 40)	34 (27, 35)	42 (35, 42)
	Normal decreasing	36 (29, 37)	30 (25, 33)	38 (33, 41)
Triangle	Constant	50 (41, 54)	39 (22, 51)	52 (45, 55)
	Polynomial increasing	53 (40, 53)	47 (31, 48)	55 (48, 55)
	Normal decreasing	50 (40, 52)	40 (27, 46)	53 (47, 55)
Total range from sensitivity analysis		(29, 54)	(22, 51)	(33, 55)

TABLE 12.4
Intervals of Weights and 95% Confidence Intervals of Occurrence Rates of AEs for Sensitivity Analyses

AE	Weight	0–30 Days	1–6 Months
Death	10	0.00% (−1.0%, 1.0%)	0.00% (−1.0%, 1.0%)
PE	8 (7, 9)	−4.00% (−7.00%, −1.00%)	−1.00% (−2.00%, 0.00%)
DVT	5 (4, 6)	0.27% (0.00%, 0.55%)	1.35% (0.00%, 2.70%)
Filter emboli	8 (7, 9)	0.11% (0.0%, 0.59%)	0.55% (0.20%, 1.20%)
IVC penetration	6 (5, 7)	0.06% (0.0%, 0.54%)	0.30% (0.10%, 0.80%)
IVC occlusion	5 (4, 6)	0.15% (0.01%, 0.48%)	0.75% (0.40%, 1.30%)
Filter fracture	4 (3, 5)	0.02% (0.0%, 0.45%)	0.10% (0.01%, 0.65%)
Filter migration	3 (2, 4)	0.15% (0.0%, 0.51%)	0.75% (0.40%, 1.40%)
Retrieval complications	3 (2, 4)	3% (2.20%, 4.10%)	3.00% (2.20%, 4.10%)

TABLE 12.5
Validation of the Original Results Using Six Additional Physicians (Phy)

Function for Occurrence Rate of PE	Function for Occurrence Rate of Other AEs	Turning Point						
		Original	Phy 1	Phy 2	Phy 3	Phy 4	Phy 5	Phy 6
Gamma	Constant	35	30	33	35	34	38	36
	Polynomial increasing	39	34	36	38	38	42	39
	Normal decreasing	36	30	33	35	34	38	36
Triangle	Constant	50	39	45	49	48	52	50
	Polynomial increasing	53	47	50	52	52	55	53
	Normal decreasing	50	40	46	49	48	53	50

method, where each weight was assumed to follow a uniform distribution on the corresponding interval and each occurrence rate was assumed to follow a Gamma or normal distribution on which the corresponding range was formulated as the 95% confidence interval.

Initially, the weights were assessed by three physicians. In order to conduct a comprehensive sensitivity analysis, we subsequently validated the results by adding six physicians (three vascular surgeons, two interventional radiologists, and one cardiologist). Among those, two physicians assigned different weights compared to their colleagues, being in opposite extremes (Table 12.5). We call one conservative and the other anticonservative. Here, conservative means that the physician is reluctant to remove the filters; hence, the assigned weights are relatively small, which leads to delayed turning points. All these differing opinions are reflected in wide intervals and were taken into account in the sensitivity analyses.

The sensitivity analyses show that the range of turning points is relatively robust, for example, from 30 to 40 days under the first scenario and from 47 to 55 days under the fifth scenario. Overall, the turning point is between 30 and 55 days. These sensitivity analyses support the robustness of the result that the net risk score reaches its minimum within the second month.

12.5 Discussion

IVC filters play an important role in the prevention of PE. However, as previously stated, the safety signal of elevated AEs with the use of these devices required a timely decision from the FDA. In the absence of complete information, a benefit–risk assessment was developed with some uncertainties. This case was considered the best approach as using a quantitative decision analysis model allowed an objective and transparent synthesis of all available information. This available information included the elicitation of weights from experts, a literature search and sensitivity analyses to account for the uncertainty in the data and for the variability of physicians' opinions about the severity of the AEs.

Without data from a well-designed clinical trial for prophylactic implantation of IVC filters, our model identified the optimal time for retrieval on the basis of the limited available information. The model suggests that, once the filter is implanted, the net risk tends to increase with time. Once the patient's transient risk for PE has subsided, the benefit–risk profile resulting from the analysis begins to favor filter removal between 1 and 2 months, assuming that retrieval is clinically and technically possible. The results provided by the model lead to a Public Health Notification that states

> The FDA recommends that implanting physicians and clinicians responsible for the ongoing care of patients with retrievable IVC filters consider removing the filter as soon as protection from pulmonary embolism is no longer needed.

The FDA is aware that the practice of leaving retrievable IVC filters in situ that could be removed could be attributed to lack of data identifying appropriate retrieval times, loss of follow-up of patients, or lack of physician initiative to consider device retrieval. Our decision analysis model not only provides insight and transparency to enable clinicians to reach an optimal and coherent clinical decision (Amin et al. 2006; Schrag et al. 1997) but also helps physicians and patients better understand the time course of risks related to implant duration and retrieval. This finding is consistent with many physicians' belief. In the situation when there was a scarcity of scientifically valid data, the proposed model fulfilled the public heath need to help physicians make decisions in a timely manner.

The analysis presented in this chapter was intended for a population-level decision and is not appropriate or sufficient for individual patient-level decisions. Although the results of this analysis may provide general guidelines for physicians, individual patient decisions should be made on a case-by-case basis, using not only the insight provided by the model but also the particular circumstances regarding each patient. Once better data for a specific patient cohort is available, the general model can be easily adopted to the specific cohort.

However, as with any model, there are limitations in the decision analysis presented here. First, the data used for the analysis were primarily obtained from single-center experiences of patients with IVC filters.

Second, to estimate the occurrence rates of AEs, we used a literature review, which bears intrinsic limitations, such as pooling data from different populations, inability to control the quality of the data, and the potential for underlying selection bias of the studies chosen for the analysis. Importantly, estimates of occurrence rates of all AEs could not be determined at all time points, with the 0- to 30-day time frame being most deficient. To mitigate this challenge, assumptions of increasing, decreasing, and constant AE density functions were made.

Third, the weights presented in the analysis were elicited from physicians with different medical specialties involved in the implantation and care of patient with IVC filters. Therefore, such weighs are subjective. Also, the model did not take into account patient preferences and weighting of severity of AEs.

Fourth, data used for this analysis of prophylactic IVC filter implantation were leveraged from studies of IVC filters in different patient populations. We recognize that among patients with short-term need of filtration, there were different subgroups of patients (i.e., trauma, bariatric, and orthopedic surgery) that have different comorbidities, demographics, and pathophysiological circumstances. Nevertheless, because of the lack of data to perform individual group analysis, those subgroups were assumed to be exchangeable, as they all had transient risk of PE.

Finally, despite differences between IVC filter designs and their failure modes, a device class approach was deemed appropriate for the purpose of this analysis since device-specific data were not available. The limitations of the available data underscore the need for additional development of high-level clinical evidence involving IVC filter implantation and retrieval.

Also, to examine whether the results of our model are robust and to evaluate the impact of the uncertainty on the assumptions and parameters, we performed extensive sensitivity analyses with respect to weights and rates of AEs. Since the weights from three physicians have been questioned to be subjective and could be biased, we later consulted six additional physicians (three vascular surgeons, two interventional radiologists, and one cardiologist) to reduce potential bias. Among those, two physicians assigned different weights compared to their colleagues, being in opposite extremes. The sensitivity analyses showed that even with variations of these parameters within stated intervals, the trend of increasing net risk with time remains the same.

To summarize, a benefit–risk assessment that employs quantitative decision analysis was used and resulted in supportive evidence to the traditionally used qualitative method. Regarding this issue, the FDA has issued two public health notifications, one in 2010 and the other in 2012. Our analysis provided supportive evidence to FDA's recommendations (FDA 2011) and the clinical community (SIR 2011).

In addition to these recommendations, several actions were taken by the relevant stakeholders. For example, the American Society of Hematology reinforced this recommendation against liberal use of IVC filters in December 2013. In July 2014, the Heart and Vascular Outcomes Research Institute has initiated a multicenter iRetrieve Study to Improve IVC Filter Retrieval Rates. A trend of removing more IVC filters in practice has been seen in the last couple of years and efforts to gather proper clinical data on the real-world use of IVC filters are being undertaken. Furthermore, the Society for Vascular Surgery and the Society of Interventional Radiology partnered to develop a clinical study to collect data on the real-world use of IVC filters, the retrieval rates, and the rates of complications associated with the use of these devices. It is designed to be the largest IVC filter study ever conducted and will provide additional insight into our understanding of the real-world use of these devices. Data from this clinical study will allow for further refinement of this mathematical model, which may ultimately help practicing physicians during the decision making as to whether or not to retrieve a given IVC filter.

12.6 Conclusion

Quantitative decision analysis affords new possibilities for regulatory decision making by weighting risks and benefits distilled from disparate sources of information to form a cohesive picture that can be used, in this case, to decide whether recommendations should be made to clinicians involved with the care of patients with retrievable IVC filters. The proposed quantitative decision analysis model sets up a quite general benefit and risk assessing template and framework. It can be easily applied to other similar situations where benefits and risks are to be weighed against each other, either with time or without time factors.

References

Amin MS, Matchar DB, Wood MA, Ellenbogen KA. Management of recalled pacemakers and implantable cardioverter-defibrillators: A decision analysis model. *JAMA* (2006);296:412–20.

Antevil JL, Sise MJ, Sack DI et al. Retrievable vena cava filters for preventing pulmonary embolism in trauma patients: A cautionary tale. *J Trauma* (2006);60:35–40.

Arcelus JI, Monreal M, Caprini JA et al. Clinical presentation and time-course of postoperative venous thromboembolism: Results from the RIETE Registry. *Thromb Haemost* (2008);99:546–51.
Aujesky D, Smith KJ, Cornuz J, Roberts MS. Cost-effectiveness of low-molecular-weight heparin for treatment of pulmonary embolism. *Chest* (2005);128:1601–10.
Bovyn G, Ricco JB, Reynaud P, Le Blanche AF. Long-duration temporary vena cava filter: A prospective 104-case multicenter study. *J Vasc Surg* (2006);43:1222–9.
Carmody BJ, Sugerman HJ, Kellum JM et al. Pulmonary embolism complicating bariatric surgery: Detailed analysis of a single institution's 24-year experience. *J Am Coll Surg* (2006);203:831–7.
Cherry RA, Nichols PA, Snavely TM, David MT, Lynch FC. Prophylactic inferior vena cava filters: Do they make a difference in trauma patients? *J Trauma* (2008);65:544–8.
Clemen RT. *Making hard decisions: An introduction to decision analysis*. 2nd ed. Duxbury Press: Independence, KY; 2012.
Decousus H, Leizorovicz A, Parent F et al. A clinical trial of vena caval filters in the prevention of pulmonary embolism in patients with proximal deep-vein thrombosis. Prevention du Risque d'Embolie Pulmonaire par Interruption Cave Study Group. *N Engl J Med* (1998);338:409–15.
Food and Drug Administration. Inferior vena cava (IVC) filters: Initial communication: Risk of adverse events with long term use. Posted online August 9, 2011. Available at: http://www.fda.gov/Safety/MedWatch/SafetyInformation/SafetyAlertsforHumanMedicalProducts/ucm221707.htm.
Gargiulo NJ III, Veith FJ, Lipsitz EC, Suggs WD, Ohki T, Goodman E. Experience with inferior vena cava filter placement in patients undergoing open gastric bypass procedures. *J Vasc Surg* (2006);44:1301–5.
Greenfield LJ, Proctor MC, Michaels AJ, Taheri PA. Prophylactic vena caval filters in trauma: The rest of the story. *J Vasc Surg* (2000);32:490–5.
Hoppe H, Nutting CW, Smouse HR et al. Gunther Tulip filter retrievability multicenter study including CT follow-up: Final report. *J Vasc Interv Radiol* (2006);17:1017–23.
Imberti D, Bianchi M, Farina A, Siragusa S, Silingardi M, Ageno W. Clinical experience with retrievable vena cava filters: Results of a prospective observational multicenter study. *J Thromb Haemost* (2005);3:1370–5.
Janne dB, Faintuch S, Reedy AW, Nickerson CF, Rosen MP. Retrievable versus permanent caval filter procedures: When are they cost-effective for interventional radiology? *J Vasc Interv Radiol* (2008);19:384–92.
Johnson ON III, Gillespie DL, Aidinian G, White PW, Adams E, Fox CJ. The use of retrievable inferior vena cava filters in severely injured military trauma patients. *J Vasc Surg* (2009);49:410–6.
Kardys CM, Stoner MC, Manwaring ML, Bogey WM, Parker FM, Powell S. The use of intravascular ultrasound imaging to improve use of inferior vena cava filters in a high-risk bariatric population. *J Vasc Surg* (2007);46:1248–52.
Karmy-Jones R, Jurkovich GJ, Velmahos GC et al. Practice patterns and outcomes of retrievable vena cava filters in trauma patients: An AAST multicenter study. *J Trauma* (2007);62:17–24.
Kaufman JA, Rundback JH, Kee ST et al. Development of a research agenda for inferior vena cava filters: Proceedings from a multidisciplinary research consensus panel. *J Vasc Interv Radiol* (2009);20:697–707.
Morales JP, Li X, Irony ZT et al. Decision analysis of retrievable inferior vena cava filters in patients without pulmonary embolism. *J Vascular Surgery: Venous and Lym Dis* 2013;1:376–84.
Oliva VL, Szatmari F, Giroux MF, Flemming BK, Cohen SA, Soulez G. The Jonas study: Evaluation of the retrievability of the Cordis OptEase inferior vena cava filter. *J Vasc Interv Radiol* (2005);16:1439–45.
Overby DW, Kohn GP, Cahan MA et al. Risk-group targeted inferior vena cava filter placement in gastric bypass patients. *Obes Surg* (2009);19:451–5.
Owings JT, Kraut E, Battistella F, Cornelius JT, O'Malley R. Timing of the occurrence of pulmonary embolism in trauma patients. *Arch Surg* (1997);132:862–6.
Piano G, Ketteler ER, Prachand V et al. Safety, feasibility, and outcome of retrievable vena cava filters in high-risk surgical patients. *J Vasc Surg* (2007);45:784–8.

Raiffa H. *Decision analysis: Introductory lectures on choices under uncertainty*. Random House: New York; 2012.

Rosenthal D, Wellons ED, Hancock SM, Burkett AB. Retrievability of the Gunther Tulip vena cava filter after dwell times longer than 180 days in patients with multiple trauma. *J Endovasc Ther* (2007);14:406–10.

Schrag D, Kuntz KM, Garber JE, Weeks JC. Decision analysis effects of prophylactic mastectomy and oophorectomy on life expectancy among women with BRCA1 or BRCA2 mutations. *N Engl J Med* (1997);336:1465–71.

Schuster R, Hagedorn JC, Curet MJ, Morton JM. Retrievable inferior vena cava filters may be safely applied in gastric bypass surgery. *Surg Endosc* (2007);21:2277–9.

Schwartz A, Bergus G. Medical decision making: A physician's guide. Cambridge University Press: Cambridge, UK; 2012.

Society of Interventional Radiology. IVC Filters: Society of Interventional Radiology Leads in Patient Care, Safety, Research. 2011. Available at: http://www.sirweb.org/news/newsPDF/Release_JVIR_IVCF_Nov11_final.pdf.

Stein PD, Matta F, Hull RD. Increasing use of vena cava filters for prevention of pulmonary embolism. *Am J Med* (2011);124:655–61.

Toro JB, Gardner MJ, Hierholzer C et al. Long-term consequences of pelvic trauma patients with thromboembolic disease treated with inferior vena caval filters. *J Trauma* (2008);65:25–9.

Vaziri K, Bhanot P, Hungness ES, Morasch MD, Prystowsky JB, Nagle AP. Retrievable inferior vena cava filters in high-risk patients undergoing bariatric surgery. *Surg Endosc* (2009);23:2203–7.

Velmahos GC, Kern J, Chan LS, Oder D, Murray JA, Shekelle P. Prevention of venous thromboembolism after injury: An evidence-based report part II: Analysis of risk factors and evaluation of the role of vena caval filters. *J Trauma* (2000);49:140–4.

13

Benefit–Risk Assessment via Case Studies

Weili He, Qi Jiang, and George Quartey

CONTENTS

ABSTRACT The development and implementation of benefit–risk assessment is multifaceted and should be done throughout the clinical development life cycle. In this chapter, we describe five real examples that regulatory agencies considered in benefit–risk evaluations, resulting in different outcomes in their approval and marketing status. These case studies illustrate a few key considerations for a full benefit–risk evaluation.

13.1 Introduction

A key element of the 2012 PDUFA (Prescription Drug User Fee Act) V reauthorization and passage of FDASIA (Food and Drug Administration Safety and Innovation Act of 2012) was the requirement for FDA to establish a structured benefit–risk (B–R) framework to improve the transparency and clarity of FDA's B–R decisions and to communicate more effectively the subjective value judgments underlying B–R determinations (Biotechnology Industry Organization [BIO] White Paper 2015; FDA 2013). As the BIO White Paper indicated, "Over the last two years, FDA has been piloting the framework and integrating it into review templates and standard operating procedures used by all drug and biologics reviewers. Starting in 2015, FDA began using the framework as part of the new molecular entity (NME) review process and plans to expand its use to all new drug applications (NDAs)/biologics licensing application (BLAs), as well as in post-approval benefit–risk decisions." By 2017, FDA requires all original NDAs to incorporate structured B–R framework in submissions (BIO White Paper 2015).

In addition, under the current International Conference on Harmonization (ICH) Guideline finalized in September 2002, Module Number 4 Efficacy, first revision (M4E, R1), medical product applicants are expected to include their conclusions about drug benefits and risks in the Clinical Overview of Module 2 of the Common Technical Document (CTD) under Section 2.5.6. In November 2014, an ICH Expert Working Group (M4E [R2]) was formed to revise Section 2.5.6 of the CTD. The work to revise CTD Section 2.5.6 is close to final at the time of this book's publication.

Taken together, it is clear that the regulators and payers are increasingly focusing on and looking for explicit elucidation of B–R profiles and trade-offs in regulatory submission packages. Sponsors are now faced with the tasks of defining key benefits and key risks of their products; describing the methodologies that are used to assess the B–R profiles; depicting strengths, limitations, and uncertainties pertaining to B–R information; and communicating the B–R evaluations with the use of summary tables and graphic displays. Given the FDA timeline for the structured B–R framework in NDAs/BLAs by 2017 and the current work on CTD Section 2.5.6 revision by the ICH Expert Working Group, sponsors will need to follow the guidance and timeline for B–R evaluation in their regulatory submission packages in the next few years.

Although in the last few years there has been a great deal of information on structured B–R assessment, there is still a paucity of real B–R case studies in literature for clinical trialists to draw best practices and lessons learned. In this chapter, we present and summarize a few real examples of B–R evaluations. Throughout this book and along with two complete real case studies in Chapters 11 and 12, we have provided the readers with a B–R evaluation toolkit for their B–R evaluations, and it is up to the practitioners to utilize these methods/tools to answer key B–R questions they face. Therefore, in our presentation of real examples in this chapter, we will not repeat the B–R analyses and results presentations that were performed for these case studies, but rather will focus on the key B–R consideration for these real cases.

In Section 13.2, we provide the background of the case studies. We describe the key B–R considerations for these case studies in Section 13.3. Section 13.4 is devoted to discussions summarizing the lessons learned from these case studies. The final section provides concluding remarks.

13.2 Description of Case Studies

In this section, we provide the background of the case studies.

13.2.1 Case Study #1: Prasugrel versus Clopidogrel in Patients with Acute Coronary Syndromes

Prasugrel, a novel thienopyridine, is a prodrug that, like clopidogrel, requires conversion to an active metabolite before binding to the platelet P2Y12 receptor to confer antiplatelet activity. The Trial to Assess Improvement in Therapeutic Outcomes by Optimizing Platelet Inhibition with Prasugrel–Thrombolysis in Myocardial Infarction (MI) (TRITON–TIMI) 38 was a phase 3 trial involving patients with acute coronary syndromes with scheduled percutaneous coronary intervention (PCI), comparing a regimen of prasugrel with the standard dose regimen of clopidogrel approved previously by the FDA. The study enrolled 13,608 patients with acute coronary syndromes (representative of the entire spectrum of those syndromes) with scheduled PCI. Patients were randomly assigned to the clopidogrel group or the prasugrel group in two strata: 10,074 patients with moderate- to high-risk unstable angina or non–ST-elevation MI and 3534 patients with ST-elevation MI. The primary efficacy endpoint was a composite of the rate of death from cardiovascular causes, nonfatal MI, or nonfatal stroke during the follow-up period. Key safety endpoints were TIMI classification system major bleeding not related to coronary artery bypass grafting (CABG), non–CABG-related TIMI life-threatening bleeding, and TIMI major or minor bleeding. Efficacy comparisons were performed on the basis of the time to the first event, according to the intention-to-treat principle. Multiplicity was controlled via the use of a closed testing procedure. The primary efficacy endpoint was analyzed in the cohort with unstable angina or non–ST-elevation MI first, and only if there was a statistically significant difference between the treatment groups was the primary endpoint analyzed in the overall cohort. Safety analyses were performed on data from patients who received at least one dose of the study drug. For more details with regard to study design and methods, see Wiviott et al. (2007).

The rate of the primary efficacy endpoint was significantly reduced in favor of prasugrel among the patients with unstable angina or non–ST-elevation MI (hazard ratio, 0.82; 95% confidence interval [CI], 0.73 to 0.93; $P = 0.002$). As prespecified, the analysis was also performed in the overall cohort of patients with acute coronary syndromes. In the overall cohort, a total of 781 patients (12.1%) in the clopidogrel group had the primary endpoint, as compared with 643 patients (9.9%) in the prasugrel group (hazard ratio, 0.81; 95% CI, 0.73 to 0.90; $P < 0.001$), supporting the primary hypothesis of superior efficacy. However, among patients treated with prasugrel, 146 (2.4%) had at least one TIMI major hemorrhage that was not related to CABG, as compared with 111 patients (1.8%) treated with clopidogrel (hazard ratio, 1.32; 95% CI, 1.03 to 1.68; $P = 0.03$). This excess of TIMI major bleeding included a higher rate of life-threatening bleeding in the prasugrel group (1.4% vs. 0.9% in the clopidogrel group; hazard ratio, 1.52; 95% CI, 1.08 to 2.13; $P = 0.01$) at the end of the study, as well as from the time of randomization to day 3 (0.4% vs. 0.3%; hazard ratio, 1.38; 95% CI, 0.79 to 2.41; $P = 0.26$) and from day 3 to the end of the study (1.0% vs. 0.6%; hazard ratio, 1.60; 95% CI, 1.05 to 2.44; $P = 0.03$). Fatal TIMI major bleeding occurred in significantly more patients treated with prasugrel (0.4%) than those treated with clopidogrel (0.1%) ($P = 0.002$) (Wiviott et al. 2007). For more details with regard to study results, see Wiviott et al. (2007).

13.2.2 Case Study #2: Dabigatran versus Warfarin in Patients with Atrial Fibrillation

Dabigatran etexilate is an oral prodrug that is rapidly converted by a serum esterase to dabigatran, a potent, direct, competitive inhibitor of thrombin. The Randomized Evaluation of Long-Term Anticoagulation Therapy (RE-LY) was a randomized trial designed to compare two fixed doses of dabigatran, 110 mg or 150 mg twice daily, each administered in a blinded manner, with open-label use of warfarin in patients who had atrial fibrillation and were at increased risk for stroke (Connolly et al. 2009). The primary efficacy study outcome was stroke or systemic embolism. The primary safety outcome was major hemorrhage. Secondary outcomes were stroke, systemic embolism, and death. Other outcomes were MI, pulmonary embolism, transient ischemic attack, and hospitalization. The primary analysis was designed to test whether either dose of dabigatran was noninferior to warfarin, as evaluated with the use of Cox proportional-hazards modeling. To satisfy the noninferiority hypothesis, the upper bound of the one-sided 97.5% CI for the relative risk of an outcome with dabigatran as compared with warfarin needed to fall below 1.46 (Connolly et al. 2009). For more details with regard to study design and methods, see Connolly et al. (2009).

A total of 18,113 patients were enrolled in the RE-LY study with a median follow-up duration of 2.0 years. Stroke or systemic embolism occurred in 182 patients receiving 110 mg of dabigatran (1.53% per year), 134 patients receiving 150 mg of dabigatran (1.11% per year), and 199 patients receiving warfarin (1.69% per year). Both doses of dabigatran were noninferior to warfarin ($P < 0.001$). The 150-mg dose of dabigatran was also superior to warfarin (relative risk, 0.66; 95% CI, 0.53 to 0.82; $P < 0.001$), but the 110-mg dose was not (relative risk, 0.91; 95% CI, 0.74 to 1.11; $P = 0.34$). The rate of major bleeding was 3.36% per year in the warfarin group, as compared with 2.71% per year in the group that received 110 mg of dabigatran (relative risk with dabigatran, 0.80; 95% CI, 0.69 to 0.93; $P = 0.003$) and 3.11% per year in the group that received 150 mg of dabigatran (relative risk, 0.93; 95% CI, 0.81 to 1.07; $P = 0.31$). Rates of life-threatening bleeding, intracranial bleeding, and major or minor bleeding were higher with warfarin (1.80%, 0.74%, and 18.15%, respectively) than with either the 110-mg dose of dabigatran (1.22%, 0.23%, and 14.62%, respectively) or the 150-mg dose of dabigatran (1.45%, 0.30%, and 16.42%, respectively) ($P < 0.05$ for all comparisons of dabigatran with warfarin). There was a significantly higher rate of major gastrointestinal bleeding with dabigatran at the 150-mg dose than with warfarin (Connolly et al. 2009). For more details with regard to study results, see Connolly et al. (2009).

13.2.3 Case Study #3: Rivaroxaban in Patients with a Recent Acute Coronary Syndrome

Rivaroxaban is an oral anticoagulant that directly and selectively inhibits factor Xa. Factor Xa initiates the final common pathway of the coagulation cascade and results in the formation of thrombin, which catalyzes additional coagulation-related reactions and promotes platelet activation. The Anti-Xa Therapy to Lower Cardiovascular Events in Addition to Standard Therapy in Subjects with Acute Coronary Syndrome–Thrombolysis in Myocardial Infarction (ATLAS ACS 2–TIMI 51) study was a phase 3 trial to evaluate twice-daily rivaroxaban at doses of 2.5 and 5 mg as adjunctive therapy in patients with a recent acute coronary syndrome, with the aim of determining a clinically effective low-dose regimen. Enrollment occurred within 7 days after hospital admission for an acute coronary syndrome. Patients were randomly assigned in a 1:1:1 fashion to twice-daily administration of either 2.5 or 5.0 mg of rivaroxaban or placebo, with a maximum follow-up of 31 months. The primary efficacy endpoint was a composite of death from cardiovascular causes, MI, or stroke (ischemic, hemorrhagic, or stroke of uncertain cause). The primary safety endpoint was TIMI major bleeding not related to CABG. As prespecified, efficacy analyses were performed with the use of a modified intention-to-treat approach (mITT), which included the randomized patients and the endpoint events that occurred after randomization and no later than the completion of the treatment phase of the study (i.e., the global treatment end date), 30 days after early permanent discontinuation of the study drug, or 30 days after randomization for patients who did not receive a study drug. Sensitivity efficacy analyses were conducted with the use of an intention-to-treat approach, which included the patients who underwent randomization and all endpoint events occurring after randomization until the global treatment end date. The primary safety analysis included all patients who underwent randomization and who received at least one dose of a study drug, with evaluation performed from the time of administration of the first dose of a study drug until 2 days after the discontinuation of a study drug. Time to event analysis with hazard ratios along with 95% CIs were used to assess the treatment effects of the study groups. Rates of the endpoints were expressed as Kaplan–Meier estimates through 24 months. Testing was prespecified to occur between the combined-dose group for rivaroxaban and placebo at an alpha level of 0.05 on the basis of the log-rank test, stratified according to the intention to use a thienopyridine. If the comparison significantly favored rivaroxaban, then each of the two doses of rivaroxaban was simultaneously compared with placebo with the use of a similar stratified log-rank test at an alpha level of 0.05 on the basis of the closed testing procedure. For more details with regard to study design and methods, see Mega et al. (2012).

The study was conducted from November 2008 through September 2011. A total of 15,526 patients were randomized at 766 sites in 44 countries. The mean duration of treatment with a study drug was 13.1 months. Rivaroxaban significantly reduced the primary efficacy endpoint of death from cardiovascular causes, MI, or stroke, as compared with placebo, with rates of 8.9% and 10.7%, respectively (hazard ratio, 0.84; 95% CI, 0.74 to 0.96; $P = 0.008$). These results were consistent in the intention-to-treat analysis ($P = 0.002$). In the analysis of the components of the primary efficacy endpoint, rivaroxaban versus placebo had a hazard ratio of 0.80 ($P = 0.04$) for death from cardiovascular causes (including hemorrhage-related deaths), 0.85 ($P = 0.047$) for MI, and 1.24 ($P = 0.25$) for stroke (including ischemic, hemorrhagic, and stroke of uncertain cause). Rivaroxaban significantly increased the rate of TIMI major bleeding that was not related to CABG, as compared with placebo, with rates of 2.1% and 0.6%, respectively (hazard ratio, 3.96; 95% CI, 2.46 to 6.38; $P < 0.001$), a finding that was also significant for the 2.5- and 5-mg doses of rivaroxaban ($P < 0.001$ for both comparisons). Also greater in the combined rivaroxaban group, as compared with placebo, was intracranial hemorrhage (0.6% vs. 0.2%, $P = 0.009$). In the comparison between the two doses of rivaroxaban, the rates of TIMI major bleeding that was not related to CABG tended to be lower in patients receiving the 2.5-mg dose than in those receiving the 5-mg dose (1.8% vs. 2.4%, $P = 0.12$).

13.2.4 Case Study #4: Natalizumab for the Treatment of Relapsing Remitting Multiple Sclerosis versus Placebo

Natalizumab (Tysabri) is a recombinant humanized monoclonal antibody produced in murine myeloma cells. Natalizumab is indicated for the treatment of patients with relapsing forms of multiple sclerosis (MS) to reduce the frequency of clinical exacerbations. MS is an autoimmune disease that damages and prevents the creation of the tissues that protect nerves, called myelin. This creates lesions or scar tissue known as sclerosis. Lesions are believed to occur when activated inflammatory cells, including T-lymphocytes, cross the blood–brain barrier. Leukocyte migration involves interaction between adhesion molecules on inflammatory cells and their counter-receptors present on endothelial cells of the vessel wall. The drug works by blocking the integrin molecule and preventing immune cells from migrating through blood vessels in the brain to areas of inflammation; however, the specific mechanism by which natalizumab exerts its effects in MS have not been fully defined.

FDA approval of natalizumab for the treatment of MS was based on two randomized, double-blind, placebo-controlled trials with more than 2000 subjects. Subjects were enrolled if they had experienced at least one relapse during the previous year and had a score of between 0 and 5 on the Expanded Disability Status Scale. In both studies, neurological evaluations were performed every 12 weeks and at times of suspected relapse. Magnetic resonance imaging (MRI) evaluations for T1-weighted gadolinium-enhancing lesions and T2-hyperintense lesions were performed annually.

In study #1, all 942 subjects enrolled had not received any interferon-beta or glatiramer acetate for at least the previous 6 months. In fact, roughly 94% had never been treated with these agents. The median age was 37, with a median disease duration of 5 years. Subjects were randomized to receive natalizumab (300 mg intravenous infusion) or placebo every 4 weeks for up to 28 months. Results showed that natalizumab reduced the risk of sustained progression of disability by 42% over 2 years (hazard ratio, 0.58; 95% CI, 0.43 to 0.77; $P < 0.001$). The cumulative probability of progression (on the basis of Kaplan–Meier analysis) was 17% in the natalizumab group and 29% in the placebo group. Natalizumab reduced the rate of clinical relapse at 1 year by 68% ($P < 0.001$) and led to an 83% reduction in the accumulation of new or enlarging hyperintense lesions, as detected by T2-weighted MRI, over 2 years (mean numbers of lesions, 1.9 with natalizumab and 11.0 with placebo; $P < 0.001$). There were 92% fewer lesions (as detected by gadolinium-enhanced MRI) in the natalizumab group than in the placebo group at both 1 and 2 years ($P < 0.001$). The adverse events that were significantly more frequent in the natalizumab group than in the placebo group were fatigue (27% vs. 21%, $P = 0.048$) and allergic reaction (9% vs. 4%, $P = 0.012$). Hypersensitivity reactions of any kind occurred in 25 patients receiving natalizumab (4%), and serious hypersensitivity reactions occurred in 8 patients (Polman et al. 2006).

In study #2, all 1171 subjects enrolled had experienced one or more relapses while on treatment with interferon beta-1a (30 μg intramuscularly) once weekly during the year before study entry. The median age was 39 years, with a median disease duration of 7 years. Subjects were randomized to receive natalizumab (300 mg intravenous infusion) or placebo every 4 weeks for up to 28 months. Subjects continued taking interferon beta-1a at their normal dosing once weekly. Results showed that combination therapy resulted in a 24% reduction in the relative risk of sustained disability progression (hazard ratio, 0.76; 95% CI, 0.61 to 0.96; $P = 0.02$). Kaplan–Meier estimates of the cumulative probability of progression at 2 years were 23% with combination therapy and 29% with interferon beta-1a alone. Combination therapy was associated with a lower annualized rate of relapse over a 2-year period than was interferon beta-1a alone (0.34 vs. 0.75, $P < 0.001$) and with fewer new or enlarging lesions on T2-weighted MRI (0.9 vs. 5.4, $P < 0.001$). Adverse events associated with combination therapy were anxiety, pharyngitis, sinus congestion, and peripheral edema. Two cases of progressive multifocal leukoencephalopathy (PML), one of which was fatal, were diagnosed in natalizumab-treated patients (Rudick et al. 2006). For more details with regard to study design and methods, see Polman et al. (2006) and Rudick et al. (2006).

13.2.5 Case Study #5: Rimonabant Weight Loss in Obese or Overweight Patients with Comorbidities

Rimonabant is a selective cannabinoid-1 CB1 receptor blocker. As of March 2007, more than 15,000 patients had taken at least one dose of rimonabant 20 mg (3478 patient-years). The Rimonabant in Obesity (RIO)-Lipids study examined the effects of rimonabant on metabolic risk factors, including adiponectin levels, in high-risk patients who are overweight or obese and have dyslipidemia (Cardiology Today 2007; Despres et al. 2005).

The RIO program is composed of four randomized, double-blinded, placebo-controlled phase 3 clinical trials recruiting more than 6000 overweight or obese patients whose weight at the start of the studies was on average 94 to 104 kg. The patients were randomly assigned to double-blinded therapy with either placebo or rimonabant at a dose of 5 mg or 20 mg daily for 12 months in addition to a hypocaloric diet (Despres et al. 2005).

Each of the four studies on rimonabant showed significant reductions in body weight and waist circumference over a 1- to 2-year period. Rimonabant also improved cardiometabolic risk factors, including triglycerides, blood pressure, insulin resistance, C-reactive protein levels, and high-density lipoprotein cholesterol concentrations in both nondiabetic and type 2 diabetic overweight/obese patients. As compared with placebo, rimonabant at a dose of 20 mg was associated with a significant ($P < 0.001$) mean weight loss (repeated-measures method, −6.7 ± 0.5 kg, and last-observation-carried-forward analyses, −5.4 ± 0.4 kg), reduction in waist circumference (repeated-measures method, −5.8 ± 0.5 cm, and last-observation-carried-forward analyses, −4.7 ± 0.5 cm), increase in HDL cholesterol (repeated-measures method, +10.0% ± 1.6%, and last-observation-carried-forward analyses, +8.1% ± 1.5%), and reduction in triglycerides (repeated-measures method, −13.0% ± 3.5%, and last-observation-carried-forward analyses, −12.4% ± 3.2%). Rimonabant at a dose of 20 mg also resulted in an increase in plasma adiponectin levels (repeated-measures method, 57.7%, and last-observation-carried-forward analyses, 46.2%; $P < 0.001$), for a change that was partly independent of weight loss alone. In conclusion, selective CB_1 receptor blockade with rimonabant significantly reduces body weight and waist circumference and improves the profile of several metabolic risk factors in high-risk patients who are overweight or obese and have an atherogenic dyslipidemia (Despres et al. 2005).

Rimonabant was generally well tolerated. The most common adverse event was nausea (13%). Later reports showed that the use of rimonabant was associated with psychiatric side effects, including anxiety, depression, and suicidal ideation. The adverse psychiatric events were observed in 26% of the participants in the rimonabant group compared with 14% in the placebo group in the same four studies, and the risk of depressive symptoms was estimated at 2.5-fold higher than that in placebo-treated patients (Cardiology Today 2007; Kang et al. 2012).

13.3 Key B–R Considerations in the Case Studies

In this section, we describe and summarize the key B–R considerations for these case studies.

13.3.1 Case Study #1: Weighing Benefits and Risks—The FDA's Review of Prasugrel

The FDA approved prasugrel on July 10, 2009. Given the superior efficacy but significant bleeding risks, the FDA grappled with a number of complex issues related to B–R (Unger 2009). We summarize the key considerations by Unger (2009) below.

The TRITON–TIMI 38 study met the primary objective with approximately 19% reduction in relative risk of death from cardiovascular causes, nonfatal MI, and nonfatal stroke. The difference was primarily driven by a reduction in the rate of nonfatal MI, including both those detected clinically and those detected solely through the measurement of cardiac enzymes (most of the latter occurred during the index hospitalization). Prasugrel reduced endpoint events but was associated with a relative increase in the risk of bleeding of approximately 30%. The frequencies of TIMI major or minor bleeding events that were not related to CABG were 4.5% with prasugrel and 3.4% with clopidogrel. Fatal hemorrhage occurred infrequently but was more common with prasugrel than with clopidogrel (0.3% vs. 0.1%). In weighing the risks and benefits, the FDA review team noted that the components of the primary endpoint represented irreversible tissue damage and concluded that the benefit of preventing such events is generally worth the risk of bleeding events that have no irreversible consequences. For each 1000 patients who were given prasugrel instead of clopidogrel, 24 primary endpoint events were prevented—21 nonfatal MI and 3 cardiovascular deaths. The cost was 10 excess major or minor bleeding events, 2 of which were fatal.

However, not all reviewers agree that the treatment effect was important, since many of the excess MI in the clopidogrel group were not manifested clinically but were merely "enzyme leaks" that were detected during routine monitoring in the peri-interventional period. The agency and the advisory committee grappled with this issue but concluded, however, that such enzyme elevations indicate tissue damage and that such damage has serious long-term consequences. With regard to concerns regarding bleeding, the FDA derived several risk-mitigation strategies in the label to ensure that prasugrel's label clearly articulates the balance between efficacy and risk—a balance that physicians will need to assess carefully when choosing treatment for individual patients.

13.3.2 Case Study #2: Anticoagulant Options—Why the FDA Approved a Higher but Not a Lower Dose of Dabigatran

On October 19, 2010, the FDA approved dabigatran for the reduction of the risk of stroke and systemic embolism in patients with nonvalvular atrial fibrillation based on the RE-LY trial. Given that both dabigatran doses met the primary efficacy and safety objective, both doses could have been approved. However, the FDA only approved higher but not a lower dose of dabigatran. We summarize the key considerations by Beasley et al. (2011) below.

Beasley et al. (2011) indicated that there were certainly reasons to approve both doses. Both doses met evidentiary standards for safety and effectiveness, with the higher dose showing clear superiority but even the lower dose proving noninferior to standard anticoagulant therapy. In addition, patients and doctors value choices that allow treatment to be individualized. For patients for whom there is reason for heightened concern about bleeding, the lower dose might have seemed desirable, even at the cost of increased risk of stroke. Moreover, many patients now refuse to take warfarin because of fear of bleeding. Whether or not it would be a rational choice, 110 mg of dabigatran might have provided an attractive option for such patients—an option clearly preferable to no treatment at all. On the other hand, nonfatal and extracranial bleeding episodes are clearly less clinically significant than strokes for most patients, and users of a lower dose would be more likely to have strokes, most likely embolic ones. The FDA review team therefore sought to identify, within RE-LY, a patient population for whom the B–R assessment of 110 mg of dabigatran suggested superiority to the 150-mg dose.

The FDA first focused on elderly patients, patients with impaired renal function, and patients with previous bleeding episodes. Since such patients would be exposed to higher dabigatran concentrations or would have a greater predisposition to bleeding episodes or both—the lower dose might offer an advantage. Among the 40% of patients in RE-LY who were 75 years of age or older (n = 7238), the rate of stroke or systemic embolism was lower with 150 mg of dabigatran (1.4 per 100 patient-years) than with 110 mg (1.9 per 100 patient-years), but the rate of major bleeding was higher (5.1 vs. 4.4 per 100 patient-years). However, most people would agree that the irreversible effects of strokes and systemic emboli have greater clinical significance than nonfatal bleeding. Any B–R assessment in which strokes and systemic emboli are given more weight than nonfatal bleeding events would find the higher dose more favorable in elderly patients. The FDA also looked at subgroups of patients with impaired renal function and patients with previous bleeding episodes. However, the superior efficacy of 150 mg of dabigatran in the impaired renal function subgroup or similar bleeding profiles in the subgroup with previous bleeding episodes could not support the approval of the lower dose.

In the end, because the FDA was unable to find any population for whom the availability of a lower dose would improve dabigatran's B–R profile, they concluded that encouraging the "play it safe" option for patients and physicians represented an undesirable stimulus to use a less-effective regimen and would lead to unnecessary strokes and disability.

13.3.3 Case Study #3: The ATLAS ACS 2–TIMI 51 Trial and the Burden of Missing Data

Although the primary efficacy endpoint was met, a substantial amount of missing data was observed. The sponsor company, Janssen Research & Development, LLC, submitted supplemental NDAs and the applications were reviewed by the FDA Cardiovascular and Renal Drugs Advisory Committee (CRDAC) on May 23, 2012, and January 16, 2014, respectively. Each time, the company failed to gain recommendation for approval by the CRDAC. We summarize the key considerations and opinions by Krantz et al. (2013) and the CRDAC reviews (FDA CRDAC 2012, 2014).

Despite seemingly robust efficacy data, several key issues were brought up during the CRDAC meeting that challenge the validity of the ATLAS ACS 2–TIMI 51 trial results (Krantz and Kaul 2013). First and foremost, an unanticipated high rate of missing data, particularly the vital status of patients, precludes reliable and valid information. Second, there was a lack of an expected dose response—the 5-mg dose did not have greater efficacy than the 2.5-mg dose of rivaroxaban. Establishment of dose or exposure response is an important consideration in regulatory decision making. Third, it is difficult to reconcile the results with the divergent impact of the two doses on the components of the primary composite endpoint of MACE—CV death, but not MI, driving the treatment benefit with 2.5 mg, whereas MI, but not CV death, driving the benefit with the 5-mg dose. The increase in bleeding with the higher dose did not account for the null effect on CV death. Fourth, there is a lack of supportive external evidence for incremental benefit associated with novel oral anticoagulants in ACS beyond standard dual antiplatelet therapy.

Although many of these issues are pertinent to the ultimate approvability and clinical utility of rivaroxaban as part of triple antithrombotic therapy, Krantz and Kaul (2013) focused on the critical issue of missing data that dominated the CRDAC panel discussion. In the ATLAS ACS 2–TIMI 51 trial, 2402 patients (15.5%) prematurely discontinued from the study, with 1294 patients (8.3%) withdrawing consent. At the end of the trial, vital status was not ascertained in 1117 of the 1294 patients who withdrew consent. By contrast, the rates of withdrawal of consent and in particular missing vital status in contemporary randomized ACS trials are appreciably lower. For example, in the PLATO trial, 3% of the subjects had incomplete follow-up, 2.9% withdrew consent, and vital status was unknown in 0.01% of subjects. Krantz and Kaul (2013) further indicated that although there is no regulatory guideline that stipulates an acceptable level of missing data, the following "rule-of-thumb" considerations proposed by Schulz and Grimes (2002) may facilitate judgments regarding the impact of "missingness" on the interpretability of clinical trial results.

1. If the loss to follow-up rate exceeds the outcome event rate, results might be questionable.
2. If missing data are <5%, the bias will be minimal; however, if they are >20%, it poses a serious threat to the validity of the study.
3. If missing data are differential by treatment group, results may be biased, especially if losses are related to treatment efficacy or tolerability.
4. If there are missing data that, when subjected to sensitivity analyses, yield different results, study conclusions are less certain.

In the ATLAS ACS 2–TIMI 51 trial, the number of patients with unknown vital status (n = 1117) exceeded the total number of primary endpoint events (n = 1002). Although the extent of missing data was <20%, there was differential missingness for MACE assessment (1.4% greater with rivaroxaban: 11% placebo vs. 12.4% combined rivaroxaban). The difference in the missing data nearly matched the difference in the primary outcome (1.2% favoring rivaroxaban: 7.3% placebo vs. 6.1% combined rivaroxaban), providing ample opportunity to amplify or obscure any true difference in endpoints.

An extension of the missing data concern is the potential to lead to "informative censoring" (i.e., patients who drop out are either more or less likely to experience the primary outcome of interest compared with those remaining in the trial in a nonrandom fashion). That concern can be compounded if the reasons for, or frequency of, dropout differs between the treatment groups. This is particularly relevant in trials of antithrombotic drugs, such as rivaroxaban, in which one expects the study agent to preferentially increase bleeding, thereby leading to greater discontinuation and dropouts relative to placebo. Because bleeding has been linked to both short-term and long-term increased risk of ischemic CV events and mortality, increased bleeding-related dropouts are likely to bias the results toward therapeutic benefit of the study drug. Not surprisingly, in the ATLAS ACS 2–TIMI 51 trial, compared to patients with complete follow-up, TIMI minor or greater bleeding rates were higher in patients with incomplete follow-up by 3-fold in the placebo group (3.1 vs. 0.9 per 100 patient-year exposure), 4.5-fold in the 2.5-mg rivaroxaban treatment group (6.3 vs. 1.4 per 100 patient-year exposure), and 5-fold in the 5-mg rivaroxaban treatment group (9.0 vs. 1.8 per 100 patient-year exposure). It is also clear that discontinuation had a differential impact among drug and placebo groups (i.e., placebo withdrawals were much less likely to have adverse bleeding events than the withdrawals in the rivaroxaban group), illustrating the potential of informative censoring to bias results in favor of active treatment.

Although, in September 2012, the sponsor submitted additional information with regard to the vital status of patients who had withdrawn from the ATLAS ACS 2–TIMI 51 trial, the FDA issued a second complete response letter in March 2013. The second FDA ACM on the same indication on January 16, 2014, failed to swing the panel in a different direction. We believe that a comment by one of the ACM panelists at the first ACM in May 2012 adequately summarized the major issue with the study design and subsequent results and conclusion. We quote the comment here: "The decision to use mITT as the endpoint, I believe, had a profound impact here. And I think what happens when you say, the primary endpoint is 30 days after you stop study drug, is you're telling the investigators and you're telling the patients that you don't care so much about what happens later on. I think that's why they had such a large withdrawal of consent rate. I think it was preordained by the use of this so-called mITT, which is really an on-treatment analysis. And so I think it colored the trial in ways we could never recover from because we're never going to ever see the ITT data."

13.3.4 Case Study #4: Weighing of Benefit and Risk: Risk Evaluation and Mitigation Strategy

The FDA initially approved natalizumab in November 2004. On February 28, 2005, the drug was suspended because of an associated incidence of PML, a rare neurological disorder. In March 2006, the Advisory Panel of the FDA voted in favor of the return of natalizumab on the market in relapsing forms of MS with a black-box warning about PML. On June 5, 2006, Biogen Idec and Elan announced the approval of a supplemental Biologics License Agreement by the FDA for the reintroduction of natalizumab as a monotherapy treatment for relapsing forms of MS. We summarize the key BR considerations by the FDA during the reevaluation below (FDA Advisory Committee Briefing Document 2006; FDA Press Release 2006).

Pressure to bring natalizumab back to the market has come from patients who believe that the drug has helped them enormously and from neurologists impressed with the superior improvements in relapse rates and disease progression. The approval for reintroduction of natalizumab was based on the review of natalizumab trial data, a revised labeling with enhanced safety warnings and a risk evaluation and mitigation strategy (TOUCH Prescribing Program) designed to inform of the potential risk of PML. The TOUCH Prescribing Program was developed by the FDA and the Marketing Authorization Holder, Biogen Idec, and is intended to make sure that healthcare professionals and patients understand the benefits and potential risks associated with the use of natalizumab, including the risk of PML. TOUCH is a distribution program designed to assess the risk of PML associated with natalizumab, minimize the risk of PML, minimize death and disability caused by PML, and promote informed risk–benefit decisions regarding natalizumab use. The risks of natalizumab treatment are addressed through the distribution program, along with education of prescribers, pharmacists, infusion center staff, and patients about potential PML infection associated with natalizumab treatment (TOUCH Risk Minimization Plan). "This is one of the very rare cases in which a drug withdrawn from the market for safety reasons has been returned to the market, after appropriate steps have been taken," said Steven Galson, who was the director of the FDA's Center for Drug Evaluation and Research at the time of the review. Before natalizumab treatment can start, patients must undergo an MRI scan. Then, patients on natalizumab are to be evaluated at 3 and 6 months after the first infusion, and every 6 months after that, with their status being reported directly to Biogen Idec. Elements of the TOUCH program include the following:

- Revised labeling with a prominent boxed warning of the risk of PML and warnings against concurrent use of natalizumab with chronic immunosuppressant therapies, and patients who are immunocompromised because of HIV and other conditions

- Mandatory enrollment for all prescribers, central pharmacies, infusion centers, and patients who wish to prescribe, distribute, infuse, or receive, respectively, natalizumab controlled, centralized distribution only to authorized infusion centers
- Mandatory FDA-reviewed educational tools for patients and physicians, including a patient medication guide, TOUCH enrollment form, and a monthly preinfusion checklist and ongoing assessment of PML risk and overall safety

From July 2006 (when marketing resumed) through January 21, 2010, there have been 31 confirmed cases of PML worldwide in patients using natalizumab. Of these 31 case reports, 10 were from patients in the United States. As of January 21, 2010, eight patients have died. In all cases, patients were receiving natalizumab as monotherapy for the treatment of MS. The overall worldwide cumulative rate of PML in patients who have received one or more natalizumab infusions is 0.5 cases of PML per 1000 patients. Since natalizumab's remarketing in the United States, there have been no cases of PML in patients treated with natalizumab for less than 12 months. The overall worldwide cumulative rate of PML in patients who have received at least 24 infusions is 1.3 cases of PML per 1000 patients. In the United States, the cumulative rate of PML in patients who have received at least 24 infusions is 0.8 per 1000 patients. Outside of the United States, the cumulative rate of PML in patients who have received at least 24 infusions is 1.9 per 1000 patients (FDA Drug Safety Communication: http://www.fda.gov/Drugs/DrugSafety/PostmarketDrugSafetyInformationforPatientsandProviders/ucm199872.htm).

On the basis of the evaluation of available data combined with the ability to manage the risk for PML with the revised label and risk management plan, the FDA believes that the clinical benefits of natalizumab continue to outweigh the potential risks.

13.3.5 Case Study #5: Weighing of Benefit and Risk: Concerns on the Safety Profile and High Dropout Rate

Rimonabant has been shown to reduce body weight and improve cardiovascular risk factors in obese patients. The drug was available in 56 countries from 2006. Despite the extensive favorable clinical data, it was not approved by the US FDA because of an increased risk of psychiatric adverse events, including depression, anxiety, and suicidal ideation. Subsequently, rimonabant was withdrawn from the European market in 2009 (Kang et al. 2012).

The FDA's Endocrinologic and Metabolic Drugs Advisory Committee in 2007 unanimously voted against approval of the proposed weight-loss drug rimonabant because of unclear safety information and data pointing to an increased risk for psychiatric and neurological adverse events. The panelists felt that additional safety information is needed before the FDA should consider approving the drug. Data from the RIO trials demonstrated that one-quarter of obese patients who were assigned to rimonabant lost 10% of their body weight after 1 year, and half lost approximately 5% of their original weight. These weight reductions were significantly greater than those among the placebo groups. However, there was serious concern about the safety profile of rimonabant. Of concern to the panel was the 5.9% incidence of psychiatric disorders, especially suicidal thinking or behavior, in patients assigned to rimonabant compared with 2.1% in those who were assigned to placebo. Patients assigned to rimonabant experienced a twofold increase in suicide or thoughts of suicide. In addition, many panelists expressed concern regarding the high number of patients who dropped out of the RIO trials. Attrition rates ranged from

32% to 49% within the first year. The lack of long-term safety data presents a serious issue since rimonabant is proposed as a lifelong weight-loss medication. There are data for 441 patients who were assigned to rimonabant 20 mg for 2 years in the clinical trials database (Cardiology Today 2007).

"The incidence of suicidality—specifically suicidal ideation—was higher for 20 mg rimonabant compared with placebo. Similarly, the incidence of psychiatric adverse events, neurological adverse events and seizures were consistently higher for 20 mg rimonabant compared with placebo," according to an FDA Briefing Document (2007). An FDA meta-analysis indicated an increased risk for suicide ideation in patients assigned to rimonabant 20 mg compared with placebo, which correlated with one additional case of suicidal thoughts or behavior per year for every 300 patients treated. There were two suicides recorded in the entire rimonabant clinical trial database. One was a patient in the RIO-North America trial who was assigned to rimonabant 5 mg, and the other was in the ongoing STRADIVARIUS trial in a patient assigned to rimonabant 20 mg (Cardiology Today 2007).

In conclusion, studies showed rimonabant helped people lose weight, but the benefits of such weight loss for reducing risks for cardiovascular and other health problems remain unproven. The drug was not approved by the FDA and was subsequently withdrawn from the European market.

13.4 Lessons Learned and Best Practices in B–R Evaluation

These five case studies demonstrated complexity and the multifaceted aspects of B–R trade-off considerations by regulatory agencies. We believe that the five case studies made clear of and showcased the following key elements in any B–R evaluations:

- Clinical impact of key benefits and key risks in B–R evaluations
- Endpoint selection, uncertainty evaluation, and weighting considerations
- Subgroup identifications
- Study design and missing data
- Evidence synthesis
- Risk evaluation and mitigation strategy

The FDA review of case study #1 focused on the key benefits and key risks of prasugrel. By identifying the key benefits and key risk factors, they focused their review on the primary efficacy endpoint of a composite of the rate of death from cardiovascular causes, nonfatal MI, or nonfatal stroke, and key safety endpoint of TIMI major or minor bleeding. Throughout their review, it was clear that the consideration of the severity and clinical impact of key efficacy and safety endpoints was important. By concluding that "… the components of the primary endpoint represented irreversible tissue damage and concluded that the benefit of preventing such events is generally worth the risk of bleeding events that have no irreversible consequences," the FDA reviewers indicated that the clinical impact of the primary efficacy events is far more important than that of TIMI bleeding events, and benefits of prasugrel outweighs its risks. We learned from this case study that for products that produce great benefits but are also associated with great risks, it is critical to focus on these key benefit and key risks with the use of appropriate B–R analysis methods along with visual displays. In this process, qualitative weighing was present, but the ultimate goal may not be to obtain numerical weights for the efficacy or safety endpoints and create a utility score. Rather, qualitative weighing or ranking was used to assist with the expert opinion on evidence synthesis. By determining that some bleeding events would have not caused irresponsible damages and thus having less weight than events that would have caused irresponsible damages, the FDA derived several risk-mitigation strategies in the label to ensure that prasugrel's label clearly articulates the balance between efficacy and risk.

Case study #2 provides a good case in study in terms of how subgroup identifications can be important for regulatory approval. As with any premarket submissions for approval, regulatory agencies often look at low doses for a safer dose, while ensuring that adequate efficacy was demonstrated. In the case of dabigatran approval, the FDA reviewers looked hard on B–R balances and trade-offs in various subgroups in the lower-dose group. The intent was to assess whether lower dose could be approved in subgroups that consisted of vulnerable patient segments. In the process, they also considered the clinical impact of key efficacy and safety endpoints and rank ordered or weighted them in a qualitative way and concluded that irreversible effects of strokes and systemic emboli have greater clinical significance than nonfatal bleeding. In the end, because the FDA was unable to find any population for whom the availability of a lower dose would improve dabigatran's B–R profile, they concluded that encouraging the play-it-safe option for patients and physicians represented an undesirable stimulus to use a less-effective regimen and would lead to unnecessary strokes and disability.

Case study #3 represents a good example of how study design and missing data played a key role in the nonapproval of rivaroxaban for the indication of ACS. The study design called for a primary analysis population of mITT, which included the randomized patients and the endpoint events that occurred after randomization and no later than the completion of the treatment phase of the study (i.e., the global treatment end date), 30 days after early permanent discontinuation of the study drug, or 30 days after randomization for patients who did not receive a study drug. In addition, more than 15% of patients prematurely discontinued from the study, and more than 8% withdrew consent. At the end of the trial, vital status was not ascertained in 1117 of the 1294 patients who withdrew consent. Further, differential dropouts in the treatment groups led to the belief that there was informative censoring with the trial, as patients who dropped out earlier might be more likely to experience the primary outcome of interest. The decision to use mITT from a design perspective had a profound impact on the trial and missing data according to one FDA ACM panel member. It was a design flaw that could never be recovered as it is impossible to collect trial data in an ITT fashion after study closure. We believe that lessons learned from this case study could be summarized as follows:

- First, for confirmatory trials, especially long-term outcome trials such as the ATLAS ACS 2–TIMI 51 trial, it is crucial to collect long-term outcome information. The ATLAS ACS 2–TIMI 51 trial was designed essentially as a trial using an on-treatment analysis to address the primary efficacy objective. For this type of trials, ITT principle should always be followed as a general rule of engagement.
- The trialists should be extremely mindful of the amount of missing data in studies. In the ATLAS ACS 2–TIMI 51 trial, the number of patients with unknown vital status exceeded the total number of primary endpoint events, providing ample opportunity to amplify or obscure any true difference in endpoints and rendering the trial results difficult to interpret.

- It was believed by the FDA ACM panels that informative censoring was likely to have occurred because of the study design flaws. Trialists should recognize the importance of study design considerations for a full B–R assessment. Safety signals often emerge with long-term follow-up. It therefore warrants considerable deliberations if trialists consider discontinuation of certain cohorts of patients earlier from the study follow-up because of lack of efficacy or serious safety concerns. Provided that it is ethically permissible and with proper mitigation plans for safety concerns, trialists should consider the discontinuation of study treatment for these cohorts of patients but continuing the study follow-up. This way, patients who were discontinued earlier for treatment but continued in the study follow-up would have their long-term efficacy and safety information captured in an ITT manner, mitigating any informative censoring concerns for these cohorts of patients.

Case study #4 also highlights the focus on key benefits and key risk considerations in bringing back natalizumab to the market for patients with relapsing forms of MS. Pressure to bring natalizumab back to the market has come from patients who believe that the drug has helped them enormously and from neurologists impressed with the superior improvements in relapse rates and disease progression. In consideration of risk assessment and mitigation strategy, FDA collaborated with the sponsors in developing a prescribing and distributing system that educates prescribers, pharmacists, infusion center staff, and patients about potential PML infection associated with natalizumab treatment. This case study provides a good example of a successful B–R evaluation.

Case study #5 offers a good example of how benefits of rimonabant in weight reduction could not outweigh the more severe risk of suicidal ideation. This is clearly the consideration of clinical impact and qualitatively ranking weight loss versus suicidal ideation at play. Although weight loss in obese subjects will improve their comorbidities and general well-being, not losing weight will not cause immediate or short-term mortality. On the other hand, depression and suicidality are severe and could lead to irreversible harm to study subjects. As shown in the rimonabant studies, patients assigned to rimonabant experienced a twofold increase in suicide or thoughts of suicide. Since the benefits of rimonabant are clearly not on the same impact scale as the risks, the product was not recommended for approval by the FDA ACM panel and was withdrawn from the EU market.

13.5 Conclusions

The development and implementation of B–R assessment should be done throughout the clinical development life cycle. This book has provided rich discussions on key considerations for B–R assessment. We argue that the issues that were revealed and identified through these case studies in this chapter will provide additional insight and bring to bear the importance of considerations in study designs, study conducts, subgroup identifications, selection of key efficacy and safety endpoints with important clinical impacts, qualitative weighting and uncertainty quantification, evidence synthesis, and risk mitigation for full B–R evaluations.

References

Beasley B, Unger E, Temple R. Anticoagulant Options—Why the FDA Approved a Higher but Not a Lower Dose of Dabigatran. *N Engl J Med* 2011; 364(19):1788–90.

Biotechnology Industry Organization (BIO) White Paper. A Lifecycle Approach to FDA's Structured Benefit–Risk Assessment Framework. Online white paper 2015: https://www.bio.org/sites/default/files/FDA_STBRA_WP.pdf.

Cardiology Today 2007. FDA panel gives thumbs down to rimonabant, http://www.healio.com/cardiology/chd-prevention/news/print/cardiology-today/%7B02a91ee3-c530-4bd9-8cf0-6f43901d517d%7D/fda-panel-gives-thumbs-down-to-rimonabant.

Connolly S, Ezekowitz M, Yusuf S, Eikelboom J, Oldgren J, Parekh A et al. Dabigatran versus Warfarin in Patients with Atrial Fibrillation. *N Engl J Med* 2009; 361(12):1139–51.

Despres JP, Golay A, Sjostrom L. Effects of Rimonabant on Metabolic Risk Factors in Overweight Patients with Dyslipidemia. *N Engl J Med* 2005; 353:2121–34.

FDA Briefing Document for February 9, 2006 Meeting of the FDA/CDER Peripheral and Central Nervous System (PCNS) Advisory Committee. http://www.fda.gov/ohrms/dockets/ac/06/briefing/20064208B1_01_04FDAClinical%20eview.pdf.

FDA Briefing Document for June 13, 2007 Advisory Committee, DA 21-888, Zimulti (rimonabant) Tablets, 20 mg.

FDA Drug Safety Communication: Risk of Progressive Multifocal Leukoencephalopathy (PML) with the use of Tysabri (natalizumab) http://www.fda.gov/Drugs/DrugSafety/PostmarketDrugSafetyInformationforPatientsandProviders/ucm199872.htm.

FDA News Release: FDA Approves Resumed Marketing of Tysabri Under a Special Distribution Program-http://www.fda.gov/NewsEvents/Newsroom/PressAnnouncements/2006/ucm108662.htm.

FDA Structured approach to benefit–risk assessment in drug regulatory decision-making draft PDUFA V implementation plan—February 2013, fiscal years 2013–2017. Silver Spring, MD: FDA; February 2013. Available at: http://www.fda.gov/downloads/ForIndustry/UserFees/PrescriptionDrugUserFee/UCM329758.pdf.

Kang J, Park C. Anti-Obesity Drugs: A Review about Their Effects and Safety. *Diabetes Metab J* 2012; 36:13–25. http://dx.doi.org/10.4093/dmj.2012.36.1.13, pISSN 2233-6079, eISSN 2233-6087.

Krantz M, Kaul S. The ATLAS ACS 2–TIMI 51 Trial and the Burden of Missing Data. *J Am Col Cardiol* 2013; 62(9):777–81.

Mega J, Braunwald E, Wiviott S, Bassand J, Bhatt D, Bode C et al. Rivaroxaban in Patients with a Recent Acute Coronary Syndrome. *N Engl J Med* 2012; 366(1):9–19.

Polman CH, O'Connor PW, Havrdova E et al. A randomized, placebo-controlled trial of natalizumab for relapsing multiple sclerosis. *N Engl J Med* 2006; 354:899–910.

Risk Minimization Plan: Summary of Touch. http://www.fda.gov/downloads/Drugs/DrugSafety/PostmarketDrugSafetyInformationforPatientsandProviders/UCM107197.pdf.

Rudick RA, Stuart WH, Calabresi PA et al. Natalizumab plus interferon beta-1a for relapsing multiple sclerosis. *N Engl J Med* 2006; 354:911–23.

Schulz KF, Grimes DA. Sample Size Slippages in Randomised Trials: Exclusions and the Lost and Wayward. *Lancet* 2002; 359:781–5.

Unger E. Weighing Benefits and Risks—The FDA's Review of Prasugrel. *N Engl J Med* 2009; 361(10):942–4.

U.S. Food and Drug Administration. May 23, 2012, Meeting of the Cardiovascular and Renal Drugs Advisory Committee. Available at: http://www.fda.gov/AdvisoryCommittees/CommitteesMeetingMaterials/Drugs/CardiovascularandRenalDrugsAdvisoryCommittee/ucm285415.htm.

U.S. Food and Drug Administration. January 16, 2014, Meeting of the Cardiovascular and Renal Drugs Advisory Committee. Available at: http://www.fda.gov/AdvisoryCommittees/CommitteesMeetingMaterials/Drugs/CardiovascularandRenalDrugsAdvisoryCommittee/ucm378911.htm.

Wiviott S, Braunwald E, McCabe C, Montalescot G, Ruzyllo W, Gottlieb S et al. Prasugrel versus Clopidogrel in Patients with Acute Coronary Syndromes. *N Engl J Med* 2007; 357(20):2001–15.

Glossary

ACO: Accountable care organization
ACR: American College of Rheumatology
AE: Adverse event
AE-NNT: Adverse Event Adjusted Number Needed to Treat
AHRQ: US Agency for Health Care Research and Quality
AL: Adaptive licensing
APPROVe: Adenomatous Polyp Prevention on Vioxx
ARRA: American Recovery and Reinvestment Act of 2009
BB: Beta-blocker
Benefit: Intended favorable effects (including the intensity, duration, and uncertainty) on a patient
BLR: Benefit-less-risk
B–R: Benefit–risk
BRA: Benefit–risk assessment
BRAMP: Benefit–risk assessment management plan
Breakthrough therapy: US FDA classification of a drug for the treatment of a serious or life-threatening condition for which there is preliminary evidence that the drug may demonstrate substantial improvement over existing therapies based on one or more clinically significant endpoints
CA: Conjoint analysis
CAD: Coronary artery disease
CBER: Center for Biologics Evaluation and Research
CDER: Center for Drug Evaluation and Research
CDM: Common data model; common model employed in distributed research networks
CDRH: US FDA Center for Devices and Radiological Health
CDS: Clinical decision support
CEC: Clinical events committee
CED: Coverage with evidence development
CER: Comparative effectiveness research
CFDA: Chinese FDA
CHMP: Committee for Medicinal Products for Human Use
CIOMS: Council for International Organizations of Medical Sciences
Claims Database: A database created to record insurance payments on behalf of individuals covered under a healthcare insurance plan
CMS: Centers for Medicare and Medicaid Services
Confounding: A situation in which the effect or association between an exposure and outcome is distorted by the presence of another variable
CTD: Common technical document
CUI: Clinical Utility Index
CV: Cardiovascular
DAS28: Disease Activity Score
DBRF: Descriptive benefit–risk framework
DCE: Discrete choice experiments
DCGI: Drug Controller General of India

DI: Desirability Index
DMARD: Disease-modifying antirheumatic drug
DMC: Data monitoring committee
DoD: US Department of Defense
DPL: A decision analysis software from Syncopation
DVT: Deep vein thrombosis
EC: European Commission
Effectiveness: Does a drug work in a real-world clinical setting?
Efficacy: Can a drug work?
e-Health: Electronic health
EHR: Electronic health record; holistic record that includes information from multiple clinical sites
EMA: European Medicines Agency
EMR: Electronic medical record; medical record from one medical system
Endpoint: A measurement of how a patient feels, functions, or survives that constitutes one of the target outcomes of the trial for its participants
ePA: Electronic prior authorization
FACIT: Functional Assessment of Chronic Illness Therapy-Fatigue scales
FDA: Food and Drug Administration
FDA AdCOM: FDA Advisory Committee
FDASIA: FDA Safety and Innovation Act of 2012
GI: Gastrointestinal
GLLMM: Generalized linear latent and mixed model
GUSTO: Global Use of Strategies to Open Occluded Coronary Arteries classification system
HAQ-DI: Health-related quality of life or disability as measured by Health Assessment Questionnaire-Disability Index
Hgb: Hemoglobin concentration
HIE: Health information exchange
HIPAA: Health Insurance Portability and Accountability Act
HOPE: Heart Outcomes Prevention Evaluation
HTA: Health technology assessment
ICH: The International Conference on Harmonisation of Technical Requirements for Registration of Pharmaceuticals for Human Use
IMI: Innovative Medicines Initiative
IMS Health: The largest vendor that provides US physician prescribing data on services and technology for the healthcare industry
IOM: Institute of Medicine
ISPOR RBMWG: International Society for Pharmacoeconomics and Outcomes Research Risk–Benefit Management Working Group
ITT: Intent to treat
IVC: Inferior vena cava
LVEF: Left ventricular ejection fraction
MAPPs: Medicines adaptive pathways to patients
MCDA: Multicriteria decision analysis
MERIT-HF: Metoprolol controlled-release randomized intervention trial in heart failure
Meta-analysis: Using statistical methods to combine quantitative evidence from two or more studies bearing on the same question
MI: Myocardial infarction
MNAR: Missing not at random

NCB: Net clinical benefit
NHS: National Health Service
NICE: UK National Institute for Health and Clinical Excellence (nondepartmental public body)
NIH: US National Institutes of Health
NMCR: Non–major clinically relevant
NNH: Numbers needed to harm
NNT: Numbers needed to treat
NSCLC: Non–small-cell lung cancer
Observational study: A study that draws inferences about the possible effect of a treatment on subjects where the assignment of subjects to treatments is not based on randomization
PAD: Peripheral arterial disease
PBRER: Periodic Benefit–Risk Evaluation Report
PBRSA: Performance-based risk sharing agreement
PCOR: Patient-centered outcomes research
PCORI: US Patient Centered Outcomes Research Institute (nongovernmental organization)
PDUFA: The Prescription Drug User Fee Act
PE: Pulmonary embolism
PHR: Personal health record
PhRMA BRAT: Pharmaceutical Research and Manufacturers of America Benefit–Risk Action Team
PMDA: Japanese Pharmaceuticals and Medical Devices Agency
PML: Progressive multifocal leukoencephalopathy
POS: Probability of success
POTS: Probability of technical success
PrOACT-URL: Problem, objectives, alternatives, consequences, trade-offs, uncertainty, risk and linked decisions
QALY: Quality-adjusted life year
QSPI BRWG: The Quantitative Sciences in the Pharmaceutical Industry Benefit–Risk Working Group
Q-TWiST: Quality-adjusted time without symptoms or toxicity
RA: Rheumatoid arthritis
RCT: Randomized clinical trial
RE-AIM: Reach the target population
Effectiveness or efficacy
Adoption by target staff, settings, or institutions
Implementation consistency, costs, and adaptions made during delivery
Maintenance
REMS: Risk Evaluation and Mitigation Strategy; drug risk management program in the United States authorized under the FDA Amendments Act of 2007
Risk: Unintended unfavorable effects (including the severity, duration, predictability, reversibility, and uncertainty on a patient)
RTM: Regression to mean
RV-NNT: Relative-value adjusted number needed to treat
SAE: Serious adverse event
SAP: Statistical analysis plan
Sentinel: Distributed network of electronic health records and medical and pharmacy claims data; created pursuant to the FDA Amendments Act of 2007

SMAA: Stochastic multicriteria acceptability analysis

Spontaneous report: An unsolicited communication of an adverse drug reaction by a healthcare professional or consumer to a company, regulatory authority, or other organization where the reaction was experienced by a patient receiving a medicinal product outside of a study or any organized data collection scheme

TIMI: Thrombolysis in Myocardial Infarction classification system

TPLC: Total product life cycle

TWiST: Time without symptoms of disease and toxic effects due to treatment

UMBRA: Universal Methodology for Benefit–Risk Assessment

Uncertainty: Uncertainty may refer to chance (random) and bias (nonrandom). The sources of such chance and bias may be attributed to inadequate sample size, measurement bias, selection process, subjectivity, and so on

Utility: A subjective measurement that describes a person's or group's preferences (satisfaction, risk attitude, etc.) for an outcome

UT-NNT: Utility- and time-adjusted NNT

VA: US Department of Veterans Affairs

Value: Cost/health outcome of interest

Value function: A function that converts observed data into a common scale. This can be subjective

Value tree: List of selected key benefits and risks, presented in a tree structure

Index

D

N

O

P

Q

S

T

U